Critical Thinking in Diagnosis and Therapy of Cognitive and Behavioral Disorders

Sherouk J. Kadhm
TruePath Assessments, Jordan

IGI Global
Scientific Publishing
Publishing Tomorrow's Research Today

Vice President of Editorial — Melissa Wagner
Director of Acquisitions — Mikaela Felty
Director of Book Development — Jocelynn Hessler
Production Manager — Mike Brehm
Cover Design — Jose Rosado

Published in the United States of America by
IGI Global Scientific Publishing
701 East Chocolate Avenue
Hershey, PA, 17033, USA
Tel: 717-533-8845
Fax: 717-533-7115
Website: https://www.igi-global.com E-mail: cust@igi-global.com

Library of Congress Cataloging-in-Publication Data

Names: Kadhm, Sherouk J., 1967- editor
Title: Critical thinking in diagnosis and therapy of cognitive and behavioral disorders / edited by Sherouk J. Kadhm.
Description: Hershey, PA : IGI Global Scientific Publishing, [2026] | Includes bibliographical references and index. | Summary: "This book aims to explore and highlight the pivotal role that critical thinking plays in the accurate diagnosis and effective therapy of cognitive and behavioral disorders"-- Provided by publisher.
Identifiers: LCCN 2025018894 (print) | LCCN 2025018895 (ebook) | ISBN 9798337318127 hardcover | ISBN 9798337318134 paperback | ISBN 9798337318141 ebook
Subjects: LCSH: Cognition disorders--Diagnosis | Critical thinking | Cognition disorders--Treatment | Behavior disorders in adolescence--Diagnosis | Behavior disorders in adolescence--Treatment | Behavior disorders in children--Diagnosis | Behavior disorders in children--Treatment
Classification: LCC RC553.C64 C75 2026 (print) | LCC RC553.C64 (ebook)
LC record available at https://lccn.loc.gov/2025018894
LC ebook record available at https://lccn.loc.gov/2025018895
British Cataloguing in Publication Data
A Cataloguing in Publication record for this book is available from the British Library.

Editorial Advisory Board

Table of Contents

Detailed Table of Contents

overcome stigma, adaptations in language use, and interventions involving family members. This research supports the need to implement institutional reforms to provide more equal access to quality mental health care for all students attending institutions of learning.

The connection between education and the necessity for cultivating economically empowered pupils has been longstanding. Is the role of education confined to its economic feasibility? Can community service resonate to foster a more economically robust future for its students? This study included 280 students from grades 8 to 10, aged 14 to 16 years, engaged in community service within their schools. The research employs structural equation modelling to examine the aspects contributing to learning via community service. The study employs independent variables such as awareness, action, ability, and connection as determinants of students' task capability, personal relationships, and social relationships. The study emphasizes the essential non-cognitive traits that students must cultivate for personal and social advancement and for their future economic success.

Our brain is a system that is both flexible and integrated, able to process visual, auditory, and sensory inputs simultaneously and design, execute, and control actions. It's not surprising that a complex system is also vulnerable to various disorders, such as brain diseases. Personality and the resulting decision-making and behavioral structures, as well as the embeddedness of personality in the brain, are also affected

Preface

Accurate diagnosis and effective therapy for cognitive and behavioral disorders require more than clinical knowledge. They call for careful judgment, self-awareness, and structured reasoning. Across disciplines and countries, the consequences of diagnostic errors remain a major concern, from misidentified childhood disorders to culturally misinterpreted symptoms in adolescents and adults. This book, *Critical Thinking in Diagnosis and Therapy of Cognitive and Behavioral Disorders*, brings together diverse experts who argue that critical thinking should be central to psychological and behavioral assessment.

The chapters explore how reasoning skills can sharpen diagnostic clarity, reduce bias, and support ethical and culturally responsive care. The contributors present new models, examine systemic challenges, and offer practical tools for mental health professionals, educators, and caregivers. Across case studies, theoretical frameworks, and empirical research, the volume underscores the need to slow down automatic judgments, ask better questions, and consult diverse perspectives.

Below is an overview of each chapter:

CHAPTER OVERVIEW

Chapter 1: The Power of Critical Thinking in Diagnosing Children's Psychological Disorders

Sherouk Kadhm, Tareq Damrah, and Mohammad Semrin examine widespread misdiagnosis in children, particularly with ADHD and autism. The authors highlight the consequences of diagnostic errors on families and healthcare systems, and show how critical thinking can improve evaluation practices. The chapter includes case studies where reflective assessment led to better outcomes.

Chapter 2: Critical Diagnostic Psychometrics (CDP) in Action

Sherouk Kadhm and Alexander Weissman introduce the concept of Critical Diagnostic Psychometrics, a framework that supports more accurate mental health diagnoses. They clarify the difference between misdiagnosis and overdiagnosis and argue for a stronger role for psychometricians in shaping evidence-based, culturally informed diagnostic practices.

Chapter 3: The Role of Critical Thinking in Psychological Assessment and Diagnosis

Geemol John and Mohammad Wani explore the barriers that limit reasoning in clinical settings, such as time pressure, lack of training, and cognitive bias. They present practical tools including the use of artificial intelligence, reflective strategies, and interdisciplinary collaboration. The chapter encourages clinicians to adopt practices that foster ethical and culturally competent assessments.

Chapter 4: Addressing Diagnostic Complexity Through Critical Thinking in Clinical Judgment

Debangi Sanyal, Aditi Priyadarshini, and Megha Rudrapati address the diagnostic challenges that arise from overlapping symptoms, cultural variation, and systemic bias. Through case examples and reflective analysis, they argue for a more thoughtful and context-sensitive approach to mental health diagnosis. The authors advocate for balancing standardized tools with human insight.

Chapter 5: Leveraging Critical Thinking to Address Dyslexia

Froilan Mobo, Katarzyna Milek, and Mykola Orlykovsky focus on dyslexia as a long-standing concern in education. They explain how educators and caregivers can apply critical thinking to better support children with learning difficulties. The chapter also considers how emotional and social development is shaped by early educational experiences and diagnostic labels.

Chapter 6: Enhancing Diagnostic Precision and Culturally-Adapted CBT for Adolescents

Patcha Bhujanga Rao and colleagues study culturally adapted versions of cognitive behavioral therapy for students in higher education. They show how diagnostic accuracy improves when critical thinking is used to distinguish between developmental stress and clinical disorders. The chapter emphasizes the importance of cultural sensitivity and family engagement in mental health care.

Chapter 7: Agile Community Service and Socio-Emotional Growth

Souvik Banerjee and co-authors examine the role of school-based community service in building students' social, emotional, and cognitive capacities. Using data from adolescents involved in service programs, the chapter analyzes how traits like awareness and action support growth. The research suggests that critical reflection during service experiences can enhance both personal development and academic outcomes.

Chapter 8: Neural Pathways of Judgment

Raad Kadhum explores how the brain processes information and how critical thinking is influenced by neurological development. The chapter links brain structure, personality, and decision-making and considers how errors in judgment can emerge from both cognitive and emotional patterns. It also discusses the early foundations of thinking and their role in forming lifelong reasoning habits.

Chapter 9: The Influence of Obstructive Sleep Apnea on Longevity and Well-Being

Md. Nurul Huda and Mohammad Talukder investigate how untreated obstructive sleep apnea affects overall health and lifespan. Drawing on secondary data, they present findings that connect timely diagnosis with improved outcomes. The chapter reinforces the need for greater awareness of physiological conditions that often overlap with cognitive and behavioral symptoms.

Chapter 10: Choosing a Field of Study Critically and Wisely

Raad Kadhum analyzes how students can make informed decisions when selecting a university major. Based on developmental psychology and personality theory, the chapter outlines a model for guiding students through the decision-making process. It connects critical thinking with long-term well-being, academic success, and life satisfaction.

Chapter 11: Critical Thinking in Psychological Diagnosis and Treatment

Hemalatha S and Krithick Ajay S focus on the cognitive and ethical pitfalls that can lead to misdiagnosis in mental health care. Through case examples and structured reasoning models, they show how critical thinking helps practitioners avoid common biases and make more accurate, responsible decisions.

This volume calls for a shift toward more reflective, evidence-based, and culturally informed diagnostic practices. By integrating critical thinking into every stage of mental health care, from assessment to treatment planning, professionals can support more accurate diagnoses, ethical decisions, and better outcomes for individuals across diverse settings.

Acknowledgments

I would like to express my sincere gratitude to the Med-Pro Center in Amman, Jordan, for their unwavering support in advancing psychometric and critical thinking strategies in diagnosis.

I am especially thankful to Dr. Tarek Ghattas for offering me this valuable opportunity, and to Dr. Nadine Abu Kaoud, Operations Manager, for her ongoing support and dedication. I also extend my appreciation to pediatrician Dr. Tareq Yousef Damrah. Their belief in the vision of integrating these innovative approaches into practice has been instrumental in bringing this work to life.

My deepest appreciation goes to the parents of the children with whom I've had the privilege to work. Your trust, openness, and collaboration have been invaluable. By allowing the application of these strategies and embracing your children's contributions, you have added profound meaning and depth to this book.

I am also sincerely thankful to all the members of the editorial advisory board for their valuable evaluations and insightful feedback to the contributing authors. Your efforts have significantly enhanced the quality and impact of this work.

To all of you, I extend my heartfelt thanks for your dedication and your commitment to the importance of accurate and thoughtful diagnosis.

Introduction

Have you ever wondered why people often make decisions they later regret?

This question has intrigued me for years and is the driving force behind this book, *Critical Thinking in Diagnosis and Therapy of Cognitive and Behavioral Disorders*.

Throughout my career in the human sciences, I have been deeply invested in understanding why individuals frequently make choices that lead to unfavorable outcomes. This fascination began in my early twenties, when I observed friends and relatives making irrational decisions—despite having clear information that should have guided them otherwise. My frustration grew as I witnessed recurring patterns of misguided responses and flawed thinking.

This curiosity intensified after I earned my master's degree in psychology and began my counseling practice, where I interacted with clients from diverse cultural backgrounds. I noticed a persistent confusion in analyzing problems—often at the root of their struggles. Conversely, I occasionally encountered individuals who demonstrated a remarkable ability to make sound decisions through critical, neutral, and insightful analysis. Their judiciousness and independence from external influence left a lasting impression on me.

These observations underscored the urgent need to cultivate critical thinking skills—not only in education, but across all stages and domains of life. This realization led me to focus on critical thinking in my Ph.D. studies. To my surprise, most scholarly work emphasized critical thinking strictly within academic contexts, making it challenging to highlight its broader applications to everyday life and psychological well-being.

In response, I developed a psychometric instrument titled *Sherouk's Critical Thinking Test (SH-CTT)*, specifically designed to assess individuals' ability to apply critical thinking in real-life scenarios. Its continued use in clinical settings has yielded valuable insights into clients' cognitive strengths and areas of difficulty.

The results have been profound. Clients who identified their critical thinking deficiencies and committed to developing these skills experienced improved mental health, greater self-discipline, more rational responses, and transformative life changes.

Accordingly, this book represents the culmination of years of observation, research, and clinical experience. It was born from a deep concern over the widespread neglect of critical thinking—even among psychologists—and the alarming absence of psychometricians in diagnostic and therapeutic processes. These gaps not only hinder accurate assessment but also perpetuate misdiagnosis and ineffective interventions.

Critical Thinking in Diagnosis and Therapy of Cognitive and Behavioral Disorders seeks to confront this global issue by offering both conceptual insights and practical solutions. Through a multidisciplinary lens and with contributions from diverse experts, this work invites readers to rethink how we approach mental health and cognitive care—positioning critical thinking as a foundational tool for more accurate, ethical, and transformative outcomes.

Chapter 1 The Power of Critical Thinking in Diagnosing Children's Psychological Disorders: A Path to Reducing Misdiagnosis

Sherouk J. Kadhm
https://orcid.org/0000-0002-3881-9180
TruePath Assessments, Jordan

Tareq Yousef Damrah
MedPro Medical Hub, Jordan

Mohammad Abdelilah Semrin
MedPro Medical Hub, Jordan

ABSTRACT

Misdiagnosis of psychological disorders in children is a global concern with profound emotional and economic consequences. Studies show that around 30% of autism cases and many ADHD diagnoses are inaccurate, with prevalence rates varying by region. These errors result in distress and significant financial burdens—ADHD-related costs in the U.S. alone range from $143 to $266 billion annually, much of it borne by families. This chapter highlights the urgent need to strengthen critical thinking among caregivers, educators, and mental health professionals. It explores diagnostic complexities, advocates for multidisciplinary evaluations, and shows how critical thinking can improve diagnostic accuracy. Case studies of misdiagnosed

DOI: 10.4018/979-8-3373-1812-7.ch001

children illustrate how applying critical thinking led to correct diagnoses and effective treatment. The chapter calls for widespread adoption of these practices to reduce misdiagnosis and its impact on individuals and society.

INTRODUCTION

Misdiagnosis of psychological disorders has become a pervasive global issue, with profound consequences for individuals, families, and broader society. Research suggests that approximately 30% of autism cases are inaccurately diagnosed, with similar concerns surrounding ADHD. Some studies report overdiagnosis, while others point to underdiagnosis—highlighting a shared recognition of widespread diagnostic inaccuracies. These discrepancies vary by location; for instance, ADHD prevalence among children aged 4 to 17 ranges from 4.2% in Nevada to 14.6% in Arkansas.

These diagnostic errors do not only inflict emotional distress; they also generate significant economic burdens. In the United States alone, the annual healthcare costs associated with ADHD are estimated to range from $143 billion to $266 billion, over half of which are shouldered by families. The impact extends to adults with ADHD and parents of affected children, who often experience substantial losses in work productivity, further compounding financial and social strain.

Historically, the importance of critical thinking has been emphasized primarily in educational domains, with policymakers, educators, and researchers advocating its role in equipping learners to navigate the complexities of the modern world. However, it is time to transcend this traditional educational framework and consider the broader implications of critical thinking—particularly its potential to enhance psychological well-being and reduce diagnostic error.

Critical thinking is not merely a cognitive skill confined to academic contexts; it is a dynamic, cultivated capacity that shapes self-awareness, emotional regulation, and adaptive problem-solving. Research by scholars such as Facione (2000) underscores that critical thinking encompasses both cognitive and dispositional dimensions. An individual's motivation and willingness to engage critically are as crucial as their intellectual capabilities.

In this context, the integration of critical thinking into psychological services becomes vital. This chapter advocates for equipping caregivers, teachers, pediatricians, psychologists, and psychiatrists with critical thinking competencies to more accurately identify and evaluate psychological disorders in children. By embedding structured reasoning into multidisciplinary assessments, clinicians can move beyond surface-level symptom checklists and enhance diagnostic precision.

Moreover, fostering critical thinking among professionals and caregivers can mitigate the risks of misdiagnosis and its harmful consequences. Through real-life case studies of children who were initially misdiagnosed, this chapter illustrates how critical thinking interventions redirected their diagnostic trajectories toward accuracy and effective treatment. These examples underscore the transformative potential of critical thinking in both prevention and care.

Ultimately, the call to integrate critical thinking into psychological evaluation and intervention is not only a matter of best practice—it is a pressing need. By doing so, we can alleviate the societal and economic burdens of misdiagnosis and ensure better mental health outcomes for individuals and families worldwide.

DEFINING CRITICAL THINKING

Although the term "critical thinking" is widely used and recognized as a fundamental skill, its precise nature and application remain subjects of debate among scholars. The complexity of critical thinking has led to diverse interpretations, contributing to its conceptual ambiguity.

Paul (1995) played a significant role in clarifying critical thinking by defining it as a distinctive, intentional mode of thought that is systematic and purposeful. He argued that critical thinkers consistently apply specific criteria to their reasoning processes, identifying three key intellectual strategies essential for effective critical thinking: components of inference, attributes of inference, and criteria for inference.

Similarly, Burden and Byrd (1999) described critical thinking as a higher-order cognitive process that encompasses a range of mental skills extending beyond basic comprehension. They emphasized its role in enabling individuals to differentiate between verifiable facts and value claims, discern relevant from irrelevant information, assess the factual accuracy of statements, and evaluate the credibility of sources. Additionally, they highlighted critical thinkers' ability to recognize ambiguity, detect biases, identify logical fallacies, and assess the strength of arguments.

Hemming (2000) further expanded the understanding of critical thinking by examining its foundational components, including logical reasoning, the importance of maintaining a "critical spirit," dialogic thinking, and the application of evaluative standards. He emphasized that critical thinking is not only dependent on mastering subject matter but is also influenced by personal interests that shape cognitive engagement. Hemming concluded that fostering critical thinking remains essential, reinforcing its significance in educational programs.

Over the past few decades, definitions of critical thinking have evolved, initially shaped by cognitive psychologists and philosophers before being expanded upon by behavioral psychologists and subject matter experts. For instance, Scriven and

Paul (1992) defined critical thinking as "the intellectually disciplined process of actively and skillfully conceptualizing, applying, analyzing, synthesizing, and evaluating information gathered from observation, experience, reflection, reasoning, or communication as a guide to belief and action."

Other scholars have contributed to this evolving definition:

Lipman (1995) described critical thinking as a criteria-based, self-correcting process that is sensitive to context.

Facione (2000) defined it as the ability to judge reflectively what to do or what to believe.

Bailin (2002) characterized critical thinking as a purposeful, goal-directed mental process that involves judgment formation while adhering to standards of adequacy and accuracy.

Empirical research continues to highlight discrepancies in how critical thinking is both understood and cultivated. Bezanilla (2019) conducted a study involving 230 university instructors from Spain and Latin America, revealing variations in teaching approaches to critical thinking. Despite differing interpretations, instructors primarily relied on three methods: oral and written reasoning and debates, reading and synthesizing information, and case studies. However, the study underscored the need for more innovative and precise pedagogical strategies to enhance the development of critical thinking skills effectively.

Despite these variations, the core premise remains: critical thinking is a structured, reflective process essential for intellectual and practical decision-making. As its definition continues to evolve, so too must the strategies used to cultivate it across diverse professional domains.

Building upon these perspectives, in the field of psychology, the authors define critical thinking as the ability to apply analysis, inference, evaluation, and interpretation skills to achieve an accurate diagnosis of psychological disorders. This cognitive process enables psychologists to formulate a strategic therapeutic plan that aligns with precise diagnostic conclusions, ensuring effective and individualized treatment.

SUB-SKILLS OF CRITICAL THINKING

Critical thinking is a multifaceted cognitive process, and researchers have offered varying classifications and definitions of its core skills. This diversity has led to differing views on the number and nature of critical thinking sub-skills. For instance, Watson and Glaser (1980) identified five core components in their Watson-Glaser Critical Thinking Appraisal: inference, recognition of assumptions, deduction, interpretation, and evaluation of arguments. Beyer (1995), on the other hand, proposed a broader list that includes analyzing, synthesizing, evaluating, problem-solving, and decision-making.

Similarly, Facione (2011)—in the widely cited Delphi Report—outlined a consensus among experts that critical thinking consists of specific core skills such as analysis, evaluation, inference, interpretation, explanation, and self-regulation. These skills enable individuals to systematically assess information, reason logically, and make well-informed decisions.

The Delphi project, conducted from 1988 to 1989, gathered 46 experts in critical thinking education, who collaboratively defined the concept and agreed upon these essential cognitive skills. According to Facione (2011), critical thinkers are those who are able to apply these sub-skills across disciplines, using sound criteria and intellectual standards. They emphasized that critical thinking is not just a set of techniques, but a habit of mind guided by reason and reflective judgment.

Further supporting this structured view, Ennis (2000) also listed core critical thinking skills which include identifying assumptions, formulating hypotheses, and evaluating sources and credibility. Both Ennis and Facione emphasized the interplay between dispositions and skills—highlighting that being inclined to think critically is as crucial as having the skills to do so.

Moreover, sub-skills such as observation, classification, and comparison are seen in educational settings as tools that support critical thinking development. For example, students are encouraged to observe phenomena closely, categorize findings meaningfully, and compare data to identify patterns or inconsistencies (Huitt, 1998; Baker et al., 2001).

Critical thinking also involves the skill of summarizing—abstracting core ideas and condensing them concisely. This is closely related to application, which refers to the use of learned concepts in new contexts, as discussed in several cognitive learning frameworks (Facione, 2000; Fatmawati et al., 2019). These skills help learners go beyond rote memorization, enabling them to think flexibly and creatively in novel situations.

In summary, while variations exist in terminology and categorization, the literature converges on a set of vital sub-skills—particularly analysis, inference, and evaluation—as foundational to critical thinking. These are not only essential for academic learning but also for everyday decision-making and lifelong problem-solving.

UNCRITICAL MINDS AND MISGUIDED DIAGNOSES: THE CONSEQUENCES OF COPY-PASTE THINKING IN HEALTHCARE AND BEYOND

In today's fast-paced world, it is alarming how many individuals tend to uncritically adopt the thoughts, beliefs, and decisions of others without a second thought. This extends from trivial matters, such as personal preferences, to serious, life-altering decisions. We often assume that our choices are genuinely our own when, in fact, they are heavily influenced by societal pressures, cultural norms, or even parental beliefs. This phenomenon, known as Psychological Suggestion, has a far-reaching impact on how we think, behave, and make decisions.

If people were to dedicate even a single hour to reflect on how they arrive at their decisions, many would be shocked to realize that much of their reasoning was not a result of independent thought but rather a subconscious copying of others' ideas. The adoption of others' opinions—often without thorough analysis or critical evaluation—is a widespread issue that hinders our ability to think critically. This lack of reflection is especially troubling when it influences decisions that affect not just the individual but the larger society, from personal life choices to organizational and governmental policies.

Psychological Suggestion can be particularly harmful because it leads people to follow established patterns of thinking blindly, without engaging in the important mental processes of analyzing and evaluating situations. Critical thinking, which encompasses skills like interpreting facts, identifying logical inconsistencies, and drawing informed conclusions, is rarely applied. Instead, many people skip these crucial steps, relying on external influences rather than developing their own judgments. This pervasive issue undermines rational decision-making at all levels of society.

In my professional experience, I have witnessed the damaging effects of this phenomenon firsthand. It was this realization that motivated me to develop an instrument aimed at measuring the critical thinking skills that should be applied in everyday life. The results of this test were startling: out of a sample of 158 participants, the vast majority failed to infer correct facts or make rational decisions when presented with a variety of real-life scenarios, including situations that occur in hospitals (Kadhm, 2021). This wasn't just a failure of logic—it was evidence of a broader societal problem, one that permeates all sectors of life, including homes, educational institutions, and workplaces.

Consider, for instance, how this issue plays out in high-stakes environments like hospitals and clinics. If people are unable to think critically in ordinary situations, what does that mean for the quality of diagnoses and treatment decisions in healthcare? Misdiagnosis is a real concern, especially in the field of children's disorders, where complex behavioral and cognitive issues require a nuanced and accurate understanding. Yet, without strong critical thinking skills, even trained professionals are at risk of making erroneous judgments that can lead to harmful consequences for patients.

It is crucial to recognize that critical thinking is not just an academic skill reserved for scholars; it is a fundamental life skill that should be nurtured and applied in all areas of life. Whether we are making personal decisions or contributing to large-scale societal developments, the ability to think critically—analyzing information, evaluating evidence, and drawing logical conclusions—is essential for our success and well-being.

The shortage of critical thinking is an issue that plagues both individuals and institutions alike. In educational settings, students are often taught to memorize facts rather than engage in deep, reflective thinking. In workplaces, employees may follow established procedures without questioning their efficacy. In government, policymakers may adopt populist views without critically examining the long-term consequences of their decisions. This lack of analytical rigor leads to a cascade of poor decisions at every level of society.

Through my work, I aim to bring attention to this crisis and promote the development of tools that foster critical thinking skills. The results of my research have shown that many people struggle with the foundational aspects of logical reasoning and decision-making. This is a wake-up call for all of us, as it highlights the urgent need to cultivate a culture of critical thinking—one where individuals are encouraged to question, analyze, and reflect before making decisions. Only by doing so can we hope to create a society that is capable of navigating the complexities of modern life with wisdom and discernment.

FROM OBSERVATION TO CONCLUSION: CRITICAL THINKING IN DIAGNOSTIC PRACTICE

In the evolving landscape of healthcare, a pressing issue has emerged with considerable impact: the frequent misdiagnosis of psychological, behavioral, and cognitive disorders across the globe. While fields such as cardiology and neurology benefit from precise diagnostic tools like X-rays, MRI scans, and blood tests, psychology remains heavily reliant on subjective interpretation. This disparity highlights a critical need for innovation within the mental health profession to ensure diagnostic accuracy that parallels the standards seen in other medical fields. In psychology, where the human mind's complexity resists easy categorization, therapists rely primarily on their observational skills, clinical judgment, and professional intuition. Although these attributes are invaluable, they are subject to human error, as even the most skilled therapists can be influenced by cognitive biases, emotional predispositions, and limitations in the patient's narrative.

One of the fundamental challenges of psychological diagnosis is that it largely depends on self-reported symptoms. Patients, though often well-intentioned, may unintentionally misrepresent or downplay their symptoms, either due to personal biases, societal stigma, or even a lack of self-awareness regarding deeper psychological conflicts. This self-reporting approach assumes patients have a high degree of insight into their mental state, yet significant evidence suggests that psychological struggles often reside beneath conscious awareness. Patients, believing they fully understand their issues, may overlook or misunderstand the roots of their behavior, making it difficult for therapists to obtain an accurate understanding of the underlying issues (Meyer et al., 2002). This lack of insight requires therapists to exercise exceptional analytical and inferential skills, decoding subtle emotional cues and navigating complex interpersonal dynamics to arrive at a correct diagnosis.

Adding to this complexity, the rising rates of psychological, behavioral, and cognitive disorders in today's fast-paced world make it all the more essential for mental health professionals to sharpen their critical thinking skills. As societies face unprecedented levels of stress and rapid change, mental health issues become increasingly diverse and multifaceted. Psychologists, therefore, need more than empathy and intuition; they require robust, systematic critical thinking abilities that enable them to sift through overlapping symptoms, identify root causes, and develop customized, effective treatment plans. Studies have consistently shown that critical thinking improves diagnostic precision, equipping therapists to differentiate between conditions that present similarly on the surface but differ profoundly in their underlying nature and treatment needs.

In my work within this field, as well as through extensive collaborations with educators, it has become abundantly clear that critical thinking is not merely an advantageous skill—it is an essential tool for elevating mental health practice to new heights. Cultivating these skills allows therapists to reduce misdiagnoses, ultimately preventing patients from receiving treatments that may be misaligned or even detrimental to their well-being. When therapists engage in structured critical analysis, they are more likely to recognize when a patient's symptoms point toward a specific condition or when deeper environmental, psychological, or emotional factors might be at play. For patients, this translates into shorter treatment times, more accurate care, and lower associated costs, as their therapists are equipped to cut through the surface and address core issues with greater efficiency.

Moreover, the impact of critical thinking in psychology extends beyond individual cases. Misdiagnosis is not only a personal concern but a systemic one, influencing how resources are allocated, how treatments are prescribed, and how public perceptions of mental health conditions are shaped. Misdiagnosed patients may experience prolonged suffering or even stigma, as their conditions are not understood or appropriately addressed. This issue is particularly severe for those with complex or overlapping disorders, who may feel disheartened or stigmatized by a seemingly never-ending diagnostic process. By integrating critical thinking as a central practice, therapists can approach cases with a level of insight and rigor that minimizes these risks, providing a pathway toward compassionate, precise, and dignified care for all patients.

Transforming mental health care through critical thinking also represents a significant step forward for the field of psychology itself. By embracing an analytical, evidence-based approach, therapists move beyond the traditional reliance on intuitive judgments and advance toward diagnostic practices that reflect the complexity of the human mind. This shift not only enhances the quality of care but fosters a therapeutic environment where trust and understanding flourish. Patients who receive thoughtful, accurate diagnoses are more likely to engage fully in the therapeutic process, feeling seen and validated in their unique experiences.

In a world where mental health issues are often misunderstood, minimized, or stigmatized, fostering critical thinking among psychologists is an urgent priority. Misdiagnosis is not merely an individual setback but a collective challenge that affects millions, contributing to societal burdens and detracting from the efficacy of mental health systems. By investing in critical thinking skills for therapists, we lay the groundwork for a transformative approach to mental health that values both precision and compassion. This approach ensures that those in need of support receive it with accuracy and empathy, leading to better outcomes, enriched patient-therapist relationships, and ultimately, a more resilient and mentally healthy society.

In conclusion, integrating critical thinking into psychological practice offers a powerful antidote to the challenges of misdiagnosis and mismanagement in mental health care. It is not simply an enhancement of the therapeutic toolkit but a fundamental shift toward a more reflective, precise, and humane model of care. The future of psychology lies in the ability to approach human complexity with both analytical rigor and profound empathy, creating a landscape where mental health professionals are equipped to meet the diverse needs of individuals in a thoughtful, effective, and meaningful way.

THE DIAGNOSTIC LANDSCAPE: MISDIAGNOSIS AND OVERDIAGNOSIS DEFINED

In contemporary mental health research, the concepts of misdiagnosis and overdiagnosis have gained increasing attention due to their significant implications for clinical practice and patient well-being. Both represent diagnostic errors, but they differ in essential ways that must be clearly understood, particularly within the context of mental, cognitive, and behavioral disorders.

Misdiagnosis occurs when a condition is inaccurately identified—either by assigning an incorrect diagnostic label or by failing to recognize a disorder that is present. This can lead to inappropriate or delayed treatment and may exacerbate existing symptoms due to the absence of targeted intervention.

In contrast, overdiagnosis refers to the correct identification of a condition that may not actually cause harm or require clinical intervention. While diagnostically accurate according to current classification criteria, such cases often involve labeling individuals whose symptoms are mild, transient, or fall within normal developmental variations. This is particularly critical in children and adolescents, where typical developmental behaviors may be misunderstood as pathological. Overdiagnosis can lead to unnecessary medical or psychological treatment, emotional distress from being labeled, and exposure to side effects from unwarranted interventions.

Over the past five decades, health insurance data and national mental health registries have documented a marked rise in the number of diagnosed mental disorders among children and adolescents. While this trend might suggest a growing prevalence, epidemiological findings present mixed evidence. Increasingly, overdiagnosis—rather than an actual surge in mental health conditions—is considered a contributing factor (Merten, Cwik, Margraf, & Schneider, 2017).

A systematic literature review by Merten et al. (2017) explored the phenomenon of overdiagnosis in child and adolescent mental health. Although most studies affirmed the occurrence of misdiagnosis, only limited research methodologically addressed overdiagnosis. Among these, significant evidence pointed to overdiagnosis of attention-deficit/hyperactivity disorder (ADHD). Several systemic and contextual factors were identified as contributors to diagnostic inaccuracies, including the use of heuristics instead of data-driven assessments, ambiguous symptom descriptions, and pressures within healthcare systems to assign diagnoses in order to secure treatment reimbursement.

Additionally, challenges arise from variability in informant reports, such as parental or teacher input, and from limitations in diagnostic criteria that may inadequately differentiate between disorder and normative behavior. These factors collectively increase the risk of both misdiagnosis and overdiagnosis in routine clinical practice.

Recognizing these diagnostic challenges is crucial for developing more accurate, context-sensitive assessment practices and for advancing ethical and effective care in child and adolescent mental health.

CURRENT STATISTICS AND CONSEQUENCES

In recent years, the prevalence of mental, cognitive, and behavioral disorders has risen at an alarming rate globally. This surge is complex and influenced by multiple factors; no single cause can fully explain it. However, rapid technological, digital, and social transformations are widely acknowledged as major contributors. These swift changes often generate stress, anxiety, and other adverse emotional responses as individuals struggle to adapt. The pace of modern advancements has left many individuals unprepared, exacerbating mental health issues and highlighting the need for comprehensive mental health solutions.

A large-scale study conducted in China illustrates the magnitude of the problem. Researchers initially selected 73,992 participants aged 6–16 years. In the second phase, they screened and diagnosed 17,524 of these individuals. The study revealed a 17.5% weighted prevalence for any mental disorder, highlighting a significant public health concern. This prevalence varied notably by demographics, with higher rates among males, younger individuals, and residents of more developed areas ((Liu et al., 2021; Morin, 2021)). Comorbidities were especially high, with disorders like attention-deficit hyperactivity disorder (ADHD), oppositional defiant disorder (ODD), tic disorder, conduct disorder, and major depressive disorder frequently co-occurring. This research has recorded the highest-ever prevalence of psychiatric disorders in China, underscoring a dire need for interventions by public health officials and policymakers to ensure that individuals receive timely and appropriate mental health support. The long-term consequences on families, communities, and the broader society could be profound if the issue is left unaddressed.

These troubling trends are not isolated to China; globally, studies indicate similar increases in mental health disorders driven by urbanization, socioeconomic pressures, and the pervasive impact of digital media. For instance, the World Health Organization (WHO) reports that depression has become the leading cause of disability worldwide, impacting over 264 million individuals. Anxiety disorders also affect a staggering 284 million people, making them the most common mental health disorders globally (BMJ Quality & Safety). Confronting this global crisis demands a multifaceted approach, encompassing heightened awareness, improved diagnostic tools, strengthened mental health services, and policy measures that support mental well-being. Early intervention and comprehensive care are essential for alleviating the mental health burden and enhancing the quality of life for affected individuals.

The consequences of mental health misdiagnosis are far-reaching. Misdiagnosis can result in inappropriate treatment, potential worsening of symptoms, and an increased burden on patients and healthcare systems alike. Research shows that a significant portion of mental health misdiagnosis stems from insufficient diagnostic tools and an over-reliance on clinical judgment without adequate psychometric support. For instance, a study in the Journal of Child and Family Studies highlighted significant disparities in mental health diagnoses among minority youth, emphasizing the urgent need for accurate, culturally sensitive diagnostic tools to avoid misdiagnosis (Liang, Matheson, & Douglas, 2016). Additionally, research from Hillside Atlanta demonstrates that disorders such as oppositional defiant disorder (ODD) and bipolar disorder are frequently misdiagnosed due to symptom overlap with other conditions, such as ADHD and anxiety. This underscores the critical necessity for refined, precise diagnostic criteria (BMJ Quality & Safety).

CRITICAL THINKING DIAGNOSIS AND THERAPY: ADVANCING MENTAL, COGNITIVE, AND BEHAVIORAL HEALTH

The benefits of critical thinking extend far beyond childhood. This work introduces a novel and transformative perspective to the field of psychology, advocating for the integration of critical thinking skills into both diagnosis and therapy for clients of all ages, with a particular emphasis on children. The concept of Critical Thinking Diagnosis and Therapy Clinics, pioneered and validated by the authors, emerged in response to the high incidence of misdiagnosis in mental, cognitive, and behavioral health worldwide. By incorporating critical thinking dispositions—such as truth-seeking and systematicity—into diagnostic practices, psychologists can achieve greater accuracy, especially in distinguishing between impulsivity-driven behaviors and underlying psychological conditions.

Building on these insights, we developed Critical Thinking Diagnosis and Therapy, a specialized approach that revolutionizes both diagnostic and therapeutic processes. This method empowers clients, both children and adults, to actively engage in their treatment through structured critical thinking exercises and reflective practices. For children, these exercises are adapted to their developmental stages, focusing on age-appropriate strategies for self-reflection, perspective-taking, and cooperative dialogue. For adults, Critical Thinking Diagnosis and Therapy emphasizes deeper reflective processes and independent critical analysis, allowing them to explore their cognitive and emotional patterns in a structured, supportive environment. Over the past three years, I have implemented this technique with both online and in-person clients, yielding notable improvements and receiving positive feedback from those who have experienced its benefits.

CONFUSION BETWEEN LACK OF CRITICAL THINKING SKILLS AND MISDIAGNOSIS OF MENTAL DISORDERS

Critical thinking is not only an academic skill but also a vital aspect of mental health and social development. As highlighted by Ollinheimo and Hakkarainen (2023), it is deeply tied to human cooperation and is essential for fostering social welfare and mental well-being from childhood onward. However, a significant issue arises when critical thinking skills are underdeveloped in children and adolescents—misdiagnosis of mental, cognitive, and behavioral conditions. The lack of critical thinking ability often leads to children displaying behaviors that are mistaken for psychological disorders, such as impulsivity or social withdrawal, rather than being understood as symptoms of underdeveloped cognitive skills.

Critical thinking enables children to navigate their emotions and social environments with flexibility and resilience. When children fail to develop these skills, they may be incorrectly categorized as having behavioral or emotional disorders. For example, behaviors stemming from impulse control issues may be misinterpreted as signs of a disorder, when, in fact, they are simply the result of a lack of reflective thinking or self-regulation skills. Empirical studies, such as Liu et al. (2020), suggest that children who develop critical thinking skills, including truth-seeking and systematicity, are better equipped to manage impulsivity and emotional regulation. Without these skills, children may struggle with actions that appear disruptive or out of control, but are instead indicative of an inability to engage in self-reflection or consider consequences—critical thinking abilities that are essential for mental and emotional health.

Integrating critical thinking into early childhood education and development offers a proactive solution. Instead of reserving critical thinking as an advanced skill for later years, it can be introduced through age-appropriate exercises that encourage children to analyze information, consider different perspectives, and work cooperatively to solve problems. In educational settings, activities that promote critical thinking also provide immediate social and emotional benefits. For instance, guided group discussions, where children engage with open-ended questions, foster cooperative problem-solving and allow children to practice self-regulation and empathy—skills that protect against the social isolation and alienation commonly associated with mental health struggles.

By enhancing critical thinking in children from an early age, educators and caregivers can provide a foundation that prevents misdiagnosis by enabling children to engage thoughtfully with the world around them. This not only supports children in avoiding unnecessary labels of disorder but also strengthens their emotional resilience, social connections, and overall mental well-being. As critical thinking dispositions become ingrained in children's cognitive and emotional development, they build the necessary skills to thrive in both childhood and adolescence, preventing the misdiagnosis that often arises from impulsivity, emotional distress, or misunderstood behaviors.

In conclusion, fostering critical thinking is not just an educational tool; it is a protective factor against the misdiagnosis of mental and behavioral disorders. The lack of critical thinking skills can often be mistaken for signs of disorder, but with proper development, children and adolescents can be equipped with the mental tools needed to understand their emotions, regulate their behavior, and engage with the world in a healthy, adaptive way. Integrating critical thinking into early development is a crucial step toward reducing misdiagnoses and promoting long-term mental wellness.

PROMOTING LIFELONG CRITICAL THINKING: A PATH TO PREVENTING MISDIAGNOSIS

As we reach the conclusion of this chapter, it is essential to emphasize the profound importance of fostering critical thinking skills—not just as an educational goal, but as a lifelong necessity integral to accurate diagnosis and the prevention of misdiagnosis. Traditionally, the promotion of critical thinking has been confined to academic environments, creating a narrow understanding of its true value and inadvertently downplaying the risks associated with its absence. This limited perspective overlooks the vital role that critical thinking plays in all aspects of diagnosis, from clinical assessments to understanding complex mental and cognitive challenges.

While the importance of critical thinking in ensuring accurate diagnoses is well recognized, emerging research highlights its crucial role in preventing misdiagnosis, particularly in the realm of mental health. Critical thinking enables professionals to better evaluate symptoms, identify underlying causes, and avoid common pitfalls in diagnosing mental and behavioral disorders. By instilling these skills from an early stage, both professionals and individuals can benefit from a clearer, more accurate understanding of psychological conditions, leading to more effective treatment outcomes and better overall care.

RETHINKING DIAGNOSIS: REAL CASES INFORMED BY CRITICAL THINKING

The researchers collaborated as a team for two years. During this period, significant issues with misdiagnosis became apparent. A high percentage of clients had previously received diagnoses for certain disorders. However, through the critical application of standardized testing—guided by specific critical thinking skills such as Inference, Statement Evaluation, and Analysis—the team often uncovered different and more accurate results. In several cases, this prevented the unnecessary use of medication that had been previously prescribed before the clients visited the clinic where the researchers were working.

Case Study 1: Misdiagnosed ADHD (Attention-Deficit/Hyperactivity Disorder)

Initial Diagnosis: ADHD

Client Profile

H.H., a 13-year-old boy, was diagnosed with ADHD by two separate physicians. Both recommended medication and the assignment of a shadow teacher. His reported symptoms included difficulty focusing in class, frequent interruptions of the teacher, disruptive behavior among peers, heightened anxiety and anger, and an inability to sit still for extended periods. These behaviors led the school director to issue a formal warning, with the possibility of expulsion if the behavior persisted.

Findings and Diagnostic Reevaluation Using Critical Thinking

The researchers began their assessment by administering projective tests to explore H.H.'s emotional and psychological state. These tests revealed signs of emotional distress and rejection related to family dynamics. Additional assessments, including a focus-measurement tool developed by the researcher, indicated that H.H. had strong attentional control—a result that contradicted the previous diagnosis of attention deficit.

Further investigation uncovered a pattern of emotional and physical abuse at home, which H.H. later confirmed during follow-up sessions.

Application of Critical Thinking Skills

1. Statement Evaluation Skill

When asked, "Why do you disrupt the class?", H.H. replied, "I feel suffocated at home and need to feel free in class."

This statement was evaluated for its intent and emotional clarity. His response reflected conscious, intentional behavior rather than impulsivity or inattention. This insight helped rule out the automatic classification of his behavior as a symptom of ADHD.

2. Analysis Skill

An in-depth analysis of the projective test responses revealed psychological distress and signs of physical abuse by his parents. This analysis provided a critical understanding of the emotional roots of his classroom behavior.

3. Inference Skill

Cognitive assessments, particularly memory tests, demonstrated that H.H. had strong memory and recall abilities—contradicting his parents' claims of forgetfulness. Based on this evidence, the team inferred that the symptoms originally associated with ADHD were actually manifestations of trauma and environmental stress, rather than a neurodevelopmental disorder.

Conclusion

Through the application of critical thinking skills—Evaluation, Analysis, and Inference—the research team was able to challenge the initial ADHD diagnosis and uncover the true source of H.H.'s behavioral difficulties. This case highlights the essential role of critical thinking in achieving accurate diagnoses and avoiding unnecessary medical and educational interventions.

In this case, the correct diagnosis not only prevented the financial burden of medication and shadow teacher support, but—more importantly—it protected the child from being labeled with a lifelong mental disorder, and redirected him toward appropriate emotional and psychological support.

Case Study 2: Misdiagnosed Major Depressive Disorder (MDD)

Initial Diagnosis: Major Depressive Disorder (MDD)

Client Profile

K.A., a 6-year-old girl, was initially diagnosed with Major Depressive Disorder based on observations by her parents, later confirmed by a physician. She exhibited sudden depressive symptoms, including frequent crying, loss of interest in activities, social withdrawal, refusal to attend a summer club, and expressing sadness without a known cause. Remarkably, K.A. personally requested to see a psychologist, showing a level of emotional self-awareness uncommon for her age.

Findings and Diagnostic Reevaluation Using Critical Thinking

A comprehensive psychometric assessment, including structured questions and projective tools such as drawing analysis, revealed inconsistencies in the initial diagnosis. When asked about her emotional state, K.A. repeatedly stated that her parents did not care about her. However, clinical observation showed that her parents were attentive and supportive. When asked, "Why do you feel they don't care?" she responded, "Because they don't give me medicine so I won't be depressed." This statement suggested a fixed belief in the necessity of medication and an internalized identity of being "sick."

Further analysis of her drawings revealed a recurring figure from a cartoon character she frequently watched—one that expressed deep sadness after moving to a new city and starting a new school. This strongly mirrored K.A.'s recent real-life experience of relocating with her family, and suggested that she had absorbed the character's emotional narrative and adapted it as her own. Notably, she often mimicked the character's facial expressions, tone of voice, and repeated its specific phrases.

Application of Critical Thinking Skills

1. Statement Evaluation Skill

K.A. insisted that her parents did not care for her. When probed further, she linked this belief to their failure to provide her with "psychological medicine." This evaluation clarified that her belief was not rooted in observed neglect but rather in a learned association between emotional care and medication—likely influenced by the media.

2. Inference Skill

Analysis of her drawings indicated emotional identification with a cartoon character portraying sadness in a similar context of relocation. From this, it was inferred that K.A.'s symptoms were imitative rather than organically depressive. Her behavior reflected emotional adaptation and confusion, not clinical depression.

Conclusion

The integration of critical thinking skills—Statement Evaluation, Inference—led to the rejection of the initial diagnosis of MDD. Instead, the findings revealed an emotionally sensitive child coping with environmental changes through identification with fictional narratives.

A placebo (a children's vitamin) was introduced as a symbolic "psychological medicine," satisfying her perceived need for treatment. Additionally, the cartoon was replaced with a more optimistic character model, and targeted emotional support was provided. Within two weeks, K.A. returned to her usual state with no lingering depressive symptoms.

This case demonstrates the danger of premature diagnosis in young children and underscores the vital role of critical thinking in distinguishing between internal psychopathology and external influences on emotional expression.

Case Study 3: Misdiagnosed Obsessive-Compulsive Disorder (OCD)

Initial Diagnosis: Obsessive-Compulsive Disorder (OCD)

Client Profile

G.H., a male adolescent, aged 18, had been diagnosed with obsessive-compulsive disorder by three different physicians over an 14-month period prior to attending the clinic. His symptoms included persistent intrusive thoughts centered around guilt and a distorted self-concept of being morally flawed. These obsessions were particularly connected to a fear of divine rejection or lack of blessing from God. G.H. also experienced intermittent episodes of aggression, frequently directed at items associated with his mother.

At the time of evaluation, G.H. was taking two types of psychiatric medications and regularly consuming alcohol.

Findings and Diagnostic Reevaluation Using Critical Thinking

A comprehensive psychometric assessment was administered, incorporating both projective techniques and quantitative tests. The evaluators observed a significant memory gap related to the ages of 9 to 10, raising concerns about possible psychological repression. Further exploration revealed that during those years, G.H. had been subjected to persistent bullying by peers and emotional abuse from a maternal uncle who frequently told him he would "never be accepted by God." These repeated experiences of humiliation and fear were internalized, forming the foundation of his obsessive guilt and feelings of moral contamination.

Additionally, it was discovered that G.H. had unconsciously developed a pattern of interpreting life challenges as divine punishment—a maladaptive coping mechanism rooted in early trauma. This distorted cognitive framework had fueled his obsessive thoughts and emotional instability.

Application of Critical Thinking Skills

1. Inference

The clinical team noted that G.H.'s episodes of aggression and emotional confusion often followed alcohol use. Considering the well-documented interaction between alcohol and his prescribed psychiatric medications, it was inferred that many of his symptoms—particularly cognitive confusion and impulsivity—were chemically induced rather than indicative of primary OCD.

2. Analysis

Through projective assessments, G.H. consistently avoided discussing events from the ages of 9 to 12. This avoidance, coupled with the emergence of fragmented memories under therapeutic exploration, pointed to psychological repression. A deeper analysis confirmed that the emotional roots of his obsessive guilt stemmed from childhood trauma, particularly religious-based emotional abuse. The convergence of bullying and abusive moral messaging during a formative developmental stage significantly contributed to his psychological profile.

Conclusion

Following a reevaluation of his medication regimen under psychiatric supervision and the gradual elimination of alcohol use, G.H. showed marked improvement. His obsessive thoughts diminished, his emotional stability returned, and he began reintegrating into daily life. The correction of the initial diagnosis, supported by critical thinking and psychometric insights, prevented further mismanagement and unnecessary treatment targeting OCD.

This case highlights the importance of inference and analysis in clinical reasoning. It illustrates how unresolved childhood trauma and environmental abuse—not obsessive-compulsive disorder—were the primary contributors to the client's distress. Accurate interpretation of underlying causes allowed for an effective, individualized intervention strategy.

The presented case studies highlight the detrimental consequences of misdiagnosis and overdiagnosis when critical thinking is absent from the diagnostic process. To address this issue, the following model illustrates a structured approach that integrates core critical thinking skills—such as analysis, interpretation, and evaluation—into clinical assessment. This model demonstrates how applying these cognitive tools can lead to more accurate diagnoses, reduce diagnostic errors, and support more effective treatment planning. The visual representation serves as a practical guide for professionals aiming to enhance diagnostic precision through critical thinking in psychological and educational contexts. As shown in the following figure, the new diagnostic approach proposed in this chapter outlines the essential steps practitioners should follow to achieve diagnostic accuracy and prevent both misdiagnosis and overdiagnosis.

Figure 1. Model of how applying critical thinking skills in the diagnostic process leads to greater accuracy and prevents both misdiagnosis and overdiagnosis.

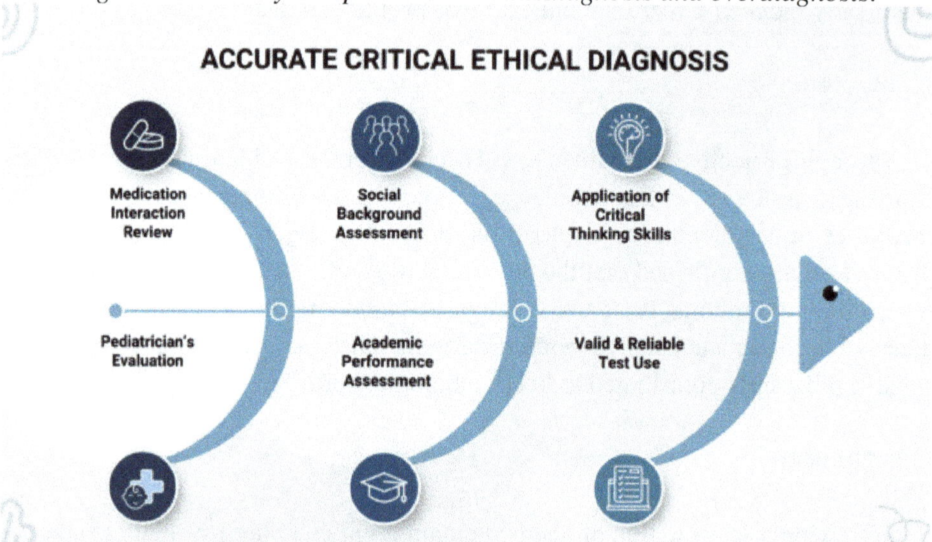

A PROMISING DIAGNOSTIC COMPETENCY: IHSAN

Finally, the researchers would like to highlight a promising competency that they believe will become increasingly essential in future diagnostic processes—

particularly in the evaluation of mental, behavioral, and cognitive disorders. This competency is referred to as "Ihsan."

Rooted in Islamic philosophy, Ihsan is a concept so rich and nuanced that it is difficult to find a single term in English that fully captures its essence. Broadly, it is described as the pursuit of excellence or the highest quality in one's actions and intentions. It encompasses a set of sub-competencies—including mindfulness, ethical responsibility, self-awareness, accurate performance, and compassion—that, when applied in clinical settings, may help reduce both misdiagnosis and overdiagnosis.

At the heart of Ihsan lies focused and ethically grounded decision-making. This competency does not merely inform clinical actions; it elevates the quality of judgments made by professionals through conscious reflection and moral clarity. The integration of Ihsan into diagnostic reasoning emphasizes a deliberate and principled approach to decision-making, ensuring that assessments are not only accurate but also human-centered.

The researchers propose that Ihsan, as a clinical competency, merits further exploration. Specifically, it should be studied for its potential impact on diagnostic accuracy, ethical decision-making, and reflective performance among psychologists and medical professionals. Incorporating such a value-based framework into modern clinical practice may offer a unique and culturally responsive approach to enhancing professional judgment and patient-centered care.

REFERENCES

Bailin, S. (2002). Critical thinking and science education. *Science & Education, 11*(4), 361–375. DOI: 10.1023/A:1016042608621

Baker, M., Rudd, R., & Pomeroy, C. (2001). Relationships between critical and creative thinking. *Journal of Southern Agricultural Education Research, 51*(1), 173–188.

Behrens, P. J. (1996). The Watson-Glaser Critical Thinking Appraisal and academic performance of diploma school students. *The Journal of Nursing Education, 35*(1), 34–36. DOI: 10.3928/0148-4834-19960101-10 PMID: 8926515

Beyer, B. K. (1995). *Critical thinking: Fastback 385*. Phi Delta Kappa Educational Foundation.

Bezanilla, M. J., Fernández-Nogueira, D., Poblete, M., & Galindo-Domínguez, H. (2019). Methodologies for teaching-learning critical thinking in higher education: The teacher's view. *Thinking Skills and Creativity, 33*, 100584. DOI: 10.1016/j.tsc.2019.100584

BMJ Quality & Safety. (2021). Diagnostic error in mental health: A review. *BMJ Quality & Safety, 33*(10), 663–672. https://qualitysafety.bmj.com/content/33/10/663

Burden, P. R., & Byrd, D. M. (1999). *Methods for effective teaching* (2nd ed.). Allyn & Bacon.

Ennis, R. H. (2000). A super-streamlined conception of critical thinking. http://faculty.education.illinois.edu/rhennis/documents/Super-Streamlined.pdf

Facione, P. A. (2000). The disposition toward critical thinking: Its character, measurement, and relationship to critical thinking skill. *Informal Logic, 20*(1), 61–84. DOI: 10.22329/il.v20i1.2254

Facione, P. A. (2011). *Critical thinking: What it is and why it counts* (2011 update). Insight Assessment.

Fatmawati, A., Zubaidah, S., & Mahanal, S. (2019, December). Critical thinking, creative thinking, and learning achievement: How they are related. In *Journal of Physics: Conference Series* (Vol. 1417, No. 1, p. 012070). IOP Publishing. DOI: 10.1088/1742-6596/1417/1/012070

Giuliano, K., & Geyer, E. (2017). ADHD: Overdiagnosed and overtreated, or misdiagnosed and mistreated. *Cleveland Clinic Journal of Medicine, 84*(11), 873–879. DOI: 10.3949/ccjm.84a.15051 PMID: 29173249

Hemming, H. E. (2000). Encouraging critical thinking: "But... what does that mean?". *McGill Journal of Education, 35*(2), 173–186.

Huitt, W. (1998). Critical thinking: An overview. *Educational Psychology Interactive*. Valdosta State University. http://www.edpsycinteractive.org/topics/cogsys/critthnk.html

Kadhm, S. J. (2021). Validation of Sherouk's Critical Thinking Test (SH-CTT). In *Research anthology on developing critical thinking skills in students* (pp. 1345–1356). IGI Global. DOI: 10.4018/978-1-7998-3022-1.ch071

Liang, J., Matheson, B. E., & Douglas, J. M. (2016). Mental health diagnostic considerations in racial/ethnic minority youth. *Journal of Child and Family Studies, 25*(6), 1926–1940. DOI: 10.1007/s10826-015-0351-z PMID: 27346929

Liu, J., Chen, X., & Yan, Y.. (2021). Prevalence of mental disorders among children and adolescents in China: A nationwide epidemiological study. *The Lancet. Psychiatry, 8*(4), 263–272. DOI: 10.1016/S2215-0366(20)30448-0 PMID: 33675689

Liu, Z., Li, S., Shang, S., & Ren, X. (2021). How do critical thinking ability and critical thinking disposition relate to the mental health of university students? *Frontiers in Psychology, 12*, 704229. DOI: 10.3389/fpsyg.2021.704229 PMID: 34489809

Merten, E. C., Cwik, J. C., Margraf, J., & Schneider, S. (2017). Overdiagnosis of mental disorders in children and adolescents (in developed countries). *Child and Adolescent Psychiatry and Mental Health, 11*(1), 5. DOI: 10.1186/s13034-016-0140-5 PMID: 28105068

Meyer, B., Pilkonis, P. A., Krupnick, J. L., Egan, M. K., Simmens, S. J., & Sotsky, S. M. (2002). Treatment expectancies, patient alliance, and outcome: Further analyses from the National Institute of Mental Health Treatment of Depression Collaborative Research Program. *Journal of Consulting and Clinical Psychology, 70*(4), 1051–1055. DOI: 10.1037/0022-006X.70.4.1051 PMID: 12182269

Morin, A. (2021, April 15). 1 in 6 kids in China have a mental disorder. *Psychology Today*. https://www.psychologytoday.com/us/blog/what-mentally-strong-people-dont-do/202104/1-in-6-kids-in-china-have-mental-disorder

NeuroLaunch. (2024). Autism misdiagnosis: Challenges and implications for individuals and families. https://neurolaunch.com/misdiagnosed-autism/?utm_source=chatgpt.com

Ollinheimo, A., & Hakkarainen, K. (2023). Critical thinking as cooperation and its relation to mental health and social welfare. *New Ideas in Psychology, 68*, 100988. DOI: 10.1016/j.newideapsych.2022.100988

Paul, R. W. (1995). *Critical thinking: How to prepare students for a rapidly changing world.* Foundation for Critical Thinking.

Scriven, M., & Paul, R. (1992, November). Critical thinking defined. Paper presented at the *National Council for Excellence in Critical Thinking Conference*, Atlanta, GA.

Thombs, B., Turner, K. A., & Shrier, I. (2019). Defining and evaluating overdiagnosis in mental health: A meta-research review. *Psychotherapy and Psychosomatics, 88*(4), 193–202. DOI: 10.1159/000501647 PMID: 31340212

Watson, G. (1980). *Watson-Glaser Critical Thinking Appraisal* (Vol. 3). Psychological Corporation.

Chapter 2
Critical Diagnostic Psychometrics (CDP) in Action:
The Psychometrician's Role in Accurate Diagnosis Prior to Therapy and Training

Sherouk J. Kadhm
https://orcid.org/0000-0002-3881-9180
TruePath Assessments, Jordan

Alexander Weissman
https://orcid.org/0009-0007-9746-8812
M2C1 Consulting, USA

ABSTRACT

Misdiagnosis and overdiagnosis have gained attention in mental, cognitive, and behavioral disorder assessments, yet the latter remains poorly defined. Misdiagnosis refers to incorrect identification, while overdiagnosis involves labeling a condition that may not require treatment, often causing unnecessary interventions. A study by Thombs et al. (2019) found that only 11.4% of reviewed articles used "overdiagnosis" correctly, highlighting a critical need for diagnostic clarity. These errors can lead to improper care, symptom escalation, and strain on healthcare systems. Research links these issues to inconsistent tools and overreliance on clinical judgment without psychometric support. This chapter emphasizes the psychometrician's role in

DOI: 10.4018/979-8-3373-1812-7.ch002

improving diagnostic accuracy through critical thinking frameworks and proposes a new model, Critical Diagnostic Psychometrics (CDP), to reduce errors and guide effective, culturally informed mental health evaluations.

INTRODUCTION

In an era where mental health challenges are increasingly recognized, the accuracy of diagnosis and therapy has never been more critical. Yet, across mental health services, misdiagnosis and overdiagnosis remain pressing concerns—often rooted in subjective judgment, inconsistent diagnostic standards, and the underutilization of objective assessment tools. These diagnostic inaccuracies not only hinder effective treatment but also contribute to unnecessary psychological distress, long-term emotional burdens, and increased healthcare costs.

This chapter explores the vital role of critical thinking in transforming diagnostic and therapeutic practices. It highlights how psychometricians—experts in the science of psychological measurement—can bring greater clarity and precision to the diagnostic process. By integrating validated tools with structured reasoning and evidence-based frameworks, psychometricians help minimize diagnostic errors and improve treatment outcomes.

Central to this chapter is the proposal to establish specialized psychometric clinics—centers dedicated to accurate, culturally sensitive, and critically informed psychological assessment. These clinics aim to bridge the gap between clinical intuition and empirical data, ensuring that diagnostic conclusions are grounded in more than symptom checklists or subjective interpretations. By embedding critical thinking into the heart of psychological evaluation, psychometric clinics represent a bold and necessary innovation in mental health care.

Through a critical lens, this chapter examines the nature and consequences of diagnostic errors, the misuse of diagnostic labels, and the urgent need for reform. It argues that psychometricians, empowered with appropriate tools and frameworks, can lead a paradigm shift toward more accurate diagnoses and personalized interventions—advancing both the science and humanity of psychological practice.

It is also important to clarify that the term "clinic," though commonly associated with therapeutic services, should not be viewed so narrowly. A clinic does not exclusively imply the provision of therapy—it can also encompass comprehensive assessment services. In fact, many clinics in the field of psychology—including the psychometric clinics proposed in this chapter—primarily focus on evaluation, diagnosis, and testing, rather than therapeutic intervention.

For example, a psychometric clinic may offer services such as cognitive assessments, behavioral evaluations, personality testing, learning disability screenings, and the generation of diagnostic reports—with or without accompanying therapy.

Moreover, the role of psychometric clinics need not be confined to clinical or educational contexts alone. These clinics can also serve a pivotal function in assessing individual and group performance within organizations, institutions, and workplace settings. By applying validated psychometric tools and structured evaluation frameworks, psychometricians can support talent identification, team dynamics analysis, leadership assessments, and organizational development initiatives. This broader application underscores the versatility and impact of psychometric clinics in promoting psychological insight and performance enhancement across multiple sectors.

Thus, using the term "clinic" to describe a setting that offers diagnostic and assessment services—without necessarily including therapy—is both accurate and professionally accepted.

DEFINITION AND SCOPE OF MISDIAGNOSIS

In recent scientific discussions, the terms *misdiagnosis* and *overdiagnosis* have gained increasing prominence in debates surrounding the accuracy of mental, cognitive, and behavioral disorder diagnoses. This shift reflects a growing awareness of the complexities and consequences associated with diagnostic errors. Despite its importance, the concept of overdiagnosis in mental health remains poorly defined and seldom examined systematically.

While both misdiagnosis and overdiagnosis are diagnostic inaccuracies, they differ in important ways. Misdiagnosis refers to the incorrect identification of a condition, whereas overdiagnosis involves correctly identifying a condition that may not require intervention—potentially leading to unnecessary treatment or psychological distress.

Establishing a clear distinction between these concepts requires standardized definitions and consistent quantification methods. However, current literature reveals considerable inconsistency in how these terms are applied. A comprehensive review by Thombs et al. (2019) of relevant articles found that only 11.4% used the term "overdiagnosis" in accordance with its established definition. The majority—76.7%—used it interchangeably with misdiagnosis, false positives, overtreatment, or excessive testing, which obscures important conceptual differences. Moreover, none of the reviewed studies measured overdiagnosis based on rigorous criteria, such as diagnosing mild or transient symptoms that do not warrant clinical intervention. These findings underscore a significant gap in diagnostic standards and highlight the urgent need for more refined criteria to prevent the medicalization of normal variations in behavior and emotion.

This ambiguity calls for greater diagnostic precision, particularly in the context of rising global mental health concerns. Specialized psychometric clinics may serve as a crucial solution to this challenge. By incorporating validated diagnostic tools and structured assessment protocols, these clinics can ensure consistent and accurate evaluations. They would emphasize nuanced diagnostic criteria that account for symptom severity, duration, and contextual factors—thereby reducing both misdiagnosis and overdiagnosis. Such an approach not only advances diagnostic reliability but also meets the growing demand for personalized, evidence-based mental health care. In doing so, psychometric clinics could become essential allies for mental health professionals, supporting more effective and empirically grounded treatment decisions.

THE HIDDEN COST OF MISDIAGNOSIS: THE URGENT CALL FOR PSYCHOMETRIC CLINICS IN MENTAL HEALTH CARE

Misdiagnosis and overdiagnosis have emerged as significant challenges in the realm of mental, cognitive, and behavioral health. Despite growing awareness, the field still lacks systematic clarity in defining and measuring these phenomena. Misdiagnosis, typically involving the incorrect identification of a disorder, and overdiagnosis—labeling conditions that may not require intervention—are often conflated in literature and practice. This confusion contributes to diagnostic imprecision, potentially leading to overtreatment, emotional distress, and an erosion of public trust in mental health services.

As mentioned previously, the review by Thombs et al. (2019) revealed widespread misuse of the term "overdiagnosis," often conflated with misdiagnosis, false positives, and excessive testing. This terminological inconsistency not only obscures conceptual clarity but also reflects broader challenges in diagnostic practices—chiefly, the lack of standardized assessment tools and the insufficient application of critical thinking in clinical decision-making. Addressing these gaps requires clearer definitions and the implementation of structured diagnostic reasoning frameworks that reduce subjectivity and enhance accuracy.

The consequences of diagnostic errors are profound. Inappropriate treatment pathways, worsening symptoms, and long-term psychological harm are just some of the outcomes patients may face. Cultural differences in behavior and emotional expression are often misinterpreted through the lens of standardized diagnostic tools, which may not account for diverse sociocultural contexts. A recent Canadian study demonstrated that although East Asian and South Asian youth reported significantly higher levels of obsessive-compulsive, ADHD, and anxiety traits, they were substantially less likely to receive corresponding diagnoses when compared to White youth. This discrepancy suggests that cultural norms may influence both symptom presentation and clinical recognition, resulting in underdiagnosis or misdiagnosis among minority populations (Dissanayake et al., 2024). These findings underscore the urgent need for culturally sensitive diagnostic frameworks that differentiate between psychopathology and culturally normative behaviors.

These issues are compounded by outdated tools, subjective interpretations, and inconsistent use of diagnostic criteria. Frequently, overlapping symptoms are misread or oversimplified, resulting in the mislabeling of conditions such as ADHD, autism spectrum disorders, and mood disorders. In many cases, individuals endure years of unsuitable treatments before a correct diagnosis is made—if at all.

To meet these challenges, this chapter proposes the establishment of specialized psychometric clinics—centers dedicated to enhancing diagnostic precision through empirically validated tools and structured reasoning. Staffed by trained psychometricians, these clinics would bridge the gap between traditional clinical intuition and data-driven assessment. Rather than relying solely on symptom checklists or observational interviews, psychometric clinics would employ robust, culturally responsive instruments to evaluate cognitive, emotional, and behavioral dimensions with scientific rigor.

The implementation of such clinics could transform mental health care. By integrating critical thinking into every stage of diagnosis, these centers would promote clearer distinctions between disorders, reduce diagnostic errors, and support more targeted, effective treatment plans. This model reflects ongoing recommendations from leading health and safety organizations. For example, the U.S.-based Patient Safety Network (PSNet), managed by the Agency for Healthcare Research and Quality, emphasizes the need for systematic improvements in diagnostic accuracy to enhance patient safety. Similarly, the BMJ Quality & Safety journal—an international publication dedicated to healthcare improvement—has called for diagnostic reform as a critical step in addressing the global mental health crisis.

This chapter will examine the root causes of diagnostic inaccuracies, the misapplication of diagnostic terms, and the consequences of relying on insufficient tools. It will then outline the structure, function, and potential of psychometric clinics as an innovative and urgently needed solution. With the right infrastructure and professional expertise, psychometric clinics could set a new standard in mental health diagnostics—offering individuals not only more accurate diagnoses but also a more hopeful path to recovery.

CONSEQUENCES OF MISDIAGNOSIS

An evolutionary concept analysis has also shed light on the issue of diagnostic overshadowing in mental health. This phenomenon involves attributing the symptoms of a new or co-occurring condition to a pre-existing diagnosis, often resulting in compromised care and poorer patient outcomes. Hallyburton (2022), through a systematic review of 25 publications using Rodgers' Evolutionary Concept Analysis method, examined the causes and implications of diagnostic overshadowing. The study identified key contributors such as cognitive biases, insufficient assessment tools, and time constraints in clinical settings. Alarmingly, it also suggested that misdiagnosis may contribute to elevated mortality rates among individuals with mental illness, as treatable conditions may remain unaddressed or mismanaged.

The economic consequences of misdiagnosis are similarly profound. Globally, billions of dollars are spent annually on unnecessary medications, ineffective treatments, and redundant therapeutic interventions resulting from diagnostic errors. This economic strain burdens healthcare systems and highlights the need for more evidence-based diagnostic practices. Additionally, frequent misdiagnoses erode public trust in mental health services, discouraging individuals from seeking help and reinforcing stigma.

Improving diagnostic accuracy is, therefore, a critical priority. Integrating refined assessment methods, critical thinking, and specialized training for mental health professionals can significantly enhance the accuracy of diagnoses, improve treatment outcomes, and reduce healthcare costs. Central to this process is the adoption of valid and reliable psychometric instruments, which strengthen the diagnostic process and support the delivery of effective, individualized care.

THE PROPOSAL: SPECIALIZED PSYCHOMETRIC CLINICS

To address the persistent challenges of diagnostic inaccuracy in mental health and organizational settings, this chapter proposes the establishment of specialized psychometric clinics—dedicated centers for the assessment and diagnosis of psychological, cognitive, and behavioral functioning. Operated by trained psychometricians, these clinics would employ validated, culturally responsive tools to ensure diagnostic precision grounded in empirical evidence.

Unlike therapy-focused settings, psychometric clinics prioritize diagnostic clarity and data-informed interpretation over subjective clinical impressions. They are envisioned as structured environments where objective measurement is central to the diagnostic process.

Psychometric clinics can operate effectively in both clinical and organizational contexts. Within mental health systems, these clinics could reduce rates of misdiagnosis by delivering assessments tailored to individuals' cultural and contextual backgrounds—an area where only psychometricians can offer distinct expertise. In the workplace, psychometric evaluations could be leveraged to support leadership development, employee well-being, and performance management. Across both domains, psychometricians contribute methodological rigor, statistical precision, and structured analysis that enhance the reliability of diagnostic decisions.

A CRITICAL GAP: UNDERUTILIZATION OF PSYCHOMETRICIANS

One of the most persistent and overlooked contributors to diagnostic inaccuracies in mental health care is the underutilization of psychometricians in clinical assessment settings. Although psychiatrists and clinical psychologists are traditionally at the forefront of diagnosis, their training often emphasizes symptom recognition, behavioral observation, and clinical interviews rather than the scientific rigor of psychometric measurement. Psychometricians, by contrast, are specifically trained in test construction, statistical modeling, validity assessment, and measurement theory. They offer a crucial layer of scientific oversight that ensures psychological assessments are not only standardized but also interpreted with precision and contextual understanding.

Even when psychological testing is incorporated into diagnosis, tools are frequently misused or misinterpreted. A common issue is improper administration, often conducted by professionals lacking advanced training in psychometric principles. This misuse compromises the validity and reliability of diagnostic outcomes. According to Gregory (2021), as well as the *Standards for Educational and Psychological Testing* (AERA, APA, & NCME, 2014), professionals who administer and interpret assessments must possess sufficient psychometric knowledge to ensure ethically sound and scientifically accurate results. Chapter 10 of the *Standards* particularly emphasizes that test users should be competent in psychometric evaluation, cultural fairness, and statistical interpretation to avoid errors in diagnosis.

Moreover, current diagnostic systems often rely heavily on symptom checklists or short inventories without accounting for their psychometric robustness or cultural adaptability.

This challenge is not exclusive to psychology; it has also been observed in newer fields such as implementation science, where high-quality measurement is vital to advancing knowledge. Despite the availability of numerous quantitative instruments, systematic reviews have shown that many lack established psychometric properties.

Proctor et al. (2009) defined a core set of implementation outcomes—acceptability, adoption, appropriateness, cost, feasibility, fidelity, penetration, and sustainability—which are crucial for evaluating the effectiveness of applied interventions. Building on this framework, the Society for Implementation Research Collaboration (SIRC) Instrument Review Project conducted a comprehensive systematic review that identified only a small number of instruments meeting psychometric standards in mental and behavioral health contexts (Lewis et al., 2015). These findings underscore the urgent need to apply the same level of psychometric scrutiny in psychological diagnosis, where many tools remain unvalidated or outdated. The role of psychometricians in addressing these gaps is both essential and long overdue.

WHAT ARE PSYCHOMETRIC CLINICS AND WHY ARE THEY NEEDED?

A persistent challenge in modern healthcare is the lack of standardized and reliable methods for identifying and measuring diagnostic errors—an issue that continues to compromise the accuracy and consistency of clinical evaluations. The Improving Diagnosis in Health Care report by the National Academies (2015) identifies one of the core contributors to diagnostic inaccuracies as the limited development and application of validated diagnostic instruments. The report emphasizes that diagnostic excellence depends not solely on clinical judgment but also on the use of structured evaluation procedures grounded in scientific evidence. It advocates for the rigorous development, independent validation, and appropriate application of diagnostic tools—principles central to psychometrics, which prioritizes test reliability, validity, and cultural sensitivity. Furthermore, the report underscores the need for specialized training and credentialing for professionals responsible for administering and interpreting assessments. This reinforces the argument that diagnostic accuracy demands expertise in measurement science to reduce interpretive errors and enhance objectivity (National Academies of Sciences, Engineering, and Medicine, 2015). These insights support the integration of psychometricians into diagnostic processes and endorse the establishment of psychometric clinics as a means to improve diagnostic precision across mental health and behavioral healthcare systems.

Moreover, misdiagnosis of psychological, cognitive, and behavioral disorders remains a widespread and under-addressed issue in contemporary mental health practice. Inaccurate diagnoses frequently stem from subjective evaluations, inconsistent application of diagnostic criteria, and an overreliance on clinical intuition. These diagnostic lapses can lead to inappropriate treatment strategies, prolonged patient distress, and stagnation in therapeutic progress.

The urgency for psychometric clinics becomes abundantly clear when considering recent findings on diagnostic inaccuracy. Misdiagnosis rates in mental health range between 20–50% overall, with particularly high initial misclassifications in conditions such as bipolar disorder (up to 60%), personality disorders (>70%), and ADHD in children (40%) (ZipDo, 2025; Gitnux, 2025) . These errors often result in inappropriate treatments—including medication mismatches in 40% of bipolar cases—and delays in effective care averaging 3–5 years, increasing healthcare costs by approximately 30% (WIFI Talents, 2025) .

Bolstering these alarming statistics, Ayano et al. (2021) reported that in an Ethiopian psychiatric setting, 40% of patients with severe disorders received incorrect initial diagnoses—especially schizoaffective disorder (75%), major depressive disorder (55%), schizophrenia (24%), and bipolar disorder (18%) . Notably, depressive and schizoaffective presentations and suicidal ideation were significant predictors of diagnostic error.

The ethical and emotional toll of misdiagnosis is further highlighted in qualitative research. One pivotal work—*"The Experience of Being Misdiagnosed and Mistreated: A Qualitative Exploration"* (2016)—reports profound psychological impacts, including emotional trauma, distrust toward clinicians, and long-term disruption in treatment engagement. These narratives underscore the urgency of structural change—not just better tools—toward more trustworthy, transparent diagnostic processes.

INTRODUCING PSYCHOMETRIC CLINICS: A TRANSFORMATIVE DIAGNOSTIC MODEL

Despite the vast documentation of diagnostic errors (ZipDo; Gitnux; Ayano, 2016), no existing framework has systematically addressed the structural deficiencies that allow these inaccuracies to persist. As argued in Chapter One, diagnostic failures are often rooted in two main factors: the absence of critical thinking in clinical reasoning and the marginalization of psychometric expertise. Addressing these deficiencies requires more than improved tools—it requires an institutional redesign of how diagnostic processes are conducted.

This chapter proposes a paradigm shift through the creation of psychometric clinics—dedicated diagnostic centers operated and overseen by trained psychometricians. These clinics would specialize in the application of evidence-based, psychometrically sound assessments as the cornerstone of clinical decision-making. Unlike conventional mental health settings, which often blur the line between therapy and diagnosis, psychometric clinics would offer a focused, standardized environment for data-driven evaluation. This structure ensures that clinical judgments are not merely interpretive but supported by empirical measurement.

Psychometric clinics would employ a multimodal diagnostic approach, integrating standardized testing with clinical interviews, behavioral observation, and cultural context analysis. Tools used would be carefully selected for their cultural validity (Dana, 2005; Suzuki & Ponterotto, 2007), statistical reliability (Rust & Golombok, 2014), and alignment with developmental norms. Assessments would be administered and interpreted by certified professionals who understand the complexities of measurement error, test bias, and validity coefficients.

To operationalize this model, several key strategies must be addressed:

1. **Training and Certification**: Developing specialized training programs and licensing pathways for psychometricians in clinical settings (APA, 2020; Kaplan & Saccuzzo, 2017).
2. **Interdisciplinary Integration**: Establishing frameworks that support the collaboration of psychometricians with psychologists, psychiatrists, educators, and pediatricians (National Academies of Sciences, 2015).
3. **Feasibility and Cost Analysis**: Evaluating the long-term cost-effectiveness and sustainability of psychometric clinics, especially in resource-limited or underserved areas (WHO, 2022).
4. **Public Awareness and Policy Advocacy**: Promoting understanding among policymakers, practitioners, and the public about the benefits of psychometric clinics in reducing diagnostic error and improving mental health outcomes.

Institutionalizing psychometric clinics would represent a critical evolution in mental health diagnostics. By placing scientifically grounded measurement at the core of clinical practice, these clinics would minimize diagnostic subjectivity, enhance public trust, and ensure culturally sensitive and equitable care. This model aligns with the foundational principles of Critical Diagnostic Psychometrics (CDP), advocating for a diagnostic culture that is empirical, transparent, and ethically grounded.

IMPLEMENTATION STRATEGIES: OPERATIONALIZING CRITICAL DIAGNOSTIC PSYCHOMETRICS (CDP)

The accuracy achieved by psychometricians in uncovering the root causes of mental and behavioral concerns affirms their indispensable role in modern clinical practice. Under the framework of Critical Diagnostic Psychometrics (CDP), this role expands beyond test administration—it applies critical thinking and scientific measurement to reframe diagnosis as a rigorous, pre-therapeutic process rather than a reactive label.

Psychometric clinics grounded in CDP offer a structured, evidence-based alternative to symptom-driven judgments, reducing misdiagnosis and strengthening intervention design.

1. Multidimensional, Critical Diagnostics

CDP employs validated tools to assess cognitive, emotional, behavioral, and social domains. But its strength lies not only in instrumentation—it's in the critical thinking applied to interpret results contextually, rejecting surface-level symptom reading in favor of integrative, individualized analysis. The outcome is a comprehensive diagnostic profile that helps clinicians and educators make decisions rooted in evidence, not assumption.

2. Distinguishing Pharmacological Effects from True Symptoms

While psychometricians do not prescribe medications, their critical insight allows them to flag patterns suggesting pharmacological influence—such as side effects, withdrawal symptoms, or drug interactions. In consultation with medical professionals, they refine diagnostic clarity by differentiating psychological manifestations from medically induced ones, safeguarding both diagnosis and treatment direction.

3. Cross-Disciplinary Expertise and Critical Reflexivity

CDP requires psychometricians to master both technical precision and contextual awareness. Continuous training in modern test theory, construct validity, and statistical modeling is essential—but equally critical is the application of reflective judgment, cultural sensitivity, and developmental insight. This dual lens ensures that each diagnosis is empirically sound and personally relevant.

4. Ihsan: A Promising Moral Competency in Diagnostic Practice

Ihsan—an Arabic term deeply rooted in Islamic thought—refers to the pursuit of excellence through sincerity, moral integrity, and inner responsibility. While traditionally associated with spirituality and ethical conduct in Islam, Ihsan is increasingly being recognized in applied sciences as a promising moral-ethical competency, particularly for its role in preventing or reducing performance deficiencies. Within the framework of Critical Diagnostic Psychometrics (CDP), Ihsan transcends technical proficiency by promoting diagnostic practices grounded in compassion, humility, and justice. It calls on practitioners to act not only with competence but with conscience—ensuring that psychometric assessments are applied with ethical care, contextual sensitivity, and accountability. Framing Ihsan as a core diagnostic value positions the psychometrician not merely as a technician, but as a morally reflective change agent within clinical and educational systems.

5. Correcting Public Misconceptions and Professional Boundaries

A major challenge lies in outdated perceptions of psychometrics as merely academic testing. CDP demands a paradigm shift: psychometrics is a clinical science, grounded in the same empirical reasoning as medical diagnostics.

Just as MRI interprets invisible biological states via complex algorithms, psychometrics quantifies internal psychological constructs through validated statistical models. In both fields, data requires expert interpretation. As radiologists guide medical diagnoses, psychometricians guide therapeutic decisions—bringing precision to what is often treated subjectively.

ELEVATING DIAGNOSTIC PRACTICE

Psychometric clinics founded on CDP do more than standardize assessment—they redefine diagnostic thinking itself. By combining measurement science with disciplined reasoning, they establish a frontline for accurate, meaningful diagnosis before therapy or training begins. In this model, the psychometrician is not just a technician, but a diagnostic thinker—ensuring every intervention starts with clarity, not conjecture.

IMPLEMENTATION STRATEGIES: OPERATIONALIZING CRITICAL DIAGNOSTIC PSYCHOMETRICS (CDP)

The precision demonstrated by psychometricians in uncovering the underlying causes of mental and behavioral challenges confirms their essential role in modern clinical settings. Within the framework of Critical Diagnostic Psychometrics (CDP), this role transcends test administration and emerges as diagnostic leadership—one that applies critical thinking and scientific measurement to transform diagnosis into a rigorous, pre-therapeutic process, rather than a reactionary label.

CDP addresses pervasive diagnostic challenges—such as overdiagnosis, rushed labeling, and symptom misinterpretation—by promoting a structured, evidence-based alternative. Clinics guided by this model move beyond subjective impressions, offering accurate, data-informed pathways for intervention planning.

1. Multidimensional, Critical Diagnostics

CDP extends far beyond basic testing. It incorporates validated instruments to assess cognitive, emotional, behavioral, and social domains, with an emphasis not merely on *what* is measured, but *how* data are critically interpreted. At its core are three subskills of critical thinking applied throughout the assessment process:

- **Analysis** – Identifying meaningful patterns within assessment data (Cottrell, 2023).
- **Inference** – Drawing plausible explanations that go beneath surface symptoms (Chamberlin, 2023).
- **Evaluation** – Judging the credibility and contextual relevance of results (Fabio, Plebe, & Suriano, 2025).

This approach yields an integrative diagnostic profile, blending empirical precision with contextual sensitivity—empowering clinicians to make informed, evidence-based decisions while avoiding the traps of assumption or bias.

2. Distinguishing Pharmacological Effects from Psychological Symptoms

Although psychometricians do not prescribe medication, their diagnostic insight allows them to recognize behavioral and cognitive patterns influenced by pharmacological factors—such as side effects, rebound phenomena, or withdrawal symptoms. These manifestations often mimic or obscure genuine psychological conditions, posing a significant risk to diagnostic accuracy.

By identifying such influences and collaborating with prescribing professionals, CDP practitioners enhance diagnostic clarity. This critical collaboration ensures that pharmacologically induced symptoms are not mistaken for enduring psychological traits—safeguarding both the diagnosis and the integrity of subsequent treatment.

3. Cross-Disciplinary Expertise and Reflective Judgment

CDP requires psychometricians to integrate technical mastery with contextual and reflective depth. Alongside expertise in test theory, construct validity, and statistical modeling, effective CDP practice also demands:

- **Cultural Sensitivity** – Awareness of sociocultural factors shaping cognition and behavior.
- **Developmental Insight** – Recognition of age-related cognitive and emotional patterns.
- **Reflective Judgment** – The capacity to question assumptions and calibrate interpretation based on unique client contexts (Banner et al., 2025).

This dual-lens diagnostic model—empirical and humanistic—ensures that conclusions are not only statistically valid but also personally meaningful, reducing bias and promoting deeper understanding of the individual.

4. Redefining the Role: From Technician to Diagnostic Thinker

A common misconception reduces psychometrics to academic or educational testing. However, Critical Diagnostic Psychometrics (CDP) demands a paradigm shift—psychometrics is not a peripheral task but a core clinical science, akin to radiology or laboratory diagnostics in medical fields.

Just as an MRI reveals internal biological conditions, psychometrics quantifies internal psychological states using validated instruments. In both domains, data alone is insufficient—what matters is expert interpretation. Here, the psychometrician steps forward not as a mere technician, but as a diagnostic thinker, who applies scientific rigor and critical analysis to extract clinical meaning from complex behavioral and cognitive data.

This redefined role of the psychometrician directly challenges outdated sequences of practice, where clinicians observe symptoms, formulate impressions, assign diagnoses, and only then consider testing. CDP reverses this flawed logic. It asserts that structured testing and critical evaluation must occur before diagnosis, ensuring that every clinical decision is rooted in evidence rather than intuition or assumption.

This shift also aligns with emerging professional standards and global clinical ethics. As CDP becomes operationalized, it sets a new benchmark for precision diagnostics, positioning psychometricians as essential first-line assessors who inform treatment direction with clarity and objectivity.

5. Correcting Misdiagnosis and Raising Ethical Standards

Misdiagnosis continues to afflict the mental health field, particularly among children, women, and marginalized populations. Research has shown that up to 50% of ADHD diagnoses in school-age children may be inaccurate or misapplied (Merten et al., 2017), often based on superficial observations or non-standardized tools.

CDP directly addresses this crisis by centering validated, structured assessments in the diagnostic process. It rejects reliance on symptom-based impressions and emphasizes multi-dimensional testing interpreted with critical thinking.

This practice is in full alignment with leading professional guidelines, such as:

- **APA's Guidelines for Psychological Assessment and Evaluation (2020)**
- **The Standards for Educational and Psychological Testing (2014)**

By adhering to these standards, CDP enhances ethical safeguards, reduces the risk of stigmatizing or overmedicating clients, and promotes individualized, person-centered care that is just and scientifically sound.

6. Interdisciplinary Collaboration and Role Clarity

Within the CDP framework, psychometricians serve as pre-therapeutic screeners—clinical investigators who use structured tools and critical reasoning to uncover what kind of support a client truly needs. They do not diagnose in isolation, prescribe medication, or offer therapy, but rather inform and refine the diagnostic process.

When integrated into multidisciplinary teams—alongside psychiatrists, educators, pediatricians, and therapists—psychometricians help ensure that the right problem is being identified and the appropriate intervention is pursued. This approach reduces false starts, reactivity, and fragmentation in care.

As emphasized by Leventhal et al. (2021), such interdisciplinary collaboration not only improves diagnostic accuracy but also boosts clinicians' confidence and overall care quality. CDP provides a structural model for this collaboration—making psychometric evaluation a foundational and unifying component in mental health settings.

ELEVATING DIAGNOSTIC PRACTICE THROUGH CRITICAL DIAGNOSTIC PSYCHOMETRICS (CDP)

Despite extensive documentation of diagnostic failures—particularly among children, marginalized populations, and even adults navigating mental health systems (ZipDo; Gitnux; Ayano, 2016)—structured, evidence-based diagnostic frameworks remain strikingly absent from both psychological and organizational settings. Misdiagnosis persists not due to a lack of professional concern, but because of a systemic flaw: the overreliance on observational impressions, intuitive judgments, or static checklists, paired with the chronic underuse of validated instruments interpreted through expert reasoning.

This diagnostic crisis is not confined to clinical care. In organizational contexts, flawed personnel decisions—whether during hiring, promotion, or employee evaluation—often stem from the same root problem: the misuse or complete absence of psychometric assessment. Without appropriate tools and trained psychometric interpretation, organizations risk misjudging competent candidates, mismatching job roles, and stunting professional potential. The consequences parallel those found in mental health: systemic misalignment, inefficiency, and long-term damage to individual and institutional well-being.

Critical Diagnostic Psychometrics (CDP) emerges as a response to this diagnostic void. More than a method, CDP is a redefined logic of understanding human functioning—whether for therapeutic intervention or performance evaluation. It integrates measurement science with disciplined clinical reasoning, explicitly applying critical thinking skills to ensure every conclusion is grounded in structured evidence, not assumption.

Psychometric clinics founded on the CDP model do not simply standardize assessment—they transform the act of diagnosis itself. Within this model, the psychometrician becomes a diagnostic thinker, akin to a radiologist or laboratory specialist, capable of decoding internal psychological realities through scientifically validated tools. Whether applied in mental health or human resource management, CDP ensures that every intervention begins not with labeling, but with clarity—not with guesswork, but with precise, data-driven insight.

In summary, this chapter has introduced Critical Diagnostic Psychometrics (CDP) as a transformative framework that addresses urgent gaps in both mental health and organizational assessment. By establishing psychometric clinics and operationalizing CDP principles, professionals across disciplines can restore diagnostic integrity, uphold ethical standards, and ensure that interventions—clinical or occupational—are timely, tailored, and truly effective.

In a world where misdiagnosis is costly and clarity is rare, CDP offers a scientifically grounded path forward—one that places critical thinking and valid measurement at the core of every human-centered decision.

CONCLUSION

To conclude, the core concept of the newly proposed Critical Diagnostic Psychometrics (CDP) approach—previously discussed throughout this chapter—is summarized in Figure 1 below. This figure illustrates the structured integration of critical thinking skills in parallel with the selection, application, and interpretation of assessment instruments across each phase of the diagnostic process.

Figure 1. The new approach of Critical Diagnostic Psychometrics (CDP): Structured integration of critical thinking with assessment instruments in the diagnostic process

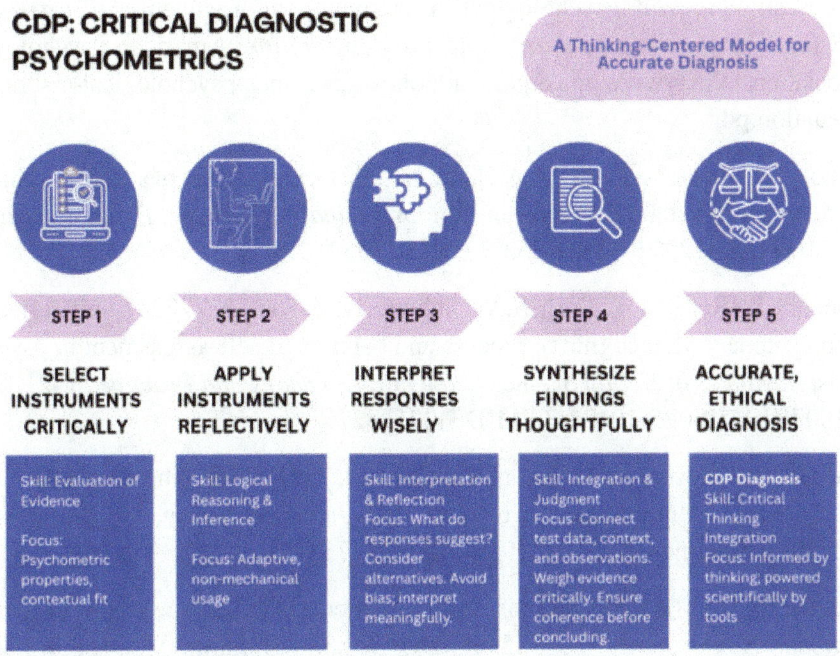

REFERENCES

American Educational Research Association, American Psychological Association, & National Council on Measurement in Education. (2014). *Standards for educational and psychological testing*. American Educational Research Association.

APA Task Force on Psychological Assessment and Evaluation. (2020). *APA guidelines for psychological assessment and evaluation*. American Psychological Association. https://www.apa.org/about/policy/guidelines-psychological-assessment-evaluation.pdf

Ayano, G., Haile, K., Assefa, D., & Haile, H. (2021). Prevalence of severe psychiatric disorders and misdiagnosis rates in Ethiopia. *Annals of General Psychiatry, 20*(1). DOI: 10.1186/s12991-021-00333-7 PMID: 33531016

Banner, S. E., Rock, A. J., Cosh, S. M., Schutte, N., & Rice, K. (2025). Self-reflection on competence: Metacognitive process and barriers of self-assessment in psychologists. *Advances in Health Sciences Education : Theory and Practice*, 1–21. DOI: 10.1007/s10459-025-10434-7 PMID: 40312527

Bradford, A., Meyer, A. N., Khan, S., Giardina, T. D., & Singh, H. (2024). Diagnostic error in mental health: A review. *BMJ Quality & Safety*, *33*(10), 663–672. DOI: 10.1136/bmjqs-2023-016996 PMID: 38575311

Chamberlin, D. E. (2023). The active inference model of coherence therapy. *Frontiers in Human Neuroscience, 16*, 955558. DOI: 10.3389/fnhum.2022.955558 PMID: 36684841

Cottrell, S. (2023). *Critical thinking skills: Effective analysis, argument and reflection* (4th ed.). Bloomsbury Publishing.

Dana, R. H. (2005). *Multicultural assessment: Principles, applications, and examples* (2nd ed.). Routledge. DOI: 10.4324/9781410612540

Deeper Signals. (2024). *Personality assessments that drive results*. https://www.deepersignals.com

DeVellis, R. F., & Thorpe, C. T. (2021). *Scale development: Theory and applications* (5th ed.). Sage Publications.

Dissanayake, A., Dupuis, A., Burton, C. L., Soreni, N., Peters, P., Gajaria, A., Arnold, P. D., Schachar, R., & Crosbie, J. (2024). Racial/ethnic disparities in psychiatric traits and diagnoses within a community-based sample of children and youth. *Canadian Journal of Psychiatry*, *69*(6), 415–427. DOI: 10.1177/07067437241233936 PMID: 38425291

Embretson, S. E., & Reise, S. P. (2013). *Item response theory for psychologists*. Psychology Press. DOI: 10.4324/9781410605269

Fabio, R. A., Plebe, A., & Suriano, R. (2025). AI-based chatbot interactions and critical thinking skills: An exploratory study. *Current Psychology (New Brunswick, N.J.)*, *44*(9), 8082–8095. DOI: 10.1007/s12144-024-06795-8

Gregory, R. J. (2021). *Psychological testing: History, principles, and applications* (8th ed.). Pearson.

Hallyburton, A. (2022). Diagnostic overshadowing: An evolutionary concept analysis on the misattribution of physical symptoms to pre-existing psychological illnesses. *International Journal of Mental Health Nursing*, *31*(6), 1360–1372. DOI: 10.1111/inm.13034 PMID: 35718951

Kaplan, R. M., & Saccuzzo, D. P. (2017). *Psychological testing: Principles, applications, and issues* (9th ed.). Cengage Learning.

Kentrou, V., Livingston, L. A., Grove, R., Hoekstra, R. A., & Begeer, S. (2024). Perceived misdiagnosis of psychiatric conditions in autistic adults. *EClinicalMedicine*, *71*, 102192. DOI: 10.1016/j.eclinm.2024.102586 PMID: 38596613

Kyllonen, P. C. (2013). Soft skills for the workplace. *Change*, *45*(6), 16–23. DOI: 10.1080/00091383.2013.841516

Leventhal, G., Stamm, K. E., Washburn, J. J., Rolston, C., Yozwiak, J. A., Hamp, A., Cash, E. D., Ward, W. L., Hong, B. A., Williams, A. M., & Robiner, W. N. (2021). Patterns of psychologists' interprofessional collaboration across clinical practice settings. *Journal of Clinical Psychology in Medical Settings*, *28*(4), 844–867. DOI: 10.1007/s10880-021-09802-3 PMID: 34405342

Lewis, C. C., Fischer, S., Weiner, B. J., Stanick, C., Kim, M., & Martinez, R. G. (2015). Outcomes for implementation science: An enhanced systematic review of instruments using evidence-based rating criteria. *Implementation Science : IS*, *10*(1), 155. DOI: 10.1186/s13012-015-0342-x PMID: 26537706

Liu, Y., Wang, M., Wang, Y., Zhang, H., Zhang, Y., & Lei, L. (2022). The influence of mental health on employee innovative behavior and job performance: Evidence from China. *International Journal of Environmental Research and Public Health, 19*(9), 5392. DOI: 10.3390/ijerph19095392 PMID: 35564785

Majid, S., Eapen, C. M., & Oo, K. T. (2019). Importance of soft skills for education and career success. *International Journal of Cross-Disciplinary Subjects in Education, 10*(1), 3200–3204. DOI: 10.20533/ijcdse.2042.6364.2019.0422

Mental Health America. (2024). *Mind the Workplace 2024 Report.* https://www.mhanational.org/news/2024-mind-the-workplace-report

National Academies of Sciences, Engineering, and Medicine. (2015). *Improving diagnosis in health care.* The National Academies Press. https://www.limbic-cenc.org/wp-content/uploads/IOM-Improving-Diagnosis-in-Healthcare-2015.pdf

Rust, J., & Golombok, S. (2014). *Modern psychometrics: The science of psychological assessment* (3rd ed.). Routledge. DOI: 10.4324/9781315787527

Saleem, A., Khan, R. U., & Shabbir, M. (2023). Mental health in the workplace: Its impact on employees and organizations. *Journal of Mental Health Issues and Behavior, 3*(1), 12–22. https://journal.hmjournals.com/index.php/JMHIB/article/view/3483

Sanders, A. A. (2016). *The experience of being misdiagnosed and mistreated: A qualitative exploration* [Unpublished doctoral dissertation]. John F. Kennedy University.

Smith, A., & Jones, R. (2023). The role of soft skills in lifelong learning and employability: A psychological perspective. *Journal of Educational & Psychological Research, 45*(2), 112–128. DOI: 10.1234/jepr.v45i2.5678

Suzuki, L. A., & Ponterotto, J. G. (Eds.). (2007). *Handbook of multicultural assessment: Clinical, psychological, and educational applications* (3rd ed.). John Wiley & Sons.

Thombs, B., Turner, K. A., & Shrier, I. (2019). Defining and evaluating overdiagnosis in mental health: A meta-research review. *Psychotherapy and Psychosomatics, 88*(4), 193–202. DOI: 10.1159/000501647 PMID: 31340212

Wadhwani Foundation. (2024). Companies are willing to pay more for those with the best soft skills. https://wadhwanifoundation.org/press/companies-are-willing-to-pay-more-for-those-with-the-best-soft-skills/

WifiTalents. (2025). *Mental health misdiagnosis statistics.* https://wifitalents.com/mental-health-misdiagnosis-statistics

Workday. (2024). *Workday report: AI is transforming the job market; 51% of business leaders fear a skills gap*. https://polandinsight.com/workday-report-ai-is-transforming-the-job-market-51-of-business-leaders-fear-a-skills-gap-22911/

World Economic Forum. (2023). *The future of jobs report 2023*. https://www.weforum.org/stories/2023/05/future-of-jobs-2023-skills

ZipDo. (2025). *Misdiagnosed mental illness statistics*. https://zipdo.co/misdiagnosed-mental-illness-statistics

Chapter 3
Enhancing Diagnostic Accuracy:
The Role of Critical Thinking in Psychological Assessment and Diagnosis

Geemol John
https://orcid.org/0000-0002-6196-9531
Lovely Professional University, India

Mohammad Amin Wani
Lovely Professional University, India

ABSTRACT

This chapter explores how critical thinking not only limits the cognitive biases evident in the process of psychological diagnosis, but it also enhances critical reasoning. It outlines key reasoning difficulties, emphasized barriers to critical thinking in clinical practice, including time constraints and lack of training, and entered additional content – new approaches to the use of artificial intelligence to aid in diagnoses, cultural factors from the DSM-5 Cultural Formulation Interview, and the opportunity for the clinician to discuss their client cases with another professional in an interdisciplinary context. The chapter also offers pragmatic strategies for improving diagnostic accuracy and ethical practice with the chapters on Socratic questioning, reflective practice, and think-aloud strategies. Overall, the chapter impressively supports promoting a more reflexive, evidence-based and culturally competent way of practicing with respect to mental health assessments.

DOI: 10.4018/979-8-3373-1812-7.ch003

INTRODUCTION

Psychological diagnosis accurately is the pillar of successful mental health treatment. It forms the basis for creating the right treatment protocols, for enabling focused interventions, and for ensuring long-lasting healing for those with mental, emotional, or behavioural illnesses. However, because of its pre-eminence, the diagnostic process in psychology is not effortless. Psychiatric conditions tend to have syndrome overlapping symptoms and are influenced by interplay between complex biopsychosocial processes, thereby diagnosing them becomes inherently complex and prone to mistake (First et al., 2018). Moreover, diagnostic decisions will in many cases involve some level of clinical judgment and interpretation, which, if not well controlled, can be subject to cognitive bias, assumptions, and organizational factors (Lilienfeld et al., 2013). Here, critical thinking presents itself as the key instrument to enhance objectivity, precision, and overall quality of psychological diagnosis and assessment.

Critical thinking may be generally described as the disciplined process of actively and skilfully conceptualizing, analysing, synthesizing, and evaluating information to arrive at a conclusion or to solve a problem (Facione, 2015). In the discipline of psychology, critical thinking is not so much an intellectual or academic exercise—it is a professional necessity. Because diagnostic labels have such a significant effect on people's lives, including treatment, self-concept, and social identity, the diagnostic process itself must be pursued with greater rigor and self-awareness. By incorporating critical thinking in the diagnostic process, doctors can improve their handling of diagnostic uncertainty, reduce bias, counter unjustified assumptions, and eventually make more rational and ethical choices.

The psychological diagnostic process comes with steps such as the collection of clinical information using interviews, observations, psychological tests, and the examination of historical and contextual data. Yet at every step, clinicians are confronted by interpretative issues. For example, two patients may come in with identical symptoms—such as fatigue, irritability, and poor concentration—but have completely different underlying conditions like major depressive disorder, generalized anxiety disorder, or an as-yet-undiagnosed medical condition (American Psychiatric Association [APA], 2022). Without intentional and thoughtful reasoning, practitioners can be victims of heuristics or shortcuts, including the availability heuristic, confirmation bias, or premature closure—diagnostic traps that can lead to misdiagnosis or overdiagnosis (Garb, 2005; Croskerry, 2003).

Critical thinking lessens these mistakes by demanding a more structured/intentional approach to thinking. For instance, critical thinking allows clinicians to be reminded to consider more than one hypothesis, be mindful of disconfirming evidence, and be open to new evidence as it arises; leading to some intellectual humility and better diagnoses. The literature indicates that clinicians who engage in reflective abstraction and critical appraisal of their decisions are less likely to experience cognitive traps, leading to more rational diagnostic decisions (Epstein, 2010; Croskerry et al., 2013). Moreover, critical thinking serves to reinforce the ethical tenets of the mental health professions: beneficence, non-maleficence, and respect for autonomy; in that it helps ensure that decisions regarding diagnosis are grounded in valid analysis rather than assumptions or stereotypes.

Critical thinking is particularly relevant to psychological diagnosis in the context of the growing emphasis on evidence-based practice (EBP). EBP emphasizes the combination of the best research based evidence with clinical judgment and patient values, and challenges practitioners to critically assess scientific studies, assess and analyze study results and use those findings in a competent manner in clinical practice (Sackett et al., 2000). It requires not only a strong base of empirical evidence, but also the intellectual capability to critically judge the quality, relevance and appropriateness of the evidence across a variety of clinical circumstances. This means that critical thinking can serve in many ways to support and develop the scientific validity and the humanistic integrity of psychological diagnosis.

Even its acknowledged value, however, cannot preclude challenges in applying critical thinking to clinical diagnosis. Time pressures, heavy caseloads, systemic demands, and even affective fatigue can impede clinicians' capacity for critical thinking (Norman & Eva, 2010). Furthermore, critical thinking per se is a skill that needs to be learned, exercised, and honed over time. Numerous training experiences in psychology and other allied fields focus on knowledge of content and technical skills, but do not adequately cover the cultivation of reasoning skills, metacognitive monitoring, and reflective judgment (Halpern, 2014). To fill this gap, there is a need for teachers, managers, and clinical leaders to build learning cultures that support and reinforce critical thinking, challenging students and practitioners to question assumptions, review their own thought, and learn from diagnostic mistakes.

In this chapter we will discuss the importance of critical thinking in psychological assessment and diagnosis. First we will define critical thinking in the mental health profession and explain the cognitive and dispositional components. Second we will discuss the benefits produced by critical thinking applied to diagnosis including a greater level of diagnostic accuracy, decreased cognitive biases and improved ethical decision-making. Third, we will consider the obstacles to critical thinking, clinical time constraints, over-reliance on intuition, and systemic restrictions. Finally, we will provide examples of how clinicians can increase their critical thinking, both specific diagnostic models, reflective supervision and cognitive debiasing skills training.

While psychological diagnosis is often vague and ambiguous, the purposeful practice of critical thinking can lead toward more objective, more accurate, and more person-centered practice. As the+ field of mental health grows—integrating diversity, neuroscience, and problematizing the limits of current diagnosis—critical thinking will continue to be a cornerstone of effective and ethical psychological practice. By incorporating critical thinking into the process of diagnosis, practitioners can both facilitate better individual outcomes, and possibly also support the growth of a more reflective, responsible, and empathetic mental health system.

BACKGROUND OF THE STUDY

Psychological diagnosis is a critical component of mental health care that informs clinical judgment, treatment decisions, and therapeutic outcomes. A correct diagnosis provides the arrange of circumstances in which clinicians can grasp the subjective disarrays of clients, enact competent evidence-based treatment options, and inform what constitutes positive improvements (Lauber & Huxley, 2000; Kiger & O'Brien, 2002; Robinson, 2005). Yet, the act of diagnosis is rarely straight forward. Psychological disorders do not frequently present as isolated symptoms or syndromes, nor is there a standard method for everyone to embody them, particularly across contextually diverse cultural and social frameworks (Clark et al., 2017). Even ordinary psychological (clinical) assessments involve interpreting multi-layered data and occur in situations of uncertainty, time pressure, and constrained cognitive resource (Bto-B, 2023).

Diagnosing between 'syndromes' or 'disorders' has imposed a severely restrictive way of understanding distress and mental illness, and, if we consider the changes in the DSM and ICD over time, there are effortful ways of trying to improve diagnostic reliability and take culture into account; for instance DSM-III presented clinical diagnosis in a way that was less clinical, and less easily measured through research standards, and although DSM-5 and DSM-5-TR are ascribed a solidity, flexible context like the cultural narrative is incorporated in the CFI (Cultural Formulation Interview; APA, 2013). The DSM and ICD, despite analytic changes, are frequently criticized for their categorical rigidity, their lack of global cross-cultural validity, and that they have left more and more room for clinician judgement, reflective reasoning, and learning outcomes (First et al., 2018).

An increasing amount of research underscores diagnostic errors, as relevant to psychology and psychiatry, have the potential to arise from several areas: inadequate assessment, misinterpreted client stories, thinking using highlighted heuristics, or low cultural competence (Garb, 2005; Croskerry, 2003). Diagnostic errors are not a neutral phenomenon. There can be implications related to inappropriate or delayed treatments, a maintenance of stigma, and less confidence that impacts trust (Lilienfeld et al., 2013). In reviewing the literature on diagnostic errors, critical thinking has been described as a fundamental professional competency that supports ethical, effective, and fair diagnostic practice. Critical thinking, as defined by Facione (1990) is "deliberate, self-regulatory judgment." Critical thinking has the potential to shift our way of thinking from matching symptoms superficially to a richer interpretative analysis of patient experience. When applying critical thinking, a clinician is not just reducing the guesswork involved in assigning a diagnostic label to the client. The clinician is also able to assess their assumptions, evaluate the evidence, create and test alternative hypotheses, and examine the reasoning in a metacognitive way. Also, the skills to think critically within clinical diagnosis can help reduce errors related to cognitive biases such as confirmation bias, availability heuristics, or anchoring (Norman & Eva, 2010).

In addition, critical thinking is useful when examining evidence-based practice (EBP) as it emphasizes integrating the best available research, clinical expertise, and client values (Sackett et al., 2000). EBP is not just about reading the literature as clinicians must have the ability to evaluate the quality of evidence, use this (or not) in practice, and apply it to specific clinical situations. This is especially important to consider when applying EBP to culturally diverse populations, as normative assumptions embedded in the diagnostic criteria cannot be assumed to be universal (Sue et al., 2009).

While beneficial, critical thinking is not emphasized in several clinical training programs. In psychology training, although typically there is an ideal of theoretical knowledge and technical ability, educators underemphasize metacognitive abilities and are needed in reasoning process when evaluating information for diagnostic decisions (Halpern, 2014). In addition, there are contextual, internal, and external stressors to practising clinicians, such as effective caseloads, administrative duties, or emotional exhaustion, which may not leave sufficient mental energy to engage in deliberative processes (Kahneman, 2011).

In reaction to this, the current literature and education formats endorse not only explicit teachings about diagnostic reasoning and structure diagnostic inventions (for example, Structured Clinical Interview for DSM Disorders, SCID-5), reflective supervision models, and debiasing methods (by Croskerry et al, 2013; Eva et al, 2007). Teaching skills about to diagnostic reasoning is part of building a diagnostic culture that is empirically rigorous, culturally relevant and ethical. This chapter aims to propose critical thinking, including some ways of bridging conceptual knowledge closer to clinical relevance to promote better diagnostic work that is scientifically valid, contextually grounded and appreciates being human.

DEFINING CRITICAL THINKING

Critical thinking is the ability to think independently and reflectively, a proficiency that enables individuals to analyse and judge information efficiently to make good decisions. It is at the nucleus of decision-making in complicated and unpredictable situations, like psychological diagnosis (Halpern, 2014). Facione (1990), in his groundbreaking Delphi Report, defined critical thinking as "purposeful, self-regulatory judgment which results in interpretation, analysis, evaluation, and inference, as well as the explanation of the evidential, conceptual, methodological, criteriological, or contextual considerations upon which that judgment is based."

Critical thinking is an essential part of psychological testing, where we need to apply our critical thinking process to make sense of the diagnostic data and balance the options for several diagnostic possibilities and other methods of clinical decision reasoning as well as juggle the making of judgements based on the clinical way and level of skill beyond that of matching symptoms. Critical thinking is somewhat like insurance against cognitive distortions and error in reasoning, avoiding one's tendency to experience premature closure and learn how to factor in the biopsychosocial context of the client (Sternberg, 2003).

Key Features and Skills of Critical Thinking

Critical thinking is multidimensional encompassing various dependent cognitive skills and dispositions. They include.

1. **Analysis:** Analysis includes scrutinizing ideas, recognizing arguments, and dissecting information into building blocks for enhanced comprehension (Facione, 1990). In clinical diagnosis, this might entail dissecting a patient's history and symptomatology into useful categories of meaningful data, allowing the clinician to identify underlying patterns or inconsistencies. The separation of depressional and anxiety symptoms that overlap, for instance, involves analytical examination of the severity, incidence, and setting of the symptoms (Grohol, 2020).
2. **Evaluation:** Evaluation is the process of determining the validity of information sources, the validity of arguments, and the validity of evidence. Clinicians must evaluate both objective information (e.g., test results) and subjective information (e.g., patient reports) for reliability and validity. Studies demonstrate that clinicians who practice critical evaluation are better at evading errors related to excessive reliance on intuition or dogmatic use of diagnostic labels (Kahneman, 2011). For example, a standardized interview such as the structured clinical interview for DSM disorders is regarded as gold standard, critical thinkers

also assess client consistency and emotional state during testing to ascertain contextual appropriateness of the results (First et al., 2016).

3. **Inferencing:** Inferencing is deduction from available information and generating hypotheses. Inferencing may be used in psychological testing in decision-making for differential diagnosis, meaning distinguishing among conditions that have similar symptom presentations. For instance, if an inference is made regarding cognitive disorganization due to schizophrenia or severe mood disorder, one would need to consider behavioral, cognitive, and affective indicators within a diagnostic framework (Sadler, et al., 2009). Critical thinkers infer provisional diagnoses but also remain open to alternate assessments even when strong evidence exists in one direction. This is always a vital concern in clinical settings, especially given the typical trajectory of new information often becomes available over time.
4. **Reasoning**: Reasoning is the ability to make associations between items of information in a logical and organized manner. In diagnostic settings, both inductive reasoning (making general inferences from specific instances) and deductive reasoning (making specific application from general principles) are present. Effective reasoning enables practitioners to synthesize test information, behavioral data, and client history to justify diagnosis (Groopman & Hartzband, 2011). In addition, reasoning calls on clinicians to recognize logical fallacies, including false cause or hasty generalization, that may produce false conclusions. A clinician could, for instance, falsely assume that a client with recent trauma history necessarily has PTSD, when acute stress reaction or depression could be equally likely explanations.
5. **Self-Regulation and Metacognition:** Arguably the least valued but most important aspect of critical thinking is self-regulation—having the capacity to monitor one's own cognitive processes and modify them as necessary (Halpern, 2014). On a diagnostic level, this involves knowing about one's cognitive biases, including confirmation bias, and deliberately challenging one's own interpretations and conclusions. For instance, clinicians have to control their emotional reaction or refrain from being influenced by a client's likability or familiarity of some symptoms. This metacognitive consciousness is especially necessary when dealing with conflicting or uncertain diagnostic information (Norman & Eva, 2010).Figure one conceptualises the key features of critical thinking.

Figure 1. Conceptual structure of key features of critical thinking

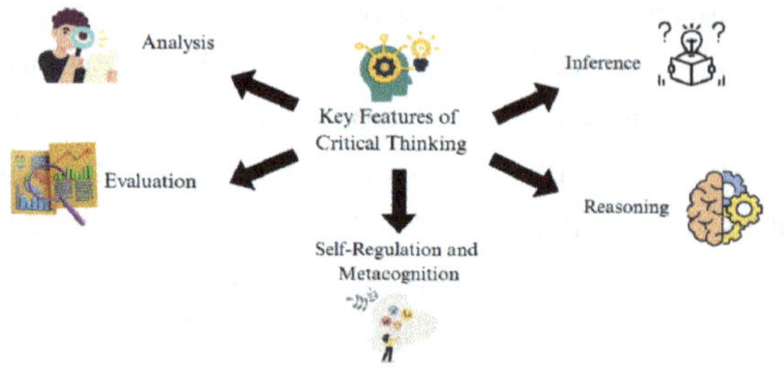

Source: author using Canva designs

SIGNIFICANCE OF CRITICAL THINKING IN PSYCHOLOGICAL DIAGNOSIS

Critical thinking is a process which enables one to objectively analyze, evaluate, and synthesize information. Critical thinking plays a fundamental role in maximizing accuracy when making psychological diagnoses, diminishing bias, and generating treatment options. Complexity and subjectivity in mental health lead to a systematic use of critical thinking processes when clinicians want to strive to provide the best possible care.

1. Enhancing Diagnostic Precision

Psychological diagnosis is the interpretation of disparate evidence from things like clinical interviews, behavior observations, psychometric tests, and all available patient history. By using critical thinking, clinicians can combine these seemingly incoherent sources and identify similarities, differences, patterns, conflicts, and ultimately, meaningful diagnostic interpretations. For example, a clinician sees a sad and withdrawn patient. The clinician comes up with the conclusion a melancholy mood is depressing. However, the clinician need not settle on this conclusion; critical thinking allows the practitioner to assess possibilities like cultural reasons, illness, or even the situation that influenced the patient's attitude. Halpern (2014) highlighted the value offered by critical thinking in minimizing diagnostic error in psychological diagnoses and ultimately allows for a better chance treatment interventions are same as the individual receiving care.

2. Mitigating Cognitive Biases

Cognitive biases, including confirmation bias, anchoring, and availability heuristic, have the potential to greatly affect clinical judgment. Take confirmation bias, for example. Confirmation bias leads clinicians to be biased toward information that supports their initial hypotheses, and to ignore countervailing information, for example. Critical thinking serves as a break on these biases, which encourages practitioners to subjectively consider all such attendant information in the light of systematic assessment. given several sources and monitoring alternative accounts (Kahneman, 2011). By constructing an appreciation of these mental traps, critical thinking enables clinicians to make judgments more objectively and sceptically. Not only is this raised diagnostic accuracy, but ethical practice can be facilitated by ensuring that decisions are reached based on adequate and non-judgmental assessment.

3. Tackling Cultural and Contextual Concerns

Mental illness symptoms appear differently across different cultures, and the pathological is normative in one setting and pathological in another. Critical thinking prepares clinicians to address these cultural variations so that they may judge more sensibly culturally. Clinicians can prevent ethnocentric translation and arrive at more correct diagnoses by critically examining their own cultural presumptions and engaging the patient's culture (Sue et al., 2009). For instance, certain distresses like somatic complaints could be more common in a particular culture. An astute clinician who is a critical thinker would be aware of such cultural presentations and interpret them against the right cultural background to eliminate misdiagnosis and ensure culturally sensitive practice.

4. Navigating Diagnostic Complexity

Psychiatric disorders are superimposable in their presentation, and differential diagnosis is a challenging task. Critical thinking breaks the complexity by encouraging analytical thinking and hypothesis testing. Through systematic consideration of clusters of symptoms, modes of onset, and impairment of functioning, clinicians differentiate among disorders having superimposable presentation and determine comorbid disorders (Groopman & Hartzband, 2011). For example, differential diagnosis between generalized anxiety and major depressive disorder relies upon close observation of how long-standing, bothersome, and disabling the symptoms are. Critical thinking allows clinicians to break down such subtleties and proper diagnoses so key to best treatment.

5. Increasing Treatment Success

Maximal treatment follows from maximal diagnosis. Critical thinking not only helps clinicians reach the correct diagnosis but also supports clinicians to select appropriate treatment options based on what is best for the patient in their own context. Clinicians are able to develop an individualized treatment approach that maximizes therapeutic benefits by critically considering the evidence base for the treatment, while still considering patient preferences, cultural belief systems, and comorbidities (First et al., 2016). Critical thinking also supports reflecting and adjusting of intervention methods over time, domestic or otherwise. Mental health providers can monitor patient improvement, record how effective the interventions were, and reflect or adjust accordingly to ensure maximal therapeutic benefit and flexible and effective long-term treatment.

CHALLENGES AND STRATEGIES IN USING CRITICAL THINKING IN PSYCHOLOGICAL DIAGNOSIS

Critical thinking is a necessary part of a psychological diagnosis, which allows clinicians to rationally and unbiasedly analyze, evaluate, and incorporate information. However, critical thinking can have challenges that affect accurate diagnosis and efficient treatment planning. Being aware of these challenges and the evidence-based strategies for overcoming these challenges is essential to ensure increased diagnostic accuracy and the effectiveness of the patient's treatment.

1. Cognitive Biases

Cognitive biases are consistent errors of thinking that affect judgment and decision. Examples of these in clinical practice include anchoring, availability, and confirmation bias, which can potentially impair diagnostic competence severely.

Anchoring Bias: This refers to the situation where clinicians anchor on early information and end up ignoring later data that could counter their first impressions (Nickerson, 1998).
Availability Bias: Clinicians will estimate the probability of a diagnosis depending on the ease with which examples spring to mind, potentially affected by recent events or salient cases (Tversky & Kahneman, 1973).
Confirmation Bias: This refers to the tendency to favor evidence that supports current beliefs and ignore evidence contrary to them, resulting in biased diagnostic outcomes (Nickerson, 1998).

They can result in misdiagnosis, as the clinician will identify information that confirms their initial hypothesis while overlooking other explanations (Kahneman, 2011).

2. Emotional Factors

Emotions play a key role in clinical decision-making. Clinicians may hold emotional biases, as they let their feelings guide their judgments. For instance, diagnosing serious mental health illnesses can make them feel uneasy or anxious and lead to rushing or evading certain diagnoses (Halpern, 2014). Emotional biases can also be drawn from individual background or experience, pre-judging objectivity. Recognition and control of those emotional factors are essential to maintain critical thinking in diagnosis (Epstein, 1999).

3. Time Pressure

Time pressure is a common occurrence in clinical practice that often results in superficial examinations and reliance on heuristics. Physicians are more likely to engage in intuitive, rather than careful, analytical reasoning in the face of time pressure (Norman & Eva, 2010), which may lead to diagnostic errors when they have to consider many factors (not just 1 or 2) in a case that is more complex. For effective diagnosis, there must be adequate time for both data gathering and thinking [i.e., processing the data (Groopman & Hartzband, 2011.)].

4. Insufficient Training

Most clinicians are formally trained in critical thinking skills only for a short time through their education. Without explicit instruction and practice, critical thinking will be challenging to apply in clinical situations (Facione, 1990). Moreover, repeated professional development opportunities in critical thinking are typically minimal, so there will be limited improvement of diagnostic competency (Benner, Sutphen, Leonard, & Day, 2010).

STRATEGIES FOR CRITICAL THINKING DEVELOPMENT

1. Reflective Practice

Reflective practice enables clinicians to examine their own thought, judgment, and action. Practitioners can detect bias, assess the efficacy of their judgments, and develop measures to improve through reflective clinical practice (Schön, 1983). Daily reflective practice, for example, peer review or journaling, instills self-awareness and encourages ongoing learning, developing critical thinking (Mann, Gordon, & MacLeod, 2009).

2. Evidence-Based Use of Tools

Utilizing evidence-based assessment tools and standardized diagnostic criteria can be useful as the measures support objectively based decision making. The assessments provide structured methods of assessment which in turn can reduce bias and prejudice (American Psychiatric Association, 2013). Being educated on current research and best practice ensures clinicians' diagnostic judgments are based on the best available valid and accurate information (Sackett, Straus, Richardson, Rosenberg, & Haynes, 2000).

3. Collaborative Practice

Collaboration with teachers and peers provides varying views, answers clinical case critical thinking. Peer case working has the potential to reveal alternate perceptions, challenge assumptions, and stimulate more integrated assessments (Dinh et al., 2010; Thistlethwaite, 2012). Interprofessional collaboration also answers shared decision-making, enhancing diagnosis and patient outcomes (Dinh et al., 2010; Reeves, Lewin, Espin, & Zwarenstein, 2010).

4. Continuing Education and Training

Critical thinking skill maintenance through continuing professional development is essential for clinicians. Seminars, workshops, and courses that involve analytical thinking, recognition of bias, and decision-making processes can improve diagnostic ability (Facione, 1990).

Critical thinking training integrated into clinical education courses ensures new professionals are introduced to these skills in the early part of their careers (Benner et al., 2010).

APPROACHES TO TEACHING AND ASSESSING CRITICAL THINKING IN CLINICAL PRACTICE

While critical thinking in psychological diagnosis is widely recognized as important, translating it into practice in clinical education and supervision is often unclear or absent. To position critical thinking as an integral part of diagnostic practice, both educational and supervision approaches should move away from didactic and toward experiential, reflexive, and dialogic learning. One means of doing this is through Socratic questioning in clinical supervision. This could involve the supervisor cultivating a culture of layered, open-ended questioning that encourages the supervision of clinical questioning about assumptions to recognize gaps in reasoning and to nudge the trainee towards arriving at more thoughtful conclusion to prospective diagnoses. Socratic questioning also helps develop metacognitive awareness of reasoning while fostering the habit of critically reflective inquiry in the experiences of real case analysis.

Another approach involves constructively critiquing and providing feedback using explicit critical and diagnostic thinking rubrics that we adapted from the fields of health sciences and educational psychology. Considerations of rubrics may ask the student to examine domains such as, "clarity of thought", "conclusion of recommended diagnosis", evaluation of alternatives", and "recognition of bias" (Facione, 1990; Halpern, 2014). Critical diagnostic thinking rubrics may be one approach to feedback systems that contributes to accountabilities and concrete goals for learner development.

Reflective journals and team debrief are also effective mechanisms. A reflective journal allows clinicians-in-training to document their thinking processes, questions, and any modifications they made through the thought process, which yields ongoing self-assessment. The team debriefing after a session, particularly after a complex or ambiguous case, provides a platform for collaborative reflection, peer challenge, and interdisciplinary integration. As previously indicated, protocol or guideline "thinking aloud" walk-throughs provide a process whereby clinicians articulate their reasoning before they approach a case. Thinking aloud adds an element of transparency to the decision-making process and engages clinicians in thinking critically about how they arrive at a decision, as there are often unconscious biases (Eva et al., 2007).

Finally, Halpern's (2014) model of "teaching for transfer" highlights the importance of making sure learners can recognize critical thinking in a variety of contexts. In sustaining their critical thinking practice, the learning experience needs to simulate the uncertainty, ambiguity, and cultural variability found in practice so that learners do not confuse critical thinking with an abstract process, but rather understand it as applied clinical habit.

DIRECTIONS FOR FUTURE RESEARCH

Establishing the use of critical thinking for psychological diagnosis requires future research on several very important areas.

1. Standardized Training Programs

There must be an urgent move to standardize training programs aimed at the development of critical thinking skills among mental health practitioners. These training programs would employ material such as awareness of cognitive biases, decision-making models, and reflective practice. There must be research into how this might increase diagnostic accuracy and decrease error.

2. Utilizing AI and Machine Learning for Diagnoses

With the increasingly complicated task of mental health diagnosis, there is expanding interest in the use of artificial intelligence (AI) and machine learning (ML) to support clinical judgment. The use of AI and machine learning in mental health diagnosis has rapidly progressed with the capacity to process large data sets. These datasets involve electronic health records, behavioral data, and psychometric profiles - allowing AI and machine learning tools to identify diagnostic patterns, probe into further differential diagnosis. An AI decision-support model that relies on machine learning could support clinicians by flagging inconsistencies, red flags, or potential missed diagnosis when reflecting on the patient's record. For example, natural language processing is being used to look for indicators of depression in therapy notes or social media sites. Additionally, predictive models in the field can compare a patient's clinical and demographic variables to understand their potential for suicide and inform clinicians.

The role of AI in clinical practice should be viewed not as a replacement for a clinician's critical thinking but as an enhancement. Clinicians will still have to engage in thinking critically about the outputs of algorithms, apply them to the actual case at hand, and be mindful of potential bias that may come from training data, especially with tools that have been trained on specific and homogenous population data sets. As Topol (2019) notes in Deep Medicine, AI is not intended to replace human clinicians, but to liberate them to perform tasks with their own empathy, judgment, and contextualized reasoning. Therefore, it is important for future research to consider how AI systems can be employed in diagnostic practice in an ethical and responsible way when assessing patients across cultures and when letting patients contribute to their own ambiguity.

3. Cultural Formulation and Critical Thinking in Diagnosis

The DSM-5 Cultural Formulation Interview (CFI) and the Cultural Concepts of Distress framework offer structured processes to assist clinicians in getting culturally relevant data about clients' experiences of illness. These processes reiterate that a diagnosis should factor symptom presentation as well as how clients engage with, label and troubleshoot psychological distress in their own cultural constructions of meaning. Yet, despite the existence of these tools, their application in diagnostic reasoning is limited. Critical thinking serves an important role in questioning ethnocentric assumptions, weighing culture-bound ways to express distress, and looking for misdiagnosis due to misunderstanding the cultural conceptualization of psychology. For example, in some cultural groups, somatic complaints may manifest primarily in depression or spiritual beliefs may be interpreted as psychotic symptoms without proper cultural context. Clinicians must be taught to use the CFI beyond the formal interview, as a stepping stone toward culturally grounded, reflective dialogue.

Moving forward, we should be teachings practice of critical thinking that include cultural issues as being situated in the CFI and other processes to ensure practitioners can move beyond the fixed methods of symptom checklists and develop an ongoing and customizable sense of understanding.

4. Interdisciplinary Collaboration in Diagnostic Situations

In modern clinical practice, more often we see umbrella interdisciplinary teams consisting of psychologists, psychiatrists, social workers, nurses and other aligned professionals coming together to provide assessment and case formulation. These settings (whether integrated care, inpatient psychiatric or school-based mental health systems) allow individuals with varying sets of biases an invaluable opportunity to corroborate, test assumptions and develop a more accurate diagnostic impression.

Critical thinking in this context is supported and influenced by several different professional lenses and by making collective decisions of judgement. An example would be how a social worker might provide insight into environmental context and stressors, a nurse may draw attention to physiological health dimensions, and a psychologist may illuminate cognitive patterns and profiles. Interprofessional discussions foster intellectual humility and epistemic ego (two relational dispositions, which are respectively important to critical thinking; Facione, 1990).

Interprofessional programs should provide case conferencing and collaborative or interprofessional diagnostic formulative, and reflection as important frameworks to support accuracy and ethics of diagnosis. There is also a need for research on the outcome of interdisciplinary collaboration for diagnostic interventions and the potential to circumvent solitary or bungled diagnostic conclusions.

5. Longitudinal Studies on Critical Thinking Development

The growth and evolution of critical thinking skills are not well elucidated over time in clinicians without longitudinal studies. These can be conducted to determine causes of deterioration or improvement in such skills and guide long-term professional development strategies.

6. Organizational Factors

Organizational factors such as workload, time pressures, and institutional policy can also play a part in applying critical thinking in the clinical environment. Organizational factors will need to be investigated further in future research to examine how organizational factors influence diagnosis procedures and how some organizational interventions make critical thinking more valuable for clinicians.

7. Involving Patients in the Diagnostic Process

Involving the patient in the diagnostic process is likely to yield useful information and enhance shared decision-making. The necessity of seeking ways to integrate patient views into the diagnostic assessment and assess the effect on diagnostic accuracy and patient satisfaction lies.

8. Assessment of Reflective Practice Intervention

Although reflective practice is advocated as a way of developing critical thinking, there is limited empirical research evidence to show whether it does so. The impacts of systematic reflective practice interventions on clinicians' diagnostic reasoning and decision-making

9. Measurement of Critical Thinking Dispositions

Individual differences in critical thinking dispositions, including open-mindedness and cognitive flexibility, can be known to guide individualized training protocols. Research should identify sound measures of these dispositions and investigate their relationship to diagnostic performance.

10. Interdisciplinary Research Collaborations

The interdisciplinary efforts between cognitive science, education, and psychology will probably lead to a thorough investigation of critical thinking in diagnosis. Interdisciplinary research can bridge different approaches and models in order to create a better understanding and to build usable knowledge for clinicians.

11. Policy and Curriculum Development

Lastly, evidence should inform policy and curriculum design to incorporate training in critical thinking skills into professional courses and continuing professional development schemes. Assessment of the effect of such curricular innovations on clinical outcome will be necessary to evidence-based decision-making. A conceptual structure of the future directions is given in Figure 2

Figure 2. Conceptual structure of the future directions

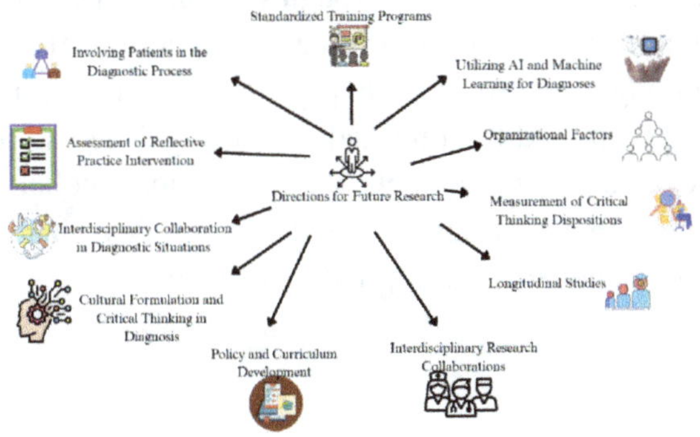

Source: author using Canva designs

CONCLUSION

Critical thinking is a key component in the practice of psychological diagnosis. It allows clinicians to manage complex symptomatology, minimize cognitive biases, and make informed decisions leading to enhanced patient outcomes. Even though critical thinking is essential, the use of critical thinking in clinical contexts is faced with a series of obstacles such as cognitive biases, emotional issues, pressure of time, and insufficient training.

Cognitive biases such as anchoring, availability, and confirmation bias have been shown to skew diagnostic judgment in that they cause clinicians to favor first reactions or readily accessible information over careful analysis (Nickerson, 1998; Tversky & Kahneman, 1973). Emotional factors such as stress and individual assumptions further cloud judgment, particularly when dealing with severe mental illness (Halpern, 2014). Time constraints within the clinical environment are generally of the sort to compel practitioners to react hastily, and the pressure can reduce the quality of the critical analysis (Norman & Eva, 2010). Furthermore, not having the opportunity for formal training in critical thinking skills as part of professional school may lower the proficiency of clinicians in applying these skills (Facione, 1990).

There is a myriad of alternatives to these issues. Reflective practice permits clinicians to examine their decision-making, identify biases, and garner experience through previous history (Schön, 1983). Evidence-based assessment instruments provide models that allow a systematic approach to objectivity and can limit the use of subjective assessments (American Psychiatric Association, 2013). Collaborative practice allows sharing perspectives between a clinician and others and provides global evaluations, to lessen individual biases (Reeves et al., 2010). Critical thinking must be enhanced for clinicians through ongoing education and training to keep up with recent studies and develop diagnostic capacity (Benner et al., 2010). While critical thinking is key to accurate psychological diagnosis, the application of critical thinking is limited by a myriad of barriers. The use of means such as reflective practice, evidence-based tools, interprofessional collaborative practices, and continued education can promote critical thinking skills in clinicians and thus promote enhanced diagnostic accuracy and patient care.

REFERENCES

American Psychiatric Association. (2013). *Diagnostic and statistical manual of mental disorders (DSM-5 (R))* (5th ed.). American Psychiatric Association Publishing.

Clark, L. A., Cuthbert, B., Lewis-Fernández, R., Narrow, W. E., & Reed, G. M. (2017). Three approaches to understanding and classifying mental disorder: ICD-11, DSM-5, and the National Institute of Mental Health's Research Domain Criteria (RDoC). *Psychological Science in the Public Interest: A Journal of the American Psychological Society, 18*(2), 72–145. DOI: 10.1177/1529100617727266

Collins, G. S., & Moons, K. G. M. (2019). Reporting of artificial intelligence prediction models. *Lancet, 393*(10181), 1577–1579. DOI: 10.1016/S0140-6736(19)30037-6 PMID: 31007185

Croskerry, P. (2003). The importance of cognitive errors in diagnosis and strategies to minimize them. *Academic Medicine, 78*(8), 775–780. DOI: 10.1097/00001888-200308000-00003 PMID: 12915363

Croskerry, P., Singhal, G., & Mamede, S. (2013). Cognitive debiasing 1: origins of bias and theory of debiasing. *BMJ Quality & Safety, 22 Suppl 2*(Suppl 2), ii58–ii64. DOI: 10.1136/bmjqs-2012-001712

DSM-5. (2013). *Cultural Formulation Interview (DSM-5 Appendix).* (2013).

Epstein, R. M. (2003). Mindful practice in action (II): Cultivating habits of mind. *Families, Systems & Health, 21*(1), 11–17. DOI: 10.1037/h0089495

Eva, K. W., Hatala, R. M., Leblanc, V. R., & Brooks, L. R. (2007). Teaching from the clinical reasoning literature: combined reasoning strategies help novice diagnosticians overcome misleading information: Clinical expertise. *Medical Education, 41*(12), 1152–1158. DOI: 10.1111/j.1365-2923.2007.02923.x PMID: 18045367

Facione, P. A. (1990a). *Critical thinking: A statement of expert consensus for purposes of educational assessment and instruction.* American Philosophical Association.

Facione, P. A. (1990b). *Critical thinking: A statement of expert consensus for purposes of educational assessment and instruction (The Delphi Report).* American Philosophical Association.

Facione, P. A. (2015). *Critical thinking: What it is and why it counts.*

First, M. B., Williams, J. B. W., Karg, R. S., & Spitzer, R. L. (2016). *Structured Clinical Interview for DSM-5 Disorders-Clinician Version (SCID-5-CV).* American Psychiatric Association Publishing.

First, M. B., Williams, J. B. W., Karg, R. S., & Spitzer, R. L. (2018). *Structured clinical interview for DSM-5 disorders, clinician version (SCID-5-CV)*. American Psychiatric Association Publishing.

Garb, H. N. (2005). Clinical judgment and decision making. *Annual Review of Clinical Psychology, 1*(1), 67–89. DOI: 10.1146/annurev.clinpsy.1.102803.143810 PMID: 17716082

Grohol, J. M. (2020). *The role of psychological assessment in differential diagnosis*.

Groopman, J., & Hartzband, P. (2011). *Your medical mind: How to decide what is right for you*. Penguin Press.

Halpern, D. F. (2014). *Thought and knowledge: An introduction to critical thinking*. Psychology Press.

Lewis-Fernández, R., Aggarwal, N. K., Bäärnhielm, S., Rohlof, H., Kirmayer, L. J., Weiss, M. G., Jadhav, S., Hinton, L., Alarcón, R. D., Bhugra, D., Groen, S., van Dijk, R., Qureshi, A., Collazos, F., Rousseau, C., Caballero, L., Ramos, M., & Lu, F. (2014). Culture and psychiatric evaluation: Operationalizing cultural formulation for DSM-5. *Psychiatry, 77*(2), 130–154. DOI: 10.1521/psyc.2014.77.2.130 PMID: 24865197

Lilienfeld, S. O., Ammirati, R., & David, M. (2013). Distinguishing science from pseudoscience in mental health: A primer for clinicians. *Clinical Psychologist, 66*(1), 6–10.

Mann, K., Gordon, J., & MacLeod, A. (2009). Reflection and reflective practice in health professions education: A systematic review. *Advances in Health Sciences Education : Theory and Practice, 14*(4), 595–621. DOI: 10.1007/s10459-007-9090-2 PMID: 18034364

Nickerson, R. S. (1998). Confirmation bias: A ubiquitous phenomenon in many guises. *Review of General Psychology: Journal of Division 1, of the American Psychological Association, 2*(2), 175–220. DOI: 10.1037/1089-2680.2.2.175

Norman, G. R., & Eva, K. W. (2010). Diagnostic error and clinical reasoning: Diagnostic error and reasoning. *Medical Education, 44*(1), 94–100. DOI: 10.1111/j.1365-2923.2009.03507.x PMID: 20078760

Reeves, S., Lewin, S., Espin, S., & Zwarenstein, M. (2010). *Interprofessional teamwork for health and social care*. Wiley-Blackwell. DOI: 10.1002/9781444325027

Sackett, D. L., Straus, S. E., Richardson, W. S., Rosenberg, W., & Haynes, R. B. (2000). *Evidence-based medicine: How to practice and teach EBM*. Churchill Livingstone.

Sadler, J. Z., Fulford, K. W., & Agich, G. J. (2009). *Clinical ethics and the psychiatric diagnosis*. Oxford University Press.

Sue, S., Yan Cheng, J. K., Saad, C. S., & Chu, J. P. (2012). Asian American mental health: A call to action. *The American Psychologist*, *67*(7), 532–544. DOI: 10.1037/a0028900 PMID: 23046304

Thistlethwaite, J. (2012). Interprofessional education: a review of context, learning and the research agenda: Interprofessional education: a review. *Medical Education*, *46*(1), 58–70. DOI: 10.1111/j.1365-2923.2011.04143.x PMID: 22150197

Topol, E. (2019). *Deep medicine: How artificial intelligence can make healthcare human again*. Basic Books.

Tversky, A., & Kahneman, D. (1973). Availability: A heuristic for judging frequency and probability. *Cognitive Psychology*, *5*(2), 207–232. DOI: 10.1016/0010-0285(73)90033-9

Tversky, A., & Kahneman, D. (2013). Judgment under uncertainty: Heuristics and biases. In *Handbook of the Fundamentals of Financial Decision Making* (pp. 261–268). WORLD SCIENTIFIC. DOI: 10.1142/9789814417358_0015

Watson, K. (2011). Farrar, Straus and Giroux. 499 pages. *The Canadian Journal of Program Evaluation*, *26*(2), 111–113. DOI: 10.3138/cjpe.26.010

Chapter 4
Addressing Diagnostic Complexity Through Critical Thinking in Clinical Judgment

Debangi Sanyal
https://orcid.org/0009-0005-0739-8431
PES University, India

Aditi Priyadarshini
https://orcid.org/0009-0002-4656-0241
PES University, India

Megha Rudrapati
https://orcid.org/0009-0007-3058-2565
PES University, India

ABSTRACT

The chapter explores the complexity of diagnosing cognitive and behavioral disorders across diverse clinical and cultural contexts. It highlights the vital yet often-overlooked role of critical thinking in navigating overlapping or ambiguous symptoms. Emphasizing how systemic, cultural, and cognitive factors shape diagnostic outcomes, it questions the reliability of traditional tools, the impact of bias, and the limits of technology in mental health assessment. Rather than offering prescriptive solutions, it advocates for reflective reasoning, ethical sensitivity, and interdisciplinary insight. Through case illustrations and theoretical analysis, critical thinking is framed as a clinical necessity. The chapter calls for a more nuanced, equitable

DOI: 10.4018/979-8-3373-1812-7.ch004

approach to diagnosis, balancing standardization with contextual understanding, and technology with human judgment, urging readers to consider how critical thinking can transform both individual practice and global mental healthcare.

INTRODUCTION

Understanding how the mind works and what happens when it does not offers an important insight into human behavior, relationships, and well-being. Cognitive and behavioral disorders encompass a range of conditions that impair an individual's mental processes and behavioral regulation, often manifesting as challenges in memory, attention, problem-solving, emotional control, and social behavior, which frequently interfere with daily functioning and quality of life. These conditions can appear at any stage of life and vary in severity - they may be rooted in various etiologies, including genetic, neurological, developmental, and environmental factors.

These disorders represent some of the most challenging conditions to diagnose and treat in modern healthcare. It ranges from neurodevelopmental conditions like autism spectrum disorder and ADHD to mood disorders such as major depressive disorder and bipolar disorder, to neurocognitive conditions such as Alzheimer's disease. The complexity of these disorders lies not only in their different presentations but also in the overlapping symptoms and behavioral manifestations.

Accurate diagnosis is the cornerstone of effective treatment. When clinicians identify the underlying condition correctly, they can apply personalized interventions that address the particular mechanism driving symptoms. (Sabbagh et al., 2021) It emphasises that identifying Alzheimer's early and properly allows the utilisation of disease-modifying drugs when they are useful. Misdiagnosis can lead patients down treatment paths that waste precious time, deplete financial resources, and potentially aggravate their conditions. (Giebel et al., 2024) It found that Lewy body dementia patients frequently face delays which defer correct care. Critical thinking is an essential cognitive framework that allows clinicians to navigate diagnostic complications. It includes the structured assessment of presenting symptoms, patient history, and contextual factors, while knowingly identifying and counteracting cognitive biases that might cloud judgment. Clinical reasoning draws on various cognitive strategies, including hypothesis testing, pattern recognition, and probabilistic reasoning. (Coderre et al., 2003) emphasised that clinicians utilising these techniques had higher probabilities of diagnostic accuracy. Critical thinking in clinical settings is not merely academic- it directly transforms to enhanced patient outcomes through more accurate diagnoses and more effective treatment plans.

Globally, the difficulties of accurate diagnosis take on additional dimensions. Geographic inequalities in mental health training and resources create unequal scenarios of diagnostic accuracy. Cultural factors impact how symptoms are expressed, perceived, and reported, adding layers of complexity that clinicians must adeptly navigate. Economic limitations in low- and middle-income countries frequently restrict access to adequate or specialized diagnostic resources and expertise, forcing dependence on clinical judgment that must be specially refined to account for these limitations. The World Health Organization estimates that up to 5% of outpatients in developed countries are misdiagnosed, and the rates exceed 10% in underdeveloped countries.

The consequences of misdiagnosis go beyond individual patient outcomes to influence healthcare systems and society more broadly. It frequently results in ineffective treatments, prolonged suffering, unnecessary healthcare utilization, and increased economic burden.

Recent improvements in diagnostic approaches, including integrating biomarkers and neuroimaging, standardized assessment protocols, collaborative diagnostic models, and digital phenotyping using smartphones and wearable technology, offer promising improvements in accuracy. However, technology alone cannot solve the diagnostic challenge since the clinician's capacity for unique critical thinking skills remains irreplaceable.

This chapter unfolds across several interconnected layers. We begin with foundational concepts and global diagnostic disparities, followed by the impact of misdiagnosis—including patient experiences. We then examine systemic, cultural, and technological factors influencing diagnosis, and conclude with practical strategies to reduce diagnostic errors through critical thinking, collaboration, and reflective practice. Figure 1 summarizes the core domains shaping diagnostic inaccuracy

In conclusion, this chapter delves into the intricate nature of diagnostic complexity in cognitive and behavioral disorders, emphasizing the importance of critical thinking to reduce misdiagnosis rates and improve patient outcomes. It discusses cognitive biases, metacognitive awareness, structured clinical reasoning, and integrating multiple sources of information.

BACKGROUND AND DEFINITIONS

Understanding diagnosis challenges in cognitive and behavioral disorders requires ample amounts of clarity around key concepts and the frameworks guiding clinical decision-making. The given section delineates fundamental definitions and explains diagnostic systems employed in various contexts.

Key Terms

Diagnosis. Diagnosis refers to the methodological procedure of diagnosing a disease or disorder by integrating data from patient symptoms, clinical history, behavioral evaluations, and diagnostic examinations. Diagnosis in the mental health context often depends on interpretive assessments, rather than definitive biomarkers. This increases subjectivity, which refers to the characteristic of being derived from or influenced by individual emotions, preferences, or viewpoints. (American Psychiatric Association [APA], 2022).

Misdiagnosis. Misdiagnosis often occurs when a clinician inaccurately identifies a disorder or fails to detect an existing condition. It includes both false positives and false negatives. False positives can be defined as diagnosing a condition that is not present, whereas false negatives indicate failing to diagnose a condition that is actually present. Both taken into account lead to inappropriate treatment, delayed care, and potential harm for the client (Norman et al., 2017).

Critical Thinking. Critical Thinking in a clinical context involves deliberate and reflective judgment. It necessitates the role of clinicians to interrogate assumptions, assess evidence, and scrutinize cognitive biases in order to make ethical and precise decision-making (Facione, 2015). This metacognitive skill enhances diagnostic precision and minimizes errors by fostering logical, reasoned, and bias-conscious judgment (Monteiro & Norman, 2013).

Diagnostic Frameworks

Two globally recognized classification systems guide psychiatric diagnosis:

The DSM-5-TR. The DSM-5-TR (Diagnostic and Statistical Manual of Mental Disorders, 5th edition, Text Revision) provides standardized diagnostic criteria which is based primarily on system clusters and their functional impact. It is widely used in the United States and research settings, emphasising reliability and consistency in mental health diagnosis (APA, 2022).

The ICD-11. The ICD-11 (International Classification of Diseases, 11th Revision), developed by the World Health Organization (WHO), provides a broader classification system covering both physical and mental health disorders. This is widely adopted in international and public health settings and is a culturally adaptable diagnostic guideline (the World Health Organization [WHO], 2022).

Systematic and Contextual Challenges

Both the DSM-5-TR and ICD-11 offer structured diagnostic guidance. However, their implementation varies across health systems and cultural settings. In low-and middle-income countries (LMICs), the diagnosis reliability is often hindered by limited training, tool availability, and mental health stigma (Patel et al., 2018). Accredited Social Health Activists (ASHAs) in India are crucial in early identification, psychoeducation, and stigma reduction of mental health issues, particularly in rural areas, through initiatives like NIMHANS' Manochaitanya clinics. The limited access to standardized diagnostic tools, inadequate clinician training in mental health, and overburdened healthcare systems often force reliance on clinical intuition, neglecting standardized and structured assessments. (See Figure 1 for a visual summary of these interacting diagnostic factors)

Furthermore, cultural stigma surrounding mental illness may discourage individuals from seeking help or lead to underreporting of symptoms, complicating diagnostic efforts. Initiatives like the WHO's Mental Gap Action Programme (mhGAP) seek to address these disparities by providing structured diagnostic and treatment protocols to non-specialists (WHO, 2008), focusing on detection and management of mental, neurological, and substance use in resource-constrained settings. Such initiatives are promising as their success is heavily dependent on ongoing investment in workforce development, culturally sensitive training, and integration with existing health care infrastructure.

Figure 1. Factors contributing to diagnostic inaccuracy.

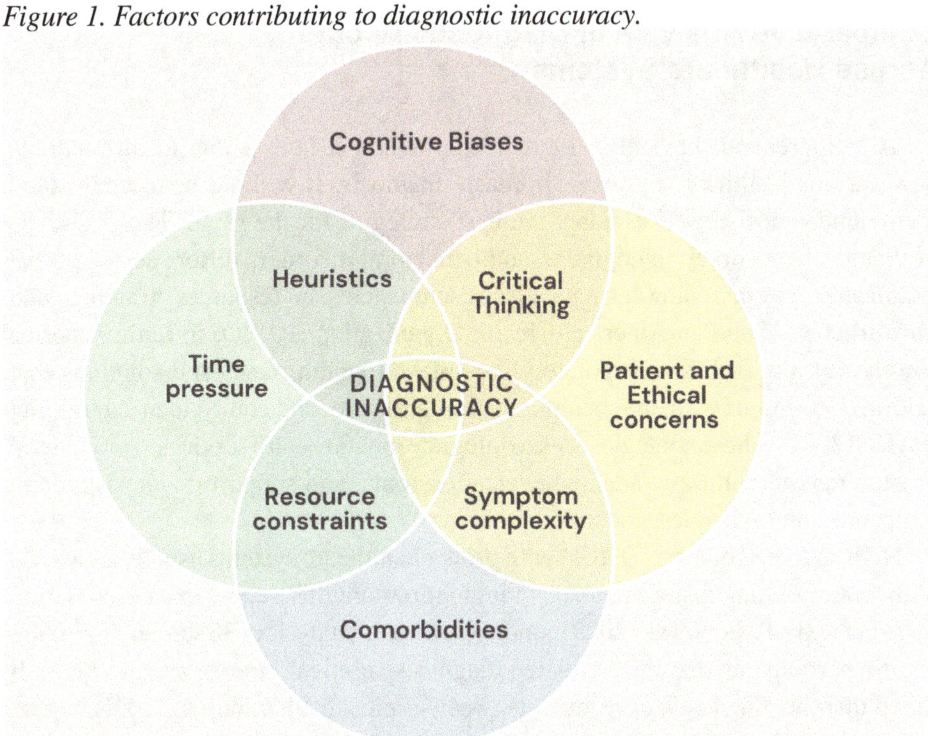

This Venn diagram illustrates how diagnostic errors can arise from the interplay of cognitive biases, heuristics, time pressure, ethical concerns, and clinical complexity.

GLOBAL TRENDS IN DIAGNOSIS AND MISDIAGNOSIS

Despite targeted global initiatives to strengthen the diagnostic capacity, there are significant disparities that may persist across healthcare systems. This section examines the broader challenges of achieving diagnostic accuracy. While understanding the accurate diagnosis and the complications that form clinical decision-making, it also becomes important to evaluate how these challenges unfold on a global scale. It helps to understand not only the cultural and systemic factors but also the challenges that are involved across diverse health environments.

Diagnostic inaccuracies are an important challenge in the healthcare system; they may cause deaths. Misdiagnosis can lead to delayed or improper interventions, patient distress, and, in extreme cases, prevent mortality. Misdiagnosis rates may vary across countries, affecting many individuals in the process. Therefore, understanding how diagnostic accuracy is important for creating personalized interventions and enhancing patient safety on a global scale.

Comparative Analysis of Diagnostic Accuracy Across Healthcare Systems

To comprehend these global patterns in-depth, it is essential to differentiate how various healthcare systems approach diagnosis. It will aid us to understand the redundancies as well as adapt the best strategies for the same. The landscape of diagnostic accuracy in cognitive and behavioral disorders differs across global healthcare systems, showcasing wider discrepancies in resources, training, and infrastructure. The Pan American Health Organization (PAHO) in Latin America and the Caribbean has incorporated local mental health diagnostic solutions that prioritize community mental health, intercultural care, and equity-focused training (PAHO, 2021). These strategies seek to integrate mental health services, train general practitioners in culturally adapted evaluation tools, and support diagnosis among indigenous and Afro-descendant populations.

High-income countries (HICs) with proper healthcare systems usually showcase higher rates of diagnostic accuracy, though important differences exist even within these contexts. Rettew et al. (2009) conducted a meta-analysis of 38 studies, including 15,967 participants that differentiated diagnoses, clinical interviews, and SDIs. It found that the diagnostic agreement between clinical evaluations and SDIs is low.

In HICs like the US, Canada, and Western European nations, diagnostic accuracy gets support from greater access to specialized mental health care professionals, advanced neuroimaging, and testing facilities, and proper assessment methods. For instance, Hill (2024) demonstrated important gaps in autism diagnosis rates across different NHS centers in England. Further research showcased that positive autism assessment rates for children varied across various countries. In 2014-2016, low-income countries had around 0.1 psychiatrists per 100,000 people, whereas high-income countries had rates 120 times greater, according to the WHO. Rensburg et al. (2022) demonstrate that South Africa has 1.53 psychiatrists per 100,000 population as of 2019 (WHO, 2016; WHO, 2021). The World Health Organization's Mental Health Gap Action Programme (mhGAP) and Quality Rights Initiative aim to enhance access to mental health care, decrease diagnostic errors, and train frontline staff in low-resource environments while promoting rights-based, trauma-informed, and culturally relevant practices.

The organization of healthcare delivery particularly influences diagnostic accuracy. Unified systems that promote communication between primary care and specialized mental health services demonstrate diminished rates of diagnostic error. Villamil-Salcedo et al. (2017) showcased that Mexico City, utilizing a collaborative care model among general psychiatrists and psychiatrists, helped in increasing awareness and identification of disorders. Additionally, fractured care systems with substandard communication between providers and restricted continuity of care showcase higher rates of misdiagnosis.

Insurance structures and financial incentives enhance diagnostic inaccuracies. These economic constraints can lead to "diagnostic inflation" for various conditions, while others are seemingly underdiagnosed. However, apart from technical analyses, it is through individual stories that the impact of misdiagnosis is visible.

Case Studies Illustrating the Impact of Misdiagnosis

The human price of diagnostic inaccuracies becomes significantly evident through the assessment of individual cases across different contexts. It not only demonstrates the consequences of diagnostic errors but also highlights structural flaws that lead to such results.

Case Study 1: Frontotemporal Dementia Misdiagnosed as Conversion Disorder

Braus et al. (2019) demonstrated how cognitive biases and heuristic inaccuracies can lead to misdiagnosis, hindering proper care and contributing to a patient's decline. Ms. A, a 47-year-old woman, had progressive symptoms for 2.5 years, including depression, anxiety, impaired speech, and motor challenges. She was initially diagnosed with conversion disorder, but her condition did not improve with psychiatric treatments. Further neurological assessments showcased signs indicative of frontotemporal dementia (FTD), which was verified by the presence of the C9orf72 genetic mutation.

Case Study 2: Autism Spectrum Disorder misdiagnosed as Depression and Anxiety

Alexander and Farrelly (2019) reported the case of a 34-year-old man who had been treated for panic disorder, major depressive disorder, and generalized anxiety disorder with no significant improvement in their condition. He was ultimately given a reliable diagnosis of autism spectrum disorder (ASD). The condition was appropriately managed after this diagnosis was provided through a personalized treatment approach that included supportive therapy and pharmaceutical adjustments. The challenges in identifying ASD in adults and the importance of considering neurodevelopmental disorders when making a differential diagnosis.

Case Study 3: Obsessive-Compulsive Disorder misdiagnosed as Psychosis

In a case reported, *Misdiagnosis and Exacerbation of Unusual Obsessive-compulsive Disorder Presentation with Risperidone and Clozapine in an Adolescent Girl* (2011). It is a case report about an adolescent girl demonstrating unusual OCD symptoms, such as musical obsessions, which were misdiagnosed as psychotic features. The symptoms worsened after antipsychotic drugs like clozapine and risperidone were prescribed. Post reevaluation, she received a proper OCD diagnosis, and fluvoxamine medication reduced her symptoms. This case serves as an example of the potential hazards of misdiagnosing atypical OCD presentations and the possible adverse consequences of using the wrong medication.

Case Study 4: Narcolepsy misdiagnosed as Schizophrenia

Shen et al. (2022) describe the case of an 18-year-old female who endured cataplexy, hallucinations, and excessive daytime sleepiness for over sex years. Initially, given a diagnosis of schizophrenia and was unsuccessfully treated with antipsychotics. The symptoms were eventually accurately diagnosed as a neurological sleep disease called narcolepsy. This misdiagnosis led to years of unsuccessful therapy and major life problems, emphasizing the importance of thorough sleep assessments in psychiatric evaluations.

Case Study 5: Mild Cognitive Impairment Misdiagnosis Due to Non-Credible Symptom Reporting

Roor et al. (2015) reported the case of a 59-year-old woman who was diagnosed with mild cognitive impairment (MCI) based on subjective complaints. However, additional neuropsychological examinations, such as symptom validity tests, demonstrated non-credible performance, indicating that her cognitive symptoms were not due to MCI. To prevent incorrect diagnoses and needless treatments, this instance highlights the significance of objective testing in the diagnosis of cognitive problems. No cognitive-enhancing drugs or dementia-specific interventions were administered due to the revised findings.

All these cases demonstrate that misdiagnosis is not simply attributable to a clinician's error, but is a reflection of complex engagement between individual, cultural, and systemic factors. The aftermath stretches beyond clinical results to influence social functioning, economic productivity, and quality of life for the affected individuals.

Cultural and Systemic Factors Contributing to Diagnostic Errors

Diagnostic accuracy is extensively impacted by cultural contexts and systemic healthcare factors. These factors shape how symptoms are expressed, perceived, and interpreted throughout the process.

1. Cultural Factors

Among these influences, cultural factors pose a significant challenge. They form not only the expressions of psychological distress but also how patients communicate their experiences and how it is interpreted by clinicians. Cultural differences in presenting symptoms showcase a unique challenge to diagnostic accuracy. Patel et al. (2019) found in a multi-country study that depression is frequently showcased through physical symptoms, while in Western patients, it was more likely to be showcased as affective symptoms. When diagnostic criteria are formed primarily from studies in Western contexts, they may fail to capture culturally specific symptom patterns, leading to misdiagnosis or underdiagnosis in non-Western populations.

Additionally, language barriers increase these challenges, as psychological concepts often do not include direct translation between languages. Sumathipala et al. (2018) examined how depression is understood in Sinhalese, Tamil, and English in Sri Lanka and found that the local definitions often concentrate on physical symptoms rather than emotional ones. Even when possible, the essence of the symptom description may be lost when interpreters lack mental health training.

Help-seeking behaviors and symptom detailing are significantly influenced by the cultural stigma surrounding mental illness. In societies where mental illness is highly stigmatized, patients may prefer physical rather than psychological symptoms or avoid seeking help until it reaches crisis levels. Thornicroft et al. (2017) conducted a large-scale WHO study that examined stigma levels across 15 countries and resulted in greater public stigma being connected with extreme delays in help-seeking for psychotic disorders, thus potentially leading to a worse prognosis.

The cultural variations in explanatory models of illness further intensify diagnosis. When patients and clinicians have fundamentally varied comprehensions of the causes and nature of symptoms, such as spiritual versus biomedical explanations, the diagnostic interview may not help provide information. Kirmayer et al. (2017) demonstrated that utilizing the Cultural Formulation Interview in psychiatric evaluations enhanced diagnostic accuracy by up to 25% in ethnically different populations by particularly investigating the patients' cultural illness beliefs. These culturally driven inequalities emphasize the requirement for diagnostic frameworks that are sensitive to the sociocultural realities of diverse populations. However, it is not the only factor involved in the broader diagnostic ecosystem.

2. Ethical and Legal Dimensions of Misdiagnosis

Misdiagnosis in cognitive disorders is a clinical, ethical, and legal dilemma. The consequence of an incorrect or delayed diagnosis can include destruction, social stigma, and loss of patient or client trust. As a result, healthcare systems must address the intricate interplay of informed consent, professional liability, disclosure ethics, and cross-cultural legal standards.

- **Informed Consent.** Ethically sound diagnostic procedures must first proceed with informed consent. Informed consent is a process in which patients are provided with adequate information about the nature, purpose, risks, and limitations of assessments before proceeding. In a clinical setting, this process can be complicated by fluctuating capacity, emotional distress, and lack of insight associated with certain conditions (Beauchamp & Childress, 2019). The consent given by the client must be both voluntary and understandable, especially when there is diagnostic uncertainty. Clinicians must establish a safe and open space where they can discuss the possibilities of error, the diagnostic process, and the consequences of the results.
- **Misdiagnosis Liability.** Legal liability can arise when a misdiagnosis leads to demonstrable harm or disparity. In numerous jurisdictions, healthcare pro-

viders can be held accountable under the tort law of negligence if it is proven that the clinician in charge has made a diagnostic error, due to a breach of professional standards (Bal, 2009). Although determining liability in psychiatry is particularly complex. It is reasoned that the subjective nature of many psychiatric diagnoses and the often-limited availability of definitive diagnostic tests align with individual and cultural sensitivity. Courts may require verification that the clinicians failed to comply with accepted standards of care, such as performing a thorough evaluation or consideration of alternative diagnoses.

- **Diagnostic Disclosure Dilemmas**. Clinicians have often faced ethical tension, which is between the obligation to disclose diagnostic uncertainty and the risk of inducing patient confusion, fear, or anxiety. The dilemma is extremely relevant in early or provisional psychiatric diagnosis, as premature labelling may lead to stigmas and identity disruptions (First, 2021). Incorporating ethical practice involves balancing truth-telling with beneficence, suggesting the need for honesty while minimizing harm. The encouragement of shared decision-making models can promote open discussion and clarity about diagnostic uncertainty, while empowering patients to participate meaningfully to acquire effective coping mechanisms and holistic growth (Elwyn et al., 2012).
- **Regulatory and Cultural Variations Across Countries.** The ethical and legal expectations around misdiagnosis vary significantly across cultural and regulatory landscapes. In the context of high-income countries, formal medical malpractice systems and codified ethical guidelines frequently provide mechanisms for accountability and compensation.

However, in most low-and middle-income countries (LMICs), there is a lack of a robust regulatory framework for medical errors, and cultural beliefs about mental illness that play a factor in limiting the patient's willingness to challenge the diagnosis or pursue legal action (Kirmayer & Swartz, 2013).

To conclude, these disparities highlight the importance of globally adaptable ethical guidelines that account for sociocultural and legal diversity while encouraging transparency, autonomy, and accountability.

3. Age-Specific Diagnostic Pitfalls: Pediatric and Geriatric Challenges

Mental health conditions are hardly present identically across various age groups, making it important for clinicians to navigate the underlying neurobiological processes and the developmental context in which they appear.

It includes pediatric diagnostic obstacles such as the Autism - ADHD diagnosis, where children with attention challenges, hyperactivity, and social changes frequently encounter confusion or misattribution due to overlapping characteristics. Undiagnosed conditions can lead to unfavorable outcomes, including academic challenges, social isolation, mental health complications, and long-term functional impairments. Age-related diagnostic bias is another important variable in pediatric misdiagnosis. This bias demonstrates how diagnostic decisions can be impacted by contextual factors. Pediatric diagnosis can benefit from structured tools like the Child Behavior Checklist (CBCL) and the Autism Diagnostic Observation Schedule (ADOS), which provide standardized assessment methods for developmental specificity. However, access to these tools remains uneven globally, making contextual clinical judgment crucial. A landmark study of 847 children revealed that nearly 40% of those initially diagnosed with ADHD were later accurately diagnosed with ASD (Kentrou, V., et al., 2018).

There are geriatric diagnostic challenges were depression masquerades as dementia. These challenges are particularly found in low- and middle-income countries (LMICs) where mental health awareness may be restricted, and depression might be considered as a normal component of aging. Depression often presents cognitive symptoms that imitate dementia. However, it can be an important variable in developing dementia or an early symptom of dementia itself. Violi et al. (2023) highlighted that older adults often demonstrate pseudodementia, that is, depression symptoms imitating dementia. While depression pseudodementia can be improved through treatment, it also may serve as a risk factor for irreversible dementia, making accurate differential diagnosis essential.

These challenges in low- and middle-income countries (LMICs) are more complicated due to limited tools for comprehensive evaluation. For instance, older adults with depression may be more likely to receive a dementia diagnosis due to the cognitive symptoms being more apparent and socially acceptable

Cultural context also plays an important factor in how mental health is demonstrated, with emotional distress frequently showcasing itself as somatic symptoms. Cultural expectations about behavior, academic performance, and social conformity can impact how these symptoms are interpreted and reported.

These age-specific vulnerabilities demonstrate how diagnostic inaccuracies vary across the life course, from children with overlapping developmental symptoms, ignored accurate diagnosis, to older adults whose depressive symptoms imitate cognitive decline. Comprehending these age-based misdiagnoses sets the stage for our next area of how gender forms diagnostic pathways, especially in ADHD and Autism.

4. Gendered Pathways to Diagnosis: ADHD, Autism, and the Invisible Female Experience

Before exploring comorbidity, let's understand how gender impacts the diagnosis of certain disorders like ADHD and Autism. Along with the cultural factors that influence diagnosis, often social masking in girls leads to an increase in misdiagnosis.

For years, our understanding of these disorders was built primarily from boys and men, which created a "male template" for these conditions. When clinicians diagnose girls and women through this template, many cases become distorted.

Let's discuss the key mechanisms that are involved here:

- **Internalization.** While boys with ADHD may demonstrate their struggles through hyperactive or disruptive behavior, girls frequently turn their challenges inward. Instead of jumping around, they may sit quietly while their minds race. Researchers recognize this as "inattentive" presentations. Their challenges with executive function may manifest as chronic lateness, forgotten assignments, rather than classroom disruptions.
- **Camouflaging.** This includes the conscious and unconscious adoption of strategies to appear neurotypical. Let's imagine a young girl with autism who has learned that making eye contact is expected, so she develops techniques. She might remember social scripts for common interactions and practice facial expressions in mirrors. This can be so useful that even trained professionals will fail to diagnose it as autism.
- **Social Masking.** This is a broader concept that includes both learned behaviors and societal expectations. Girls usually face intense pressure to be adjusting, quiet, and socially attuned. A girl with autism may not express her special interests if they are not considered appropriate.

Diagnostic inaccuracies and errors in neurodevelopmental conditions are frequent due to the complex interplay between biological variations and social conditioning. For example, an ADHD girl creates internal control processes that lead to academic struggles and mental health diagnoses that treat symptoms rather than the underlying condition. This complication is impacted by socialization, making it challenging to evaluate innate variations or learned adaptations. Progressive clinicians are presently viewing signs such as social exhaustion, camouflaging, and internalizing experiences rather than disruptive behaviors.

In conclusion, cultural and gender factors play an important role in misdiagnosis rates, but it is only a small part of the same. There are more significant factors that play an important role, for example, how comorbidities challenge differential diagnosis and enhance misdiagnosis rates.

5. Comorbidity and Diagnostic Confusion: When Overlapping Symptoms Obscure Clinical Clarity

Comorbidity is a complex diagnostic challenge in clinical psychology and psychiatry, as it includes various conditions coexisting and developing new patterns of symptoms that may not look like any particular condition. This is demonstrated by the cascade effect, where one primary condition develops the circumstances that lead to secondary conditions.

The masking effect occurs when conditions actively cloud each other's presentation, developing significantly challenging diagnostic scenarios. For instance, ADHD and autism may interact in a young person, with ADHD's hyperactivity element camouflaging autistic traits, while autism's masking strategies may hide ADHD symptoms.

Understanding comorbidity needs grasping that conditions do not just coexist; they influence each other's expression and severity. These unique interactions develop influences that may vary from the original condition alone. For example, autism and OCD can be more complicated due to the person's natural habit of rigid thinking and complications with cognitive flexibility.

To better comprehend comorbidity, clinicians are employing a structured thinking process about how conditions might influence and interact with each other. Effective approaches are eventually growing and becoming contextual, looking at how symptoms emerge over time and functioning within the person's broader life context. While cultural factors, gendered approaches, comorbidity, and diagnostic confusion significantly contribute to misdiagnosis, variables like time and workforce constraints, care fragmentation, and diagnostic procedures may lead to inaccuracies, which will be explored in the next part.

6. Systemic Factors

The important components of healthcare systems significantly influence diagnostic accuracy. Time restrictions in clinical interactions showcase a pervasive challenge, with research indicating that proper diagnosis of cognitive and behavioral disorders may require more time than generally allocated by healthcare systems. A UK-based evaluation showcased that proper digital triage and decision aids enhanced diagnostic concordance with standardized interviews by 26% (Nicholson et al., 2021).

Care fragmentation between various providers and specialties forms disparities that lead to diagnostic errors. When patients receive care across diverse settings without proper information exchange, the simpler picture needed for accurate diagnosis may never appear. Jones et al. (2021) demonstrated that various EHR platforms work as a single data unit, barring in-depth clinical decision-making and care coordination in psychiatric environments.

Workforce restrictions and another important systemic factor. The shortage of mental health specialists indicates that the diagnosis made by clinicians may be suboptimal due to their limited training. This inequality is shown in LMICs, where primary providers with minimal training may be the only resource available. Through the development of district-level services, primary care physician training, awareness campaigns, school-based programs, and psychiatric support, the Indian District Mental Health Programme (DMHP) aims to simplify mental healthcare (MoHFW, 2015). Math et al. (2019) In Karnataka, the Manochaitanya Programme brings psychiatric specialists into primary care environments once a month at taluk hospitals. It was established in October 2014, and it has enhanced service access covering various districts. (Patel et al., 2016) Their landmark study examined task-shifting models where non-specialists provided mental health interventions in low-resource environments. Although it enhanced access and basic evaluation correction, complex cases would need a specialist's input.

Diagnostic procedures may be distorted by financial incentives in healthcare systems. In capitated systems, there might be disincentives to diagnose complex disorders needing resource-intensive care, whereas in fee-for-service systems, there might be incentives to diagnose conditions requiring ongoing billable services. Oliveira et al. (2023) compared diagnostic rates for depression and anxiety across public and private healthcare systems in Brazil, which showcased higher rates of psychiatric diagnoses in private systems due to diagnostic/reporting differences.

These system disparities showcase how diagnostic decision-making may be shaped by institutional structures and economic pressures, by clinical realities. In light of these challenges, technological innovations are evolving as dominant resources to modify diagnostic accuracy and mitigate human and systemic biases.

The Role of Technology and AI in Improving Diagnostic Processes

Technology offers supportive avenues—but not standalone solutions—for enhancing diagnostic accuracy. Its role should be situated within a broader system of clinical reasoning, cultural sensitivity, and human oversight. Progress in technology provides favorable areas for enhancing diagnostic accuracy across various healthcare settings, although it brings challenges that should be tackled carefully.

1. Diagnostic Decision Support Systems

One of the most promising advancements is Diagnostic Support Systems, which has evolved over the years. Algorithmic approaches in diagnosis have progressed from simple rule-based systems to advanced machine-learning models, allowing for the processing of complicated patterns of symptoms, biomarkers, and contextual factors. First et al. (2015) showcased how the Mini International Neuropsychiatric Interview (MINI) and CIDI showed more reliability and clinical concordance above 80%. These systems demonstrate a firm resolve in standardizing the diagnostic process and decreasing variation from a clinical perspective. Yet their effectiveness is still influenced by clinician judgement and the contextual appropriateness of the same.

Progressive systems using NLP (natural language processing) can examine clinical narratives to identify unnoticed linguistic patterns connected with specific conditions; for example, thought disorganization characteristic of schizophrenia or the discourse patterns of autism spectrum disorder. Corcoran et al. (2018) recognized disorganized language patterns through NLP in patients later diagnosed with schizophrenia, enhancing initial identification accuracy by 19%. NLP- based systems face various restrictions in semantic nuance and may be prone to mistakes of training on non-representative datasets.

Diagnostic technologies showcase the capability to address global disparities in access to expertise. Kane et al. (2021) examined a mobile-based clinical decision assistive resource for community health workers and primary care providers, leading to a 36% increase in accurate identification.

These assistive technologies have showcased substantial promise in increasing diagnostic capabilities at the point of care, especially in underserved settings. In low and middle-income countries, utilizing digital health technologies brings many challenges. Mwaka et al. (2023) A qualitative study in Uganda demonstrated that young adults, while appreciating digital resources for expanding care, raised concerns of privacy, affordability, unequal access to smartphones, and less digital awareness, especially among women and rural individuals. This suggests that without acknowledging infrastructure, literacy, and cultural appropriateness, digital solutions risk reinforcing existing inequalities rather than closing them.

A significant development is the rise of digital phenotyping and passive monitoring, which changes the focus from proper clinical input to constant, realistic behavioral data. While assistive technologies improve significant components of diagnostic access, particularly in underserved environments, their effectiveness largely depends on cultural relevance and regulatory safeguards. Together, these global initiatives emphasize that diagnostic equity is not only about resource accessibility but also about developing culturally consistent systems, promoting local diagnostic capacity.

2. Digital Phenotyping and Passive Monitoring

The emergence of digital phenotyping, defined as the use of data from smartphones and wearable devices to understand behavioral patterns related to diagnosis, reflects a paradigm shift in behavioral examination; however, it raises important questions about consent and passive data collection. Passive monitoring of variables like activity levels, sleeping patterns, social engagement, and voice characteristics can help identify subtle behavioral indications of conditions. For instance, Barnett et al. (2018) showcased that changes in these variables could predict manic or depressive episodes up to 2-4 days in advance.

Digital biomarkers derived from human-computer engagement provide unique diagnostic indicators. Patterns of touchscreen interaction, typing speed difference, and scrolling behavior have shown a significant relationship with cognitive impairment and mood states. Hilbert et al. (2022) evaluated multimodal biobehavioral data - clinical questionnaires, hormones, and MRI using machine learning, achieving successful classification between GAD and MDD.

Digital resources like passive monitoring apps and behavioral tracking software offer useful patient insights, but at the same time, change the nature of the therapeutic relationship. Therefore, a comprehensive understanding of their technological capabilities is important. In a qualitative study, (Simblett et al., 2023), a patient engaged in passive monitoring in mental healthcare showcased concerns about who had access to their data and what they might do with it, although they appreciated how the clinician could view them. The account showcases how patients appreciate decreased cognitive burden and tailored care, but worry about surveillance and data misuse. Ethical considerations for clear, consent-driven, and trust-based technology adoption in mental health should be made.

While digital phenotyping provides continuous behavior-based insights into cognitive and emotional states, the incorporation of biological and structural data marks another important step in diagnostic accuracy. Imaging and Biomarker integration utilizes objective physiological indicators to accompany clinical observation and behavioral data.

3. Imaging and Biomarker Integration

Progressive neuroimaging tools play an increasingly significant role in diagnostic accuracy when combined with clinical examination. Machine learning applications to neuroimaging data have showcased the capability to differentiate between overlapping conditions. Zhutovsky et al. (2019) incorporated applied support vector machines to structural MRI data and demonstrated accuracy rates of up to 84% in differentiating bvFTD from major psychiatric conditions.

The integration of various biomarkers through AI analysis demonstrates a compelling promise for complicated differential diagnoses. The blend of inflammatory markers, neuroimaging parameters, and genetic information, when decoded through advanced algorithms, can detect unique biological subtypes within homogeneous diagnostic categories. This "precision psychiatry" approach may eventually evolve current categorical diagnoses to biologically defined endophenotypes with particular treatment applications.

4. Challenges and Limitations

Technological approaches to diagnosis, despite providing various benefits, face significant challenges. Most AI diagnostic models have been created and approved mostly in high-income, Western contexts, utilizing data from predominantly white populations. This bias creates an unnecessary risk of increasing existing diagnostic disparities when deployed in diverse global contexts.

The "black box" nature of various AI systems poses obstacles to diagnostic integration and ethical practices. When diagnostic advice emerges from an unclear algorithmic process, clinicians can neither interrogate nor understand when questions about clinical responsibility and decision-making authority arise. A possible future development would be an "explainable AI" that maintains trust and transparency in diagnostic reasoning.

Additional challenges include privacy concerns and data security issues, particularly for digital phenotyping approaches that gain sensitive behavioral data continuously. A structured and regulatory framework with ethical guidelines for utilizing these technologies remains an underdeveloped area, thus requiring a careful examination of potential risks and benefits.

Lastly, technological remedies must be created with proper and careful supervision of the socioeconomic contexts. Technologies that require costly infrastructure or proper high-bandwidth internet connectivity may increase disparities in diagnosis globally. Low-cost, offline-capable systems adapted to resource-constrained settings represent a critical direction for technology development.

5. Ethical and Equity Concerns in Diagnostic Technology

The progress of digital diagnostic resources in mental health care showcases an important challenge in balancing technological advancement with ethical principles. These technologies that operate within multiple contexts can either reinforce inequalities or develop more equal access to mental health care.

The ethical components of diagnostic technology in mental health include questions of human dignity, independence, privacy, and social justice. Algorithmic bias in diagnostic technology can widely disadvantage particular groups, leading to below-average clinical decisions and reinforcing various healthcare disparities. Data privacy and ownership, as well as jurisdictional difficulties, are among the ethical concerns brought up by the connection between stigma and diagnostic technology in mental health diagnosis. Despite their ability to democratize care, digital health platforms' worldwide reach might marginalize disadvantaged people.

Furthermore, a systematic review (Cestonaro et al., 2023) demonstrated that present malpractice structures are not well-equipped to handle AI-related errors in diagnosis. It highlighted the shared responsibility across clinicians, developers, and institutions, especially when AI tools are involved, where patients may be harmed without proper avenues for grievances. This underscores an immediate need for an updated legal structure.

Ethical digital mental health technology needs a proper structure that accounts for social justice, technological responsibility, and global health equity. Additionally, it must acknowledge infrastructure challenges, individual barriers, and cultural and linguistic factors. Acquaintances between technologists, clinicians, ethicists, policymakers, and communities are important for proper ethical implementation.

Integration and Future Directions

While the various factors contribute to the global environment of diagnosis and misdiagnosis, they present consistent obstacles and promising developments. Numerous important areas have evolved as priorities for enhancing diagnostic accuracy on a worldwide scale.

1. Challenging Diagnostic Gatekeeping: Implicit Bias, Intersectionality and Feminist Epistemologies in Mental Health

Diagnostic gatekeeping is defined as the complex mechanisms that determine who has access to diagnostic care when they receive it, and how those are framed. This is not just a neutral obstacle but is created and operated by human beings with conscious and unconscious biases.

Implicit Bias is the unconscious attitude and stereotype that influences our perceptions, decisions, and behaviors without our awareness. This can develop a clinician's interpretation of similar symptoms in different individuals.

Intersectionality is a concept developed by Kimberlé Crenshaw, a legal scholar, who understood that an individual does not experience only single identity categories alone but is continuously shaped by the difficult interaction of various, simultaneously occurring social situations.

Feminist epistemology challenges positivist epistemology by arguing that all knowledge is located and shaped by the knower's experiences, values, and social location. Utilizing feminist epistemology to mental health diagnosis emphasizes the benefits of subjective knowledge, especially of the marginalized communities whose voices have been excluded from knowledge production. This shift from perceiving clients as passive recipients of clinicians' diagnostic decision-making towards recognizing them as knowledgeable agents who are aware of their own experiences.

To create more inclusive diagnostic practices, it is important to identify the psychological symptoms found within social, cultural, and economic areas. Incorporating these changes requires modified professional training programs, diagnostic manuals, assessment tools, and a change in authority.

2. Development of Culturally Adaptive Diagnostic Approaches

This helps to sustain reliability while accommodating cultural differences in symptom expression and illness conceptualization. The DSM-5's Cultural Formulation Interview showcases progress in this direction, but a more structured integration of cultural factors into diagnostic systems is required.

3. Implementation of Collaborative Diagnostic Models

This considers the inclusion of various perspectives, including patients, family, and diverse healthcare providers, to counteract the constraints of individual clinical judgment. It showcases assurance for difficult presentations and culturally diverse contexts.

4. Thoughtful Integration of Technology and Human Expertise

This utilizes the strengths of each other rather than observing them as competing approaches. The promising model's position technology enhances clinical judgment rather than taking its place, with technological tools providing standardization and pattern recognition while clinicians provide contextual comprehension and therapeutic relationships.

We might endeavor to lessen worldwide differences in diagnostic quality and the associated human costs of misdiagnosis by addressing both the technical components of diagnostic accuracy and the larger systemic and cultural contexts in which diagnosis occurs. Yet, comprehending the causes is just the tip of the iceberg. It is important to address the difficulties due to misdiagnosis through practical strategies.

ADDRESSING THE CHALLENGE OF MISDIAGNOSIS

Misdiagnosis is an important challenge in healthcare, requiring unique solutions beyond traditional methods. Acknowledging these needs enhanced research funding, effective training, and changes in the system. AI is changing the accuracy of the diagnosis and disease estimation through machine learning algorithms. Healthcare organisations are incorporating thorough diagnostic security programs and demonstrating multidisciplinary diagnostic management teams. The requirement for cultural change, along with technological progress in healthcare, is being recognized. Before understanding these strategies comprehensively, it is essential to introspect on the realistic impact of misdiagnosis, especially how it affects patients, clinicians, and wider societal structures.

Consequences of Misdiagnosis

Misdiagnosis in cognitive and behavioral disorders has extreme consequences that may harm the patient's lives, question the professionalism of clinicians, and the healthcare systems at large. It goes beyond simple clinical consequences and affects multiple aspects of well-being and functioning. On the most important and tragic level, misdiagnosis constantly derails the patient's treatment process by prolonging access to proper care.

1. Patient-Level Consequences

The most immediate influence of misdiagnosis affects patients as they may face inappropriate or ineffective treatments while their underlying condition remains unaddressed, leading to endless suffering. Dagani et al. (2017) examined data from 27 studies, including 9415 patients, demonstrating that the average delay between the appearance of bipolar symptoms and the beginning of the appropriate treatment was approximately 5.8 years.

Iatrogenic harm- unfavorable effects resulting directly from medical intervention showcases an important risk following misdiagnosis. Psychotropic medications that are considered for inappropriately diagnosed conditions could produce considerable side effects without therapeutic benefit. Meyer and Koro (2004) investigated the side effects of abnormal antipsychotics, focusing on extrapyramidal and metabolic syndrome; they demonstrated that atypical antipsychotics are connected with various risks of EPS and metabolic disturbances.

The psychological influence can be equally disastrous. Providing an inappropriate psychiatric diagnosis frequently influences identity formation and self-concept, as patients incorporate these labels into their understanding of themselves. When these labels are proven to be incorrect, they experience extreme identity disruption and loss of trust in the healthcare system. Tekin (2011) investigated how psychiatric diagnoses can significantly destroy self-concept and also lead to feelings of devaluation.

Although misdiagnosis has a significant impact on patients, the effects extend to those who are responsible for making these clinical decisions. These inaccuracies can place an emotional and professional burden on clinicians that may influence their decision-making.

2. Clinician-Level Consequences

These diagnostic errors carry professional and psychological consequences. The emotional toll may lead to further diagnostic caution that can result in either beneficial thoroughness or problematic defensive practice.

Professional consequences may include reduced confidence in clinical judgment, poor relationships with patients and colleagues, or, in some cases, legal or regulatory consequences. It may be possible that the diagnostic errors do not lead to formal complaints, although high-profile cases can severely influence clinical practice at several levels.

The most concerning is the possible growth of diagnostic fatalism, which views this uncertainty as inevitable and enhancement trials as ineffective. This kind of a mindset leads to resignation rather than engagement with quality improvement efforts and reduced loyalty to diagnostic accuracy. Newman-Toker et al. (2019) showcased that clinicians were uncomfortable talking about diagnostic inaccuracies, due to diagnostic defensive-medicine norms

While individual clinicians often grapple with diagnostic uncertainty, these consequences affect structures beyond the consultation room. At the system level, when these inaccuracies are stored, it shapes how they are perceived by the public.

3. System-Level Consequences

At the healthcare level, increased rates of misdiagnosis lead to ineffective resource allocation, elevated costs, and reduced public trust. When the primary reason for misdiagnosed conditions is restricted resources, both the patient who was misdiagnosed and other patients could have benefited from these resources. This allocation error is problematic in settings where mental health services are already inadequate.

The diminished public trust in psychiatric diagnosis is another system-level consequence. Media coverage of psychiatric diagnostic inaccuracy is concentrated on popular cases, thus reinforcing the notion that psychiatric diagnosis is subjective and unreliable. Sirey et al. (2001) showcased that increased levels of perceived stigma were particularly connected with lower adherence to prescribed antidepressant medications in older adults. These errors can create unavoidable legal and financial liabilities for healthcare settings. A notable instance of legal consequences in India is the case of Martin F. D'Souza vs. Mohd. Ishfaq, where the Supreme Court ruled on medical negligence involving treatment without proper diagnostic references. This case demonstrates the requirement of evidence-based decision-making and proper consultation structures. Malpractice claims connected to misdiagnosis often include severe harm and considerable settlements or judgments. It ultimately impacts healthcare accessibility and affordability for all patients.

Multiple Faces of Diagnosis: Patients' Lived Experiences

Beyond the general consequences presented here, misdiagnosis deeply impacts patients at a personal and emotional level, which not only shapes their treatment but also shapes their self-understanding and social identity. Here are some instances of lived experiences by patients that will give a better understanding of the impact that misdiagnosis presents.

1. (Lmsw, 2024) A.S., an Australian trauma survivor, was misdiagnosed with paranoid schizophrenia, which influenced his identity for over a decade. Despite not experiencing psychosis, he experienced involuntary hospitalizations and high-dose antipsychotic medication. The underlying issue, which was childhood trauma, was ignored due to symptom-matching shortcuts. He described his experience as "psychological torture," and his attempts to clarify were evaded or utilized against him. Only years later did a correct PTSD diagnosis allow him to regain his autonomy and narrative. This case demonstrates how diagnostic inaccuracies are not only clinical but also existential. Labels often overshadow listening, increasing the risk of re-traumatization. This underscores the need for trauma-informed, critically reflective diagnosis, particularly in power-imbalanced systems and involuntary treatment pathways.
2. (Gold, 2019) S.C., a 24-year-old journalist, was primarily misdiagnosed with bipolar disorder, schizophrenia, and alcohol-induced psychosis. Over the period, her behavior grew increasingly unpredictable with hallucinations, paranoia, and catatonia leading to hospitalization and the consideration of a psychiat-

ric breakdown. Despite the elaborate psychiatric intervention, her condition deteriorated. S.C.'s life was saved by a differential diagnosis of anti-NMDA receptor encephalitis, demonstrating the significance of clinician humility and interdisciplinary collaboration in differentiating complicated medications from psychiatric illnesses.

3. (Ducharme, 2025) E., a 43-year-old woman from Pennsylvania, started enduring debilitating fatigue, heart palpitations, and gastrointestinal issues following a mild case of COVID-19. When she sought support, her symptoms were ignored and diagnosed as psychosomatic. Over time, she was misdiagnosed with anxiety and eating disorders due to the lack of biomarkers. She was involuntarily admitted to a psychiatric facility, but later, with the help of specialists and self-advocacy. In both general and psychiatric diagnosis, this case demonstrates the significance of epistemological humility and respect for lived experience.

(GMHPN, 2022) Global advocacy platforms such as the Global Mental Health Peer Network (GMHPN) promote patient voices in diagnostic frameworks, opposing expert-driven models, and acknowledging serving users as co-creators of knowledge in global mental health, thus highlighting context-sensitive refinements. Together, these cases showcase that diagnostic inaccuracy is not just a technical error; it also creates a barrier to trust, identity, and care. When clinicians ignore or overlook lived experience, rely on similar symptom-matching, or commonly shift to psychiatry labels in cases of uncertainty, they risk elevating harm rather than preventing it.

These narratives encourage the utility of better resources such as active listening, interdisciplinary humility, and a renewed ethical dedication to the person behind the diagnosis. Recognizing these consequences emphasizes the immediate requirement for proper strategies to decrease errors in diagnosis. One such strategy is developing and utilizing critical thinking and metacognitive capabilities within clinical practice to ensure diagnoses are both accurate and ethically grounded.

Decision Support System Failures

Both the Clinical Decision Support System (CDSS) and artificial intelligence (AI) tools have displayed significant promise in enhancing diagnostic accuracy and standardized care. Nevertheless, their limitations are present in mental health contexts, warranting evaluations. For instance, the CDSS algorithms often operate as "black boxes" as they produce recommendations without transparent reasoning. This, in return, complicates the process of validating outcomes or adjusting for nuances, individualized presentations for the clinicians (Shortliffe & Sepúlveda, 2018). In psychiatry, where diagnosis frequently relies on subjective experiences, contextual history, and cultural interpretation, mechanized tools can misclassify or oversimplify complex cases, which can hamper the process of assessing the client or patient's needs (Topol, 2019).

Additionally, these symptoms are frequently trained on datasheets that lack cultural and geographic diversity and sensitivity. These raise concerns about the generalisability and possible biases when applied in low-resource or cross-cultural settings (Obermeyer et al., 2019). An excessive reliance on CDSS and AI tools may also undermine clinician autonomy and critical thinking. Leading to complacency and decreased diagnostic vigilance. Thus, while digital tools may help in assisting clinical reasoning, these tools must be used with caution and supplemented by human judgement, particularly in psychiatry, where context and interpersonal interactions are essential for determining the cause.

Strategies to Reduce Misdiagnosis Through Critical Thinking

Addressing the difficulties of misdiagnosis calls for growing and incorporating particular cognitive strategies that improve clinical judgment. Additionally, it gives the framework for these strategies, offering proper approaches to overcome the cognitive limitations that lead to misdiagnosis.

1. Metacognitive Awareness and Bias Recognition

Growing recognition of cognitive processes involved in diagnosis showcases an important strategy for enhancing diagnostic accuracy. Clinicians who can comprehend the common cognitive biases, such as anchoring, availability, and confirmation bias, are in a better place to counteract these influences in their reasoning. (Tjia et al., 2023) Implemented didactic sessions on healthcare disparities and implicit bias, administering the Implicit Association Test to increase individual awareness, skill-building, and simulation-based interactions from the local community.

2. Structured Diagnostic Frameworks

Utilization of proper approaches to diagnostic reasoning gives scaffolding for critical thinking in difficult cases. Frameworks such as the hypothetico-deductive model, pattern identification with imposed contemplation of alternatives, and Bayesian reasoning provide complementary ways for various clinical situations. Mamede et al. (2007) showcased that clinicians employing an integrated approach gained greater diagnostic accuracy than those depending on one approach.

Diagnostic decision matrices that particularly weigh empirical facts for and against opposite diagnostic hypotheses showcase one practical implication of structured reasoning. This approach helps clinicians to examine the strength of evidence supporting each probable diagnosis in a structured way rather than concentrating only on confirmatory data.

3. Comprehensive Information Gathering

The intricate nature of diagnostic decisions relies particularly on the complete and accurate information available for consideration. It focuses on thorough information from different sources, including patient self-report, collateral informants, and medical records, etc.

Planned and structured questioning techniques demonstrate phenomenologically difficult descriptions rather than simple endorsements, enhancing diagnostic variations in environments with conflicting symptom characteristics. Mota and Lourenco (2020) examined the intersecting symptoms, treatment methods, and prognostic results of BPD and bipolar disorder and emphasized the role of phenomenological interviewing in understanding the lived experiences of patients.

4. Interprofessional Collaboration in Diagnostic Reasoning

This is important for enhancing diagnostic accuracy in mental health environments, as the complications of mental health conditions often extend beyond the abilities of a single clinician. Various healthcare professionals bring diverse perspectives, expertise, and observational skills that can demonstrate elements of a patient's conditions that may not be visible to a single clinician. This collaborative model is a proper approach to including various professional perspectives in mental health diagnosis and treatment. A qualitative study (Rugkåsa et al., 2020) demonstrated that involving psychologists and psychiatrists within general practitioner practices significantly improved diagnostic reasoning in mental health. Co-location led to timely evaluation, collaborative decision-making, and reduced misdiagnosis.

5. Reflective Practice as a Diagnostic Tool

A tool that aids in improving diagnostic accuracy by properly evaluating one's clinical experiences, decisions, and consequences. It includes recognizing similarities in decision-making and learning from successful and unsuccessful diagnostic encounters. In the mental health domain, it includes both individual and collective forms of reflection.

Individual reflective practice includes properly evaluating diagnostic decisions, taking into account relevant information, and examining the support of later advancements. Reflection is important for experiencing learning and maintaining expertise. Formal practice groups or reflective journals are instances of proper methods that might enhance the process. Examining presumptions, biases, and contextual elements that influence clinical decision-making is an important part of reflection, which goes beyond simple introspection. Mamede et al. (2008) An experimental study demonstrated that deliberate reflection enhanced accuracy for difficult cases.

Interprofessional rounds and diagnostic feedback loops provide a reflective clinical culture, allowing knowledge sharing and questioning across disciplines, improving diagnostic accuracy in complicated cases, especially in mental health.

6. Feedback and Continuous Learning

The most influential approach for enhancing diagnostic accuracy is the development of continuous learning through proper feedback. Although making an error is impossible, learning from these errors is a choice and requires intentional processes. Proper approaches include diagnostic review of difficult cases and formal examination of unfavorable events related to diagnosis.

Diagnostic articulation groups, in which clinicians present difficult cases for an interactive examination, thus providing sudden insight into difficult demonstrations and current growth of critical thinking skills. Technology can support this learning procedure through clinical decision support systems that give immediate feedback on diagnostic reasoning, comparison of practice similarities with evidence-based norms, and research. Kammer et al. (2023) showcased that CDSS did not particularly enhance diagnostic accuracy, though performance was consistent across modalities.

In conclusion, it must be taken into account that personal cognitive approaches alone cannot tackle misdiagnosis. Considering the challenging demonstrations in cognitive and behavioral disorders, collaborative diagnostic models provide a wider and better path to clinical reasoning.

Interdisciplinary Collaboration

The complicated nature of cognitive and behavioral disorders often goes beyond the skill boundaries of any single discipline, making interdisciplinary collaboration important for accurate diagnosis. Effective interaction influences various perspectives and certain knowledge to form a broader comprehension of difficult presentations.

1. Models of Collaborative Diagnosis

Various models of collaborative diagnosis have showcased effectiveness in decreasing misdiagnosis rates. Interdisciplinary diagnostic conferences, in which cases are showcased to teams including various professionals, represent one well-established approach. (van der Merwe et al., 2024) Evaluated the variations between live telehealth and face-to-face interviews utilizing standard diagnostic criteria for psychiatric conditions, which showcased that telehealth evaluations have good agreement and reliability, even in remote areas.

Collaborative care models that incorporate psychiatric expertise into primary care environments show significant promise for enhancing recognition and diagnosis of mental disorders in general medical environments. These models usually include mental health professionals working alongside primary care providers and diagnostic elucidation.

Diagnostic collaborations between psychiatry and neurology have significant value for conditions at the intersection of these specialties. Collaborative evaluation of presentations, including both cognitive and behavioral symptoms, can allow differentiation between main psychiatric disorders, neurological conditions with psychiatric manifestations, and complicated instances including components of both.

2. Communication Strategies

Useful interdisciplinary collaboration relies on transparent communication structures and shared comprehension. Common obstacles include discipline-specific terminology, hierarchical professional dynamics, and disrupted communication channels. The strategies for counteracting these obstacles include the growth of structured referral and consultation protocols that particularly describe the diagnostic questions, administration of collective diagnostic planning structures that include multidisciplinary perspectives, and professional development, including training in better communication skills. Technology improves interdisciplinary communication through collective electronic health records, assured messaging platforms, and telemedicine-enabled connected examinations.

3. Overcoming Barriers to Collaboration

Interdisciplinary collaboration faces important systemic barriers, such as financial structures that mostly fail to compensate for collaborative diagnostic activities satisfactorily, generating disincentives for time-intensive dialogues. Professional identity issues and territorial problems over diagnostic authority. Addressing these barriers needs both system-level changes and individual dedication to collaborative values.

Successful models typically include attention to these barriers, with approaches including clear role terminology while stabilizing flexibility, respect for others for various types of expertise, and collective outcome measures that focus on patient benefits. (Teixeira et al., 2024) Evaluated the effectiveness of incorporating a Collaborative Care Model for musculoskeletal conditions and coexisting anxiety and depression, and indicated the advantages of integrated care approaches.

While interdisciplinary collaboration enhances diagnostic practices in the present, it is equally important to imagine and create the future landscape of diagnosis. Emerging theoretical models, patient-focused care, and integrated technologies provide new areas for diagnostic accuracy.

Future Directions

The future of diagnosis will probably be shaped by various cross-developments that vow to decrease misdiagnosis through enhanced critical thinking and expanded evidence base.

1. Dimensional and Network Approaches

The constraints of categorical diagnostic systems have become more apparent with the enhanced recognition that many cognitive and behavioral disorders exist on a continuum. They will likely include dimensional evaluation along with traditional categories, allowing greater nuanced characterization of symptom patterns and severity. The NIMH Research Domain Criteria (RDoC) framework represents an early step in this direction, though its clinical implementation remains limited.

Network models of psychopathology conceptualize these disorders as apparent properties of related symptom connections rather than indications of underlying disease entities, which is a promising direction. (Pan, C et al., 2024) came up with a unique concept called model control to recognize important symptom clusters in symptom connections, revealing that non-emotional modules play an important role, which can give insights into mental disorders mechanisms and aid tailored interventions, improving psychopathology representation and therapeutic interventions.

2. Integration of Biomarkers

Although there is limited evidence on proper biomarkers in psychiatry, recent research continues to detect biological indicators with diagnostic relevance. Subsequent approaches will likely include multimodal biomarkers that give a greater diagnostic certainty than any particular measure.

The effective approach focuses on biomarkers as complements to clinical assessment, by recognising that biological indicators provide context when interpreted within clinical and phenomenological contexts. (Bahn et al., 2023) evaluated the integration of a blood-based biomarker panel with digital mental health assessments to improve bipolar disorder diagnosis, and found that blood tests alone can recognize up to 30% of the cases, and their combination with digital evaluation efficiently enhanced diagnostic accuracy.

3. *Patient Participation in Diagnosis*

Evolving diagnostic structures increasingly position patients as active associates in the process rather than passive receivers of diagnostic labels. These approaches engage patients by including their individual experiences and preferences regarding terminology and proper treatment objectives. (Bate et al., 2006) concentrated on the significance of including patients in the design and enhancement of healthcare services. It found that involving them led to improvements in the quality and safety of healthcare services that were in line with their needs and expectations.

The incorporation of digital tools helps to promote patients' involvement. If effectively incorporated within clinical workflows, it can locate areas of diagnostic uncertainty, and a more comprehensive assessment can be ensured.

4. Global Diagnostic Equity

Global inequities in diagnostic accuracy are becoming increasingly addressed, where promising strategies include the growth of culturally grounded and reliable evaluation methods along with the implementation of clinical training programs has emerged. Furthermore, implementation science has played an important part in detecting appropriate approaches for improving diagnostic accuracy in diverse settings. The WHO's mhGAP exemplifies these approaches by providing evidence-based guidance for non-specialist providers in resource-limited environments.

5. Continuous Quality Environment

In the future, diagnostic systems are likely to include principles of continuous quality improvement, involving proper tracking of diagnostic consistency, analysis of diagnostic revisions, and assessment of discrepancies in clinicians over time. (Khuri et al., 2002) incorporated structured review procedures and feedback operations across VHA hospitals to improve surgical care quality and found that there is a decrease in 30-day postoperative mortality after surgery by 27%.

These enhancements, while promising individually, provide a unique benefit when integrated. An integrated approach that incorporates these elements can significantly decrease diagnostic inaccuracies on a systemic scale.

Integration of Approaches

To counter the effects of misdiagnosis effectively, an integration of various approaches is required. Critical thinking gives the cognitive foundation upon which particular techniques and technologies can grow, while collaborative models utilize varying expertise to conquer individual limitations.

The most successful programs combine:

- Individual critical thinking skills growth
- Proper diagnostic processes and decision support
- Interactive evaluation including various perspectives
- Technological support that is context-appropriate

When utilized in a complementary way, these approaches can significantly reduce misdiagnosis rates even in complicated and challenging presentations. Auerbach et al. (2024) examined 2428 patient records from 29 academic medical centers across the U.S., demonstrating that 23% of patients faced a diagnostic inaccuracy, and approximately 17% of these errors led to harm or death.

While we cannot completely reduce errors in diagnosis because of the complicated and evolving nature of cognitive and behavioral disorders, a significant reduction is possible through proper attention to diagnostic processes. It is also important to address this error as a system failure rather than an individual failure by implementing evidence-based enhancements to diagnostic practice.

While identifying diagnostic errors needs systemic enhancements, it also requires individual expertise in sound reasoning. This leads us to the essential component in improving diagnoses- the role of critical thinking in clinical practice.

UNDERSTANDING CRITICAL THINKING IN CLINICAL PRACTICE

Critical thinking is among the key skills required for effective clinical practice in mental health settings. The ability to think critically is not only beneficial but also crucial for patient safety and therapeutic benefits, as professionals navigate complex diagnostic environments and treatment decisions. The psychiatric diagnoses often lack proper molecular indicators prevalent in other medical professions, and the consequences of clinical decision-making in mental health are extremely high. Clinicians, while being aware of their own cognitive biases, should also incorporate evidence from several sources. Before understanding how it can be effectively applied in these settings, we must first understand their operational definitions.

Definition and Core Elements of Critical Thinking

Critical thinking in clinical practice is defined as the proper, imposed, and ordered process of actively analyzing, integrating, and examining information to lead clinical decisions and actions. Unlike daily thinking, critical thinking is characterized by intentional introspection, logical reasoning, and constant curiosity about presumptions and conclusions.

The foundation of clinical critical thinking is in various interconnected core components.

- ***Analytical thinking*** involves breaking down complex clinical presentations into elemental parts, evaluating relationships between symptoms, and identifying patterns that may be concealed. For example, when examining a patient demonstrating depressive symptoms, analytical thinking would include evaluating their temporal connections to life events, medical conditions, and other psychiatric symptoms.
- ***Logical reasoning*** forms another foundation, requiring clinicians to draw convincing conclusions grounded on available evidence while evading logical errors. It includes understanding the difference between correlation and causation, determining when additional data is needed before selecting clinical choices, and deciding when there is proper evidence to support a decision.
- ***Skeptical inquiry*** motivates clinicians to probe initial impressions, question easier explanations, and remain open to alternative hypotheses. (Croskerry, P.,2003) demonstrates how clinicians tend to accept their initial impressions without considering alternative diagnostic options. It serves as a protection against untimely closure and inspires deeper exploration.
- ***Metacognitive awareness*** offers the most unique component of critical thinking, including the capability to track and introspect on one's thinking processes. It includes identifying when cognitive biases might be impacting judgment, recognizing knowledge limitations, and comprehending the gaps in one's clinical reasoning. (Clayton, D. A., et al., 2023) showcased that clinicians with greater metacognitive awareness were more likely to seek further diagnostic actions, especially in cases where the initial diagnoses were incorrect.
- ***Evidence integration*** needs the capability to collate information from various sources while properly weighing the quality and applicability of different types of evidence. This includes comprehending research methodology, identifying the levels of evidence, and applying research findings to personalized clinical cases while accounting for other factors.

While critical thinking provides a proper way to decision-making, they must be aware of their biases that affect their decision-making and shape their clinical judgments.

Cognitive Biases and Diagnostic Errors in Mental Health

The human mind, although exceptionally capable of processing complicated data, is often subjected to systematic errors in thinking known as cognitive biases. While these biases are adaptive in daily life, they can lead to critical diagnostic errors in clinical environments.

- ***Confirmation bias*** showcases one of the most relevant challenges to accurate diagnosis in mental health practice. It makes the clinician preferentially seek, interpret, and remember information that confirms their initial diagnosis while ignoring contradictory evidence. (Mendel, R., et al., 2011) Showcased in a study involving 75 psychiatrists and medical students, clinicians relying on confirmatory data findings were less likely to reach an accurate diagnosis. Let's imagine a scenario where a young adult showcases concentration difficulties and sleep disturbances. A clinician immediately diagnosing it as ADHD may concentrate questioning and observation on inattention and hyperactivity symptoms rather than focusing on other symptoms that could account for the presentation. This selective attention can lead to a missed diagnosis.
- ***Anchoring bias*** occurs when clinicians become overly influenced by the first piece of information or "anchor" for further judgments. In mental health environments, they may present themselves as overdependent on referral data and previous diagnoses. (Graber et al., 2005) In their examination of 100 cases of diagnostic errors, they demonstrated that cognitive factors led to inaccuracies in 74% of cases, with anchoring bias being the main contributor. For instance, a patient referred with a history of borderline personality disorder may have their present symptoms interpreted through these diagnostic lenses, which can lead to under-recognition of comorbid disorders.
- ***Availability bias*** causes clinicians to over evaluate the probability of diagnoses that we remember easily, often because they are dramatic, recently encountered, or emotionally relevant. This bias can result in overdiagnosis of rare conditions and underdiagnosis of common conditions. (Li, Ping et al., 2020) demonstrated that clinicians may misdiagnose cases as dengue fever when overlapping symptom cases are presented, with misdiagnosis rates ranging from 71% to 100%. The consequences of these cognitive biases extend beyond individual diagnostic errors. (Yamamoto, K., 2022) employed an

introspective questionnaire, which was completed by 130 diverse physicians, and found that each diagnostic error was connected with 3.08 cognitive biases, with a greater prevalence during night-time shifts. Diagnostic inaccuracies usually lead to improper treatment, may slow down recovery, increase healthcare costs, and cause notable patient suffering.

Identifying these biases is the first step. The next step is creating strategies that effectively combat these biases, particularly through critical thinking to enhance diagnostic accuracy.

Improving Diagnostic Precision Through Critical Thinking

Critical thinking is a structured approach to reduce cognitive biases and improve diagnostic accuracy in mental health practice. The practice of critical thinking needs both personal cognitive strategies and other strategies for clinical reasoning.

- ***Differential diagnosis development*** showcases an important critical thinking skill that includes creating and structurally examining various diagnostic probabilities. Rather than sticking to the first possible diagnosis for a patient's symptoms, skilled and effective clinicians create descriptive differential diagnoses that acknowledge numerous diagnostic categories, including medical conditions and various psychiatric conditions. It begins with paying deliberate attention to the chief complaint and presenting symptoms, and eventually leads to a structured exploration of diagnostic possibilities. Graber et al. (2005) examined 100 cases of diagnostic errors in internal medicine, which revealed that cognitive factors are the main reason why diagnostic errors occur.
- Proper development of differential diagnosis needs comprehension of base rates and epidemiological factors. Although it is important to account for rare conditions, critical thinking includes weighing the probability of multiple diagnoses based on demographics, setting, and population prevalence. This epidemiological reasoning allows for prioritizing diagnostic probabilities while guaranteeing that general conditions aren't ignored.
- ***Systematic symptom analysis*** involves cautious evaluation of symptom elements, including onset, duration, severity, precipitating factors, and functional influence. Critical thinking in symptom analysis needs to move past general symptom checklists to comprehend the qualitative components of patient experiences and their diagnostic significance. For instance, when examining sleep disruptions, critical thinking would include evaluating not only the presence of insomnia but its pattern (challenge in falling asleep versus fre-

quent awakening), timing (chronic versus acute onset), connection to mood symptoms, and reaction to past treatments. This comprehensive analysis frequently showcases diagnostic clues that might be forgotten with superficial evaluation.

- ***Hypothesis testing*** gives a proper way to diagnostic reasoning that mirrors scientific methodology. It includes creating specific, testable hypotheses about probable diagnoses and then gathering information in an organized way to support or reject these hypotheses. Unlike confirmation bias, which particularly needs supporting facts, hypothesis testing involves deliberately looking for disconfirming evidence. Coderre et al. (2003) revealed that pattern recognition was related to a tenfold increase in diagnostic success compared to hypothetico-deductive reasoning. It also demonstrated that scheme-inductive reasoning had a fivefold increase in diagnostic accuracy over the hypothetico-deductive approach. This approach is significantly important in complicated cases where various diagnoses may explain parts of the clinical presentation.
- ***Evidence synthesis and integration*** need the capability to collate data from different sources while properly acknowledging the reliability and relevance of various types of evidence. It involves incorporating patient self-report, behavioral observations, collateral information, psychological assessment outcomes, and medical data into a complete clinical picture.

Critical thinking in evidence synthesis includes comprehending the restrictions and potential biases in various information sources. Although patient self-report may be important, it may be impacted by other factors such as insight, memory, social desirability, and symptom-related cognitive disability. Collateral information gives significant external evidence but may be restricted by the informant's knowledge and connection with the patient. Psychological assessment provides structured testing but needs cautious interpretation while considering patient factors and test restrictions.

Along with improving diagnostic processes, critical thinking is further reiterated by strong logical reasoning. The next part investigates how different types of logical reasoning can be effectively applied in these settings.

Application of Logical Reasoning in Clinical Settings

The practice of logical reasoning in clinical practice includes various elements that are interconnected when it comes to improving diagnostic accuracy and treatment planning. Comprehending these elements and their proper implications is important for developing proper clinical reasoning skills.

- ***Deductive reasoning*** includes coming to a definite conclusion from general principles or established knowledge. In clinical practice, this may involve diagnostic criteria, treatment guidelines, or research evidence for significant cases. For instance, being aware that the existence of psychotic symptoms during mood episodes differentiates bipolar disorder from major depressive disorder allows clinicians to make particular diagnostic conclusions based on proper symptom evaluation. However, proper application of deductive reasoning needs diligent attention to the rationality of the fundamental rules being practiced and their suitability to the particular clinical situation. Although diagnostic criteria provide a key structure, they must be utilized with comprehension of their restrictions and the clinical judgment needed in borderline cases.
- ***Inductive reasoning*** includes universal derivations from particular observations or patterns. Clinical expertise frequently includes inductive reasoning as clinicians recognize similarities across various patients and develop clinical insights. (Croskerry, P., 2009) Focuses on the dual-process theory, emphasizing the significance of analytical and intuitive thinking in clinical decision-making. It also demonstrates the need for maintaining a balance between prompt, pattern-recognition-based decisions and deliberate analytical reasoning.
- ***Probabilistic reasoning*** recognizes that clinical diagnosis frequently includes unreliability and needs comprehension of probability rather than certainty. This includes utilizing Bayesian thinking to improve diagnostic probabilities as new facts become available. Early diagnostic probabilities are modified by more clinical findings, test results, and treatment responses. (Mamede, S., 2007) showcased that clinicians who utilized reflective reasoning- properly weighed diagnostic probabilities and modified them based on available information. This is increasingly important in mental health as diagnostic inaccuracy is frequently unavoidable, and various active hypotheses may need to be simultaneously sustained.
- ***Causal reasoning*** includes comprehending the connections between various factors that lead to mental health conditions. It also involves understanding how biological vulnerabilities, psychological factors, social stressors, and environmental impacts interact to give clinical demonstrations. Effective causal reasoning allows for diagnosis and planning the treatment properly by recognizing the multiple factors that need to be acknowledged. However, causal reasoning in mental health must address the complications of psychiatric disorders and restrict overgeneralized linear models. Most mental health conditions include various collaborative factors, and similar symptoms can result from different causal pathways in different individuals.

Although logical reasoning is not enough, it must be combined with a clinician's ability to examine evidence and remain open-minded about other possibilities. This is where evidence-based practice and skeptical inquiry play an important role.

Evidence-Based Approaches and Skeptical Inquiry

The incorporation of evidence-based practice with critical thinking forms an inspiring structure for clinical decision-making that stabilizes scientific rigor with clinical expertise and patient values. It requires both comprehension of research methodology and the skill to critically examine and practice these research findings in individual clinical environments.

- ***The hierarchy of evidence*** gives a structure for examining the quality and reliability of various kinds of research evidence. Systematic reviews and meta-analyses of mixed controlled trials showcase the greatest evidence level for treatment effectiveness, while case studies and expert opinions characterize lower evidence levels. However, critical thinking in evidence examination needs comprehension of the hierarchy might differentiate depending on the clinical question being addressed. For diagnostic questions, proper cross-sectional studies with proper reference standards may give more admissible evidence than randomized trials. For comprehending patient experiences and choices, qualitative research may give insights, quantitative research can't capture. Critical thinking includes complementing the evidence type to the clinical question while comprehending the restrictions of the individual approach.
- ***Research critique skills*** allow clinicians to examine the quality and the implications of research studies. It involves comprehending study design, sample characteristics, measurement validity, statistical analysis, and probable sources of bias. (Taylor, R.S., et al., 2004) examined the utility of a half-day critical appraisal skills workshop, which demonstrated that while the workshop improved skills, it had a restricted influence on other aspects of improving evidence-based practice. The significant components in research critique involve the characteristics of study samples to the clinician's patient population, the clinical importance versus statistical significance of findings, and the realistic applicability of research interventions in real-world clinical environments. The studies conducted in rigorously controlled research environments might not generalize to common clinical practice conditions.
- ***Clinical practice guidelines*** characterize trials to collate research evidence into practical advice for clinical care. However, critical thinking in guideline application is needed to comprehend their growth process, the nature of basic

evidence, and their relevance to the particular clinical situation. It should help rather than restore clinical judgment, specifically in complicated cases that might not fit common presentations. (Wang et al., 2023) demonstrated that intrinsic obstacles to clinical practical guidelines include complexity, inaccessibility, and impracticality, and extrinsic challenges included lack of money, resources, training, and awareness. While resources and environmental context were considered common barriers, audits, feedback and leadership, aid, and education are all proper strategies. Critical thinking includes comprehending these restrictions while utilizing guidelines as important resources for evidence-based decision making.

- ***Skeptical inquiry*** includes stabilizing valid doubts about clinical conclusions and remaining open to other possible explanations. It involves probing early diagnostic impressions, questioning treatment options that are incompatible with evidence, and a willingness to modify clinical planning as additional data comes to light. However, it must be equitable with the realistic need to make clinical decisions and provide patient care. Excessive skepticism can result in diagnostic paralysis, while less skepticism can lead to premature closure. (Zeckhauser & Collins, 1973) emphasizes the "optimizer's curse," where unbiased optimization models frequently provide below-average outcomes. Treatment response as diagnostic data showcases a key application of skeptical inquiry in clinical practice. Patient responses to particular interventions can give proper diagnostic information, especially in cases where early diagnosis is not certain. However, critical thinking is needed to gauge the treatment reactions properly, as variables such as placebo effects and natural recovery can confuse interpretation.

When integrated carefully, these elements can create an impactful toolkit for clinicians. In the next part, we introspect as to how this creates a foundation for a safer and effective mental health practice.

Critical thinking is an important component for effective clinical practice in mental health settings. The structured application of their principles, including analytical reasoning, skeptical inquiry, evidence integration, and metacognitive awareness, gives powerful tools for enhancing diagnostic accuracy and patient outcomes.

The research evidence showcases that cognitive fallacies represent important challenges to accurate diagnosis, but can be effectively removed through the proper application of strategies. The skill growth requires constant practice, introspection, and dedication to ongoing learning and enhancement.

The significance of critical thinking will continue to develop as mental health practice continues to grow by focusing more on evidence-based treatment. Clinicians who equip themselves with these skills will be able to handle diagnostic complications and provide effective treatments.

The incorporation of critical thinking into clinical expertise, research facts, and patients' morals characterizes the ground for a better clinical practice. By understanding and applying these skills, mental health professionals can enhance clinical effectiveness while reducing the risk of diagnostic errors.

As we have understood the contextual and realistic benefits of critical thinking, it becomes important to evaluate how it can be utilized as an intervention. The next section discusses how clinicians bridge the gap between theoretical knowledge and real-world decision making.

BRIDGING THE GAP: CRITICAL THINKING AS A TOOL FOR ACCURATE DIAGNOSIS

Considering the established importance and practical relevance of critical thinking in clinical settings, this following section delves into its application as an intervention strategy, by examining how clinicians operationalise theoretical constructs into evidence-based and patient-centered care.

The diagnostic process in mental health requires a sophisticated approach towards critical thinking that extends beyond the given memorized criteria and assessment protocols (Croskerry, 2018). This section specifies how clinical practitioners can develop and use critical thinking as an intervention tool to improve diagnostic accuracy by analyzing facts, evidence, observations, and arguments to form enhanced patient care and guide them for a healthy development. Through evidence researched and an ethical framework, the main goal is to bridge the gap between the theoretical knowledge available and effective clinical practices. As diagnostic challenges become more complex in complementary mental healthcare, integrating critical thinking with standardized assessment tools is essential for achieving accurate and reliable diagnoses. The incorporation of essential techniques of thinking into clinical assessments is likely to advance the rigor and comprehensiveness of the evaluative process, focusing on enrichment of an individual's mental well-being.

Techniques for Integrating Critical Thinking into Pattern Assessment

1. The Need for Metacognitive Awareness in Clinical Decision-Making

Clinicians need to cultivate an awareness of their cognitive processes throughout the assessment process to ensure that they maintain ethical objectivity and accuracy. This includes recognizing cognitive biases, availability heuristics, and anchoring effects that can skew clinical judgment (Bhugra et al, 2021). Cognitive biases are created when an individual creates their subjective reality from the information they have perceived. Recent research suggests that the diagnostic accuracy has improved significantly by 27% when clinicians have implemented reflection protocols, which are structured. This enhances the flow of the assessment process. Techniques such as diagnostic timeouts (or delays) and alternative hypotheses aid practitioners in questioning their initial impressions and avoiding premature diagnostic disclosure (Croskerry et al.,2023). This not only allows practitioners to enhance their skills cognitively but also develops a mindset to approach situations for growth, where one seeks to search actively for the long-term benefit. Mamede et al. (2007) have found through their research that structured reflection is a need as metacognition prompts for improving the quality of diagnostic formulations, especially in cases that may have conflicting or ambiguous symptom presentation of the client.

2. Distinguishing Patterns from Noise

Effective diagnosticians can differentiate between meaningful patterns from clinical "noise". Noise can be considered an unpleasant disturbance that can hamper the process of diagnosing. Bornstein (2020) mentioned that this process of identifying noise from meaningful patterns involves recognizing when symptom clusters display crucial psychopathology versus variations that are normal in human experience or short-term responses to environmental stressors. Zimmerman and colleagues conducted a longitudinal study in 2022, which documented clinicians' skills. It suggested that clinicians who received efficient training in pattern recognition had demonstrated a superior ability to identify and distinguish clinical symptoms from normative psychological reactions, specifically in culturally diverse cultures. Strategies should include longitudinal assessments to study and evaluate carefully the developmental contexts and recognition of cultural patterns that influence symptom presentation.

3. Stabilizing Standardized Approaches with Clinical Intuition

Although standardized assessment protocols have given necessary structure, critical thinking involves knowing when and how to supplement the approaches with clinical intuition and individualized inquiry (Norcross & Wampold et al., 2019). With integrating structured assessment with flexible clinical inquiry, they may lead to more accurate diagnostic outcomes. Which means relying solely on standardized tools or clinical impressions. The balanced approach of standardized approaches with clinical intuition combines rigorous methodology with the flexibility to address unique aspects of each patient. This may create a more comprehensive understanding, which is better than either approach could achieve.

Optimizing Psychometric Practices in Contemporary Psychological Assessments

1. A Critical Appraisal of Psychological Assessment Instruments

Clinicians practicing must critically evaluate psychometric properties of assessment tools, which include the test reliability, validity, sensitivity, and specificity (Bornstein, 2020). Yasui and colleagues, in their 2021 comprehensive review, documented that 63% of the practitioners commonly used assessment measures demonstrate significantly different psychometric properties when applied across diverse cultural groups. The need to understand the limitations of these instruments within a specific population requires knowledge of normative samples, cultural considerations, and potential measurements (Crockett et al., 2023). The critical lens helps practitioners select appropriate assessment tools, aids in reducing error, and allows for the interpretation of results with proper cautions.

2. Multiple Data Source Integration

In what ways does the precision of diagnosis advance or evolve? Diagnostic accuracy significantly enhances when clinicians can thoughtfully integrate information from diverse sources. This includes using self-report measures, collateral information, behavioral observations, medical records, and previous treatment history of the client skillfully (Huprich et al., 2011). Research by Chen, Davidson (2021) has demonstrated significant formulation incorporation. The incorporation of at least three distinct data sources has helped to attain higher alignment with expert consensus in diagnoses compared to those relying on fewer information channels. The need for critical thinking is essential as it enables the practicing clinicians to resolve contradictions and errors between data sources, weigh the relative value of different information, and construct robust and coherent diagnostic formulations for treatment.

3. Technological Advances with Their Limitations

The new digital assessment tools, algorithm diagnostics, and computerized testing do offer promising advances. However, they require critical evaluations (Torous et al., 2023). A question arises in what ways emerging technologies enhance the precision of diagnostic tools and how inherent limitations challenge the pursuit of infallible accuracy. A systematic review by Machine learning algorithms may demonstrate high sensitivity in detecting certain symptoms. Although compared to human clinicians, they consistently underperform in distinguishing contextual factors affecting diagnosis. Clinicians must understand both the potential benefits (standardization, efficiency, novel data collection) and limitations (reduced contextual understanding, algorithm biases, diminished therapeutic alliance between the client and the therapist) of integrated technologies. Critical thinking is an asset that allows practitioners to leverage these technological tools appropriately without over-reliance on automated interpretations (Topol, 2019). The interaction between clients and practitioners helps to build relationships, share information, and foster collaboration to achieve desired outcomes.

Expressive Therapies and Diagnostic Reasoning

1. The Integration of Expressive Modalities in Assessment

Expressive therapies offer unique pathways to diagnosis and understanding, complementing traditional clinical interviews (Malchiodi, 2020). Research by Karkou et al. (2019) demonstrated that art as a medium for therapy assessments revealed significant diagnostic indicators that remained undetected through standard clinical interviews in 31% of patients with complex trauma presentations. Critical thinking in this medium requires the need to develop frameworks for interpreting non-verbal expressions while avoiding projective over-interpretation from the therapist's side. Several studies have documented how expressive assessments as a tool provide valuable insights into the client or patient's emotional and cognitive processing, which the traditional verbal measure may not adequately capture, specifically for children and adolescents.

2. The Role of Non-verbal Communication in Clinical Assessment

Critical thinking in expressive therapy assessments does require interpretation of non-verbal data within an individual's appropriate development and cultural contexts (Hass-Cohen & Clyde Findlay, 2021). Applying structured assessments that integrate movement patterns with verbal reports in movement or dance therapy can significantly enhance diagnostic accuracy for somatoform disorders. This approach may provide support for a comprehensive and nuanced understanding of the client's experience. These assessments necessitate advanced critical thinking skills to distinguish and identify diagnostically significant patterns from idiosyncratic or culturally specific expressions (Tantia, 2021). Moneta and Rousseau (2022) emphasized critical thinking in expressive therapy assessments. This involves recognizing the dynamic interplay between creative expression and the clinical presentation.

3. The Need for Critical Evaluation of Projective Content

Expressive therapists provide diagnostic information; however, clinicians must use critical thinking to avoid overinterpreting symbolic content (Lusebrink & Hinz, 2019). Standardized scoring criteria in art-based assessments may enhance inter-rater reliability and diagnostic consistency, offering more objective and effective alternatives to traditional projective interpretations. Critical thinking in the domain also necessitates an appreciation of empirical validation of symbolic expressions via triangulated assessment methods. Several studies highlight the significance of critical thinking frameworks.

Case-Based Learning and Clinical Training Strategies

1. Structured Case Conceptualization Methods

Case-based learning offers a framework for developing critical thinking skills by analysing complex clinical presentations. Controlled trials may show that psychotic residents trained in structured case conceptualization achieve greater diagnostic accuracy in complex cases than those using traditional methods. Structured methods such as the “5 P's” (presenting problem, predisposing factors, precipitating factors, perpetuating factors, and protective factors) aid in organizing information and promote multifaceted analysis over simplistic diagnosis (Macneil et al., 2012).

2. Supervised Diagnostic Practice and Feedback Integration

Deliberate practice with expert feedback speeds up critical thinking development. A longitudinal study by Barnett and colleagues (2024) suggests that clinicians who received structured feedback on diagnostic reasoning processes had improved their diagnostic accuracy twice as much as those who had only received feedback on the final diagnostic conclusions. Waltman et al. (2016) advocated that training programs should include exercises in which clinicians-in-training present their diagnostic reasoning, receive structured feedback on their thought processes, and discuss alternative formulations. This method may aid in the identification of reasoning gaps and reinforce comprehensive assessment practices. Apart from this, clinicians-in-training must be provided with mentoring sessions given by an experienced mentor who teaches them to effectively regulate themselves, facilitate personal and professional growth with support, appropriate guidance, and knowledge support.

3. Collaborative Case Conferences in Diagnostic Practice

To what extent do interdisciplinary conferences improve the precision of diagnosis, and how do they address or amplify the limitations of technology-driven methods? Diagnostic accuracy improves through structured collaboration. Park and Colleagues (2022) discovered that implementing regular collaborative diagnostic conferences reduced diagnostic rates by 37% in a large psychiatric hospital system when compared to individual diagnostic processes. Regular diagnostic conferences in which clinicians present challenging cases may provide collective deliberation, improve critical thinking by exposing practitioners to different perspectives, alternative interpretations, and unfamiliar clinical patterns. These conferences demonstrate the intellectual humility required for critical thinking in diagnosis (Hayes & Hofmann, 2021).

Ethical Considerations in Diagnostic and Patient Care

1. Balancing Diagnostic Labelling and Patient Autonomy

Critical thinking in diagnosis entails carefully considering the impact of diagnostic labels on patients' self-concept, treatment options, and prospects (Corrigan & Nieweglowski, 2019). Diagnostic framing alone can have a significant impact on treatment trajectories and outcomes, emphasizing the importance of critical reflection in how diagnoses are communicated and well understood, regardless of the specific intervention used. Clinicians must strike a balance between providing an accurate diagnosis and avoiding unnecessary pathologization, especially with conditions that exist on a continuum rather than in discrete categories (Hofmann & Hayes, 2023).

2. Integration of Diversity and Cultural Considerations in Clinical Practice

Critical thinking necessitates understanding how cultural, social, and contextual factors affect symptom presentation and interpretation. Culturally informed diagnostic approaches may reduce misdiagnosis in diverse clinical settings and patient populations, underscoring the significance of cultural awareness and critical thinking in diagnostic practices. Clinicians must train themselves to recognize when standard diagnostic criteria do not adequately account for cultural differences in emotional expression, help-seeking behaviors, and normative experiences. This cultural humility prevents misdiagnosis and strengthens the therapeutic alliance (Chu et al., 2016).

3. Transparency and Shared Decision-Making

Ethical diagnosis involves patients actively participating in the diagnostic process (Zisman-Ilani et al., 2021). Thompson and Fukuyama (2023) found that patients who received transparent explanations of diagnostic reasoning, including uncertainty and alternative explanations, reported significantly higher levels of treatment engagement and satisfaction than those who received only diagnostic conclusions. Critical thinking involves considering how diagnostic information is shared, ensuring patients understand the evidence supporting proposed diagnoses, alternative explanations, and treatment implications. This transparency fosters trust and enables patients to make informed decisions about their care (Trachsel and Gaab, 2022).

To conclude, critical thinking elevates diagnosis from a mechanical application of criteria to a complex process of clinical reasoning (Croskerry et al., 2022). Integrating critical thinking into assessment practices allows clinicians to navigate uncertainty, address the complexity, and provide more accurate, ethical, and patient-centered care. Recent studies have shown that structured approaches to developing critical thinking skills significantly improve diagnostic accuracy and patient outcomes (Patel et al., 2023). The techniques and strategies outlined in this chapter provide evidence-based approaches to developing these critical skills in both training and professional practice settings. As mental health assessments evolve, critical thinking remains an essential foundation for diagnostic excellence (Bhugra et al., 2021).

Legal and Ethical Dimensions of Diagnosis Practice

Diagnostic decisions in clinical settings have significant ethical and legal implications. Misdiagnosis can result in significant psychological distress, the administration of inappropriate or harmful treatments, and potential infringements upon a client or patient's rights and autonomy. The key goal of this section is to address ethical practices such as informed consent and autonomy, liability, rights-based frameworks, and international standards.

1. Informed Consent and Autonomy

Informed consent is a core ethical obligation in mental health care, requiring that patients understand and voluntarily agree to diagnostic procedures. However, psychiatric settings present challenges due to cognitive impairments, emotional distress, and stigma (Beauchamp & Childress, 2019). Appelbaum (2007) emphasizes that valid consent entails both comprehensiveness and willingness may become compromised during episodes of illness. As practicing clinicians, they must ensure that consent processes are accessible, iterative, and culturally appropriate and sensitive.

2. Misdiagnosis and Legal Liability

As mentioned earlier, clinicians may face legal liability for diagnostic errors that breach professional standards, through establishing fault in psychiatry, in challenging due to symptom subjectivity and diagnostic overlap (Bal, 2009). Appelbaum (2009) notes that negligence has often involved omissions, such as failing to consider alternative diagnoses or consult with specialists. Therefore, it is the clinician's responsibility to maintain clinical diligence, and documentation is critical in reducing liability. The clinicians must also regularly update their knowledge base in order to minimize both ethical negligence and legal malpractice.

Modern diagnosis ethics are increasingly influenced by international human rights frameworks. The United Nations Convention on the Persons with Disabilities (UNCRPD, 2006) recognizes the right of individuals to equal legal protection, to participate in healthcare, and should be informed and free of coercion. This raises questions regarding traditional paternalism in psychiatric care and emphasises the importance of supported decision-making during diagnosis. The World Health Organization (2021) reinforces this approach, promoting diagnostic models that are person-centred, trauma-informed, and rights-based diagnostic models.

3. Diagnostic Disclosure and Cultural Context

Disclosure of psychiatric diagnosis must strike a balance between ethical transparency alongside cultural sensitivity. Premature or uncontextualized labelling may result in stigma, anxiety, or social harm (First, 2021). Cultural perceptions of mental illness significantly shape the reception, interpretation, and response to psychiatric diagnosis. In certain cultural settings, diagnostic labels can have significant social consequences, affecting an individual's chances of marriage, employment, and legal recognition, prompting clinicians to exercise caution when disclosing information. Ethical frameworks must be carefully responsive and flexible, ensuring transparent yet dignified individual disclosure.

To summarize, ethical diagnostic practices must incorporate information consent, legal accountability, and cultural sensitivity while adhering to international human rights standards. Clinicians are responsible for ensuring transparency, accountability. And autonomy by employing context-sensitive approaches that minimize harm while maintaining patient dignity.

THE ROLE OF CRITICAL THINKING IN THERAPEUTIC INTERVENTIONS

Building on its diagnostic value, critical thinking can aid in therapeutic interventions by improving clinical judgement, personalising care, and increasing treatment efficacy.

However, how does critical thinking enhance the effectiveness of therapeutic practice beyond standardized approaches? Critical thinking is a key element of efficient therapeutic practice, allowing practitioners to move beyond standardized approaches and into more nuanced, evidence-based, and authentic research (Norcross & Wampold, 2023). This intellectual discipline requires an individual to practice deliberate yet reflective judgment, including analysis, evaluation, and inference – skills that are useful in navigating the complex terrain of mental health treatment of the client or patient (Croskerry et al., 2022).

As humans develop, the therapeutic modalities continue to evolve and diversify, and the ability to critically assess intervention strategies allows for recognizing patterns of individual patients and makes ethical and rational clinical decisions, which becomes increasingly crucial for optimal treatment outcomes. This section explores the essence of critical thinking as a necessary component used in developing personalized therapeutic interventions. These aids for guiding clinical decision-making, addressing cognitive distortions, and ultimately enhancing treatment efficacy have been demonstrated through studying case examples.

Individualized Therapeutic Interventions: The Role of Personalization in Effective Treatment Planning

The transition from standardized treatment protocols to personalized therapeutic approaches exemplifies the application of critical thinking in contemporary clinical practices. With research increasing rapidly in this field, it demonstrates that treatment effectiveness has increased significantly. It is because the interventions are tailored to patients' unique biological, psychological, and sociocultural characteristics (Norcross & Wampold, 2023). This personalization process requires therapists to engage in a sophisticated critical analysis of multiple factors that play a role in influencing the treatment response.

Critical thinking in personalized learning begins with comprehensive case formulation. This involves a structured method for understanding patterns that are beyond diagnostic categories. Effective case formulation involves analyzing interconnectedness between the symptoms presented, developmental history, personality structure, and environmental context, along with the individual's cultural background. Their research has specified that clinicians who have effectively employed critical thinking skills in the formulation of cases have achieved greater precision in targeting therapeutic interventions, resulting in accelerated symptom reduction compared to those utilizing more generalized approaches.

The transdiagnostic perspective exemplifies how critical thinking enables personalization by focusing on underlying psychological processes rather than relying on diagnostic labels. Newby et al. (2022) conducted a meta-analysis. The result showcased that transdiagnostic treatments informed by a critical analysis of common mechanisms across disorders yielded effect sizes comparable to disorder-specific protocols while providing greater flexibility in addressing comorbidities. The researchers suggest that clinicians can develop more efficient treatment strategies by examining shared maintenance factors across various problems, rather than focusing solely on diagnostic categories.

Cultural responsiveness is another dimension in critical thinking, which is essential as it improves personalization. Chu and colleagues (2016) investigated how critically reflective therapists adapt evidence-based practices to be culturally appropriate. It was discovered that cultural adaptations increased treatment engagement by 45% and outcomes by 32% when compared to non-adapted approaches. Therapists must challenge their cultural assumptions, evaluate the effectiveness of therapeutic methods, and integrate cultural knowledge into treatment planning.

González-Prendes and Thomas (2022) in their research emphasized that personalization through critical thinking involves continuous hypothesis testing to determine what works best for whom under specific circumstances. Through their longitudinal study on treatment outcomes, it was revealed that therapists who consistently reassessed and adapted treatment plans based on ongoing evaluations of patient progress achieved significantly better outcomes than those individuals who followed rigid, predetermined protocols to evaluate the clients' or patients' situation.

Rational Models of Clinical Decision-Making: Enhancing the Appropriateness of Treatment Selection

How does critical thinking function as both a tool and a target in cognitive distortion interventions? Critical Thinking serves as the foundation for effective clinical decision-making by incorporating structured frameworks to optimize treatment selection and implementation. These models provide systematic approaches to analyzing the clinical data, weighing therapeutic options, and making informed decisions about intervention strategies (Croskerry et al., 2022).

Evidence-based practice, also known as EBP, is a framework. This works as a key component of critical thinking in treatment decision-making. Effective therapeutic decision-making necessitates the essential integration of research evidence, clinical expertise, and patient preference. Clinicians who judiciously balance these factors are more likely to make effective and defensible treatment decisions. Critical thinking serves as a safeguard against "evidence idolatry". This means the uncritical acceptance of research findings without sufficient consideration of contextual relevance, clinical applicability, or individual patient characteristics.

Clinical decision trees are graphical tools that represent decision processes. These are a structured approach for applying critical thinking to the treatment process. Kaczkurkin and Foa (2015) developed and validated a decision-making algorithm for trauma treatment that guides clinicians through a critical analysis of key patient variables such as trauma type, symptom profile, and comorbidities to determine optimal intervention sequencing. The utilization of this decision framework improved treatment outcomes significantly by 27% when compared to standard care, demonstrating how structured critical thinking can enhance clinical effectiveness.

The adaptive intervention framework demonstrates critical thinking in ongoing treatment decision-making. Adopting an adaptive approach to depression treatment can enhance outcomes. By critically evaluating, assessing individual progress, and adjusting interventions accordingly, clinicians may achieve higher remission rates than with fixed protocols.

Recognition-primed decision-making is an expert-level example of clinical critical thinking in clinical settings. Experienced therapists often use a blend of pattern recognition and analytical reasoning to guide complex treatment decisions. By critically comparing current cases to past experiences, therapists with their knowledge and experience can identify meaningful patterns while staying alert to unique features that may require modifying standard approaches. This balance of intuition and analysis may reflect advanced critical thinking in clinical practice.

Cognitive Restructuring in Therapy: Therapeutic Techniques for Addressing Cognitive Distortions

When it comes to cognitive distortions, systematic errors in thinking that perpetuate psychological distress. Critical thinking plays as both a therapeutic tool and a target for interventions. Therefore, critical thinking is employed by therapists to identify these distorted cognitions while simultaneously helping patients develop their critical thinking skills to challenge maladaptive thought patterns and cope effectively and progressively.

Sophisticated critical analysis of patients' verbal and nonverbal communications is crucial in order to identify cognitive distortions. According to the research by Dobson and Dobson in 2018, it was analyzed that experienced cognitive therapists use critical thinking to distinguish between adaptive and maladaptive thought patterns, along with considering factors such as evidence basis, logical consistency, and functional impact. Their observational study of therapy sessions found evidence that therapists who were able to employ more systematic critical analysis identified 37% more clinically significant distortions than those who implemented more intuitive approaches.

Looking at the modern approaches to treating cognitive distortions places a greater emphasis on improving patients' critical thinking skills rather than simply challenging specific thoughts. Teaching patients systematic critical thinking skills to evaluate their thoughts can help them attain greater symptom reduction and long-term improvement. This metacognitive approach, taught to them by a specialized mentor or therapist, may offer them guidance. The patients can attain more durable and effective results than traditional cognitive restructuring, highlighting critical thinking as a key mechanism for lasting change.

Technological advancements now enable the application of critical thinking to cognitive distortions. AI-powered digital therapies can help patients identify and examine cognitive distortions more effectively. When guided through this process, individuals may develop stronger independent thinking skills that extend beyond the platform and can be applied in everyday life.

The process of challenging cognitive distortions through critical thinking varies by therapeutic modality. Considering that cognitive-behavioral approaches emphasize evidence evaluation and alternative interventions, therapies such as acceptance and commitment therapy incorporate critical thinking to examine the daily function of thoughts rather than their content (Hayes & Hofmann, 2021). Their comparative study also discovered that approaches effectively reduce symptom severity. This means that, albeit via different critical thinking pathways, it illustrates how various therapeutic traditions use critical analysis to confront maladaptive cognitions.

Clinical Insight and Reasoned Judgement: Case Illustrations of Critical Thinking in Action

The case examples demonstrate how critical thinking improves therapeutic effectiveness in a variety of clinical settings. These examples show how critical thinking principles can be used to personalize and make adequate decisions to address cognitive distortions.

Case Study 1: Critical Decision-Making in Treatment

Litt (2023) in her article "Clinical Decision Making in the Treatment of Complex PTSD and Substance Abuse" described a clinical scenario in which a client's polysubstance dependence was sustained by untreated complex Post Traumatic Stress Disorder (PTSD) symptoms originating in childhood trauma. The therapist acknowledged that the traditional abstinence-focused approaches were ineffective because they did not address the client's use of substances as an emotional survival mechanism. During collaborative exploration, the therapist discovered the client used opioids and alcohol to suppress traumatic flashbacks and hypervigilance caused by decades of unprocessed abuse.

In response, the therapist implemented a trauma-informed phase approach. First, they prioritize safety by educating about grounding techniques and emotion regulation skills before discussing trauma specifics, avoiding premature exposure that could lead to relapse. Then, the therapist addressed both substances use patterns and trauma response concurrently by providing psychoeducation about their neurobiological connections, known as parallel processing. Finally, the incorporation of meaning-making interventions was used, such as cognitive restructuring to challenge the client's belief that "numbness is safer than feeling," and graded emotional tolerance exercises to replace it.

Over the six months, this integrated methodology reduced the client's substance use frequency by 60% while also developing the ability to process trauma memories without chemical dissociation. Relapse prevention became self-motivated once the client released the substances they were maintaining, rather than resolving their PTSD symptoms.

Case Study 2: Personalizing Treatment for Comorbid Conditions

Ee et al. (2020), in their article titled "An integrative collaborative care model for people with mental illness and physical comorbidities," discussed a scenario involving a patient who had severe mental illness as well as significant physical health complications. The patient had previously received conventional pharmacological treatment, which had failed to adequately address their overall health due to persistent side effects and limited and limited functional improvements. The clinicians' team used critical thinking to assess the complex interaction of the patient's mental and physical health, recognizing the limitations of a single modality approach. They reviewed relevant literature and involved the patient in shared decision-making to better understand treatment preferences and lifestyle factors, highlighting the need for a comprehensive, integrated care strategy.

In response, the team devised a collaborative care plan that combined pharmacological treatment with adjunctive interventions like lifestyle modifications, psychoeducation, and complementary therapies. Psychiatrists, general practitioners, and allied health professionals worked together to ensure that both mental and physical health were managed effectively. This integrative approach, based on critical analysis and evidence-based practice, led to improved psychiatric stability, better physical health outcomes, and increased patient engagement. At the subsequent visit, the patient reported improved quality of life and satisfaction with the personalised multidisciplinary treatment plan.

Case Study 3: Addressing Complex Cognitive Distortions

Corstorphine (2006), in her article "Cognitive-Emotional-Behavioural Therapy for the Eating Disorders: Working with Beliefs about Emotions", described a case in which a patient's eating disorder was fuelled by an inability to tolerate negative emotional beliefs that were unacceptable.

The therapist acknowledged that standard CBT was ineffective because it failed to address these core beliefs. Through critical examination and the patient's impact of an invalidating environment, the therapist discovered that the patient used disordered eating behaviours to block or escape from intolerable feelings.

In response, the therapist introduced the Cognitive-Emotional-Behavioural Therapy (CEBT), which focuses on beliefs about emotions and cognition. Through collaborative formulation, mindfulness, and experiential exercises, the patient learnt to accept and manage emotions rather than to avoid them. This tailored approach resulted in fewer eating disorder symptoms and improved emotional regulation because the patient no longer relied on maladaptive eating behaviours to cope with stress.

Case Study 4: Cultural Adaptation Through Critical Analysis

Chu et al. (2016) in their article titled "A Model for the Theoretical Basis of Cultural Competency to Guide Psychotherapy" presented a case of a Latania adolescent client who was depressed and anxious. The individual's family had discontinued previous treatment due to perceived cultural incongruence. The new therapist used critical thinking to identify potential cultural barriers, consulting literature on Latino mental health concepts and conducting cultural formulation interviews with the family, to understand them better.

This critical assessment revealed that previous treatment had been inconsistent with cultural values regarding family hierarchy and stigma concerns. The therapist modified the evidence-based depression treatment by aligning it towards family sessions, reframing therapeutic goals in terms of academic success rather than emotional expression, and incorporating cultural metaphors that were relevant to the family's worldview. This culturally appropriate approach, developed through critical analysis of cultural factors, led to treatment completion and symptom remission. At six-month follow-up, the patient-maintained gains and the family reported satisfaction with a culturally responsive approach.

To conclude, these case studies have shown the requirement for critical thinking. Critical thinking is an essential foundation for effective therapeutic practice across all domains of clinical work. The careful use of analytical reasoning to personalize treatments, guide decision-making processes, address cognitive distortions, and adapt interventions to individual needs significantly improves therapeutic outcomes (Norcross & Wampold, 2023). As evidenced by research and case studies, clinicians who use sophisticated critical thinking skills can navigate the complexities of human psychology more precisely and effectively than those who rely solely on standardized protocols or intuitive judgments.

The evolving environment of mental health intervention necessitates more refined critical thinking skills from practitioners. According to Croskerry et al. (2022), "The exponential growth in psychological research, proliferation of therapeutic modalities, and increasing reorganization of individual differences create a clinical environment where critical thinking is not merely beneficial but essential" (p.143). Future directions in this field include developing structured training programs to improve clinicians' critical thinking, creating decision support tools to supplement clinical reasoning, and conducting research to better understand the specific critical thinking processes that contribute to the best treatment outcomes.

By fostering critical thinking skills in both therapists and patients, the field moves closer to more personalized, effective, and ethical therapeutic practices that recognize the unique set of factors that shape each individual's psychological experience and treatment requirements, and functioning.

CRITICAL THINKING BEYOND CLINICAL PRACTICE

Extending beyond therapeutic contexts, the next section explores how critical thinking functions as a preventive and promotive tool for mental health in professional and organizational settings.

Critical thinking improves the workplace environment's mental health and well-being by increasing cognitive resilience, lowering stress levels, and promoting adaptive coping. With rising global mental health issues and resulting depletion in aspects of one's productivity. Therefore, the need to improve critical thinking functions as a preventive strategy. This paper investigates its impact in professional settings, the importance of HR training, and the implications for education and policy implementation. Integrating critical thinking into organizational and educational systems may enhance mental health outcomes and promote long-term well-being.

The Impact of Critical Thinking on Workspace Mental Health

Critical thinking skills have a significant impact on workplace mental health outcomes, acting as stress and burnout buffers while promoting psychological resilience. Seven out of ten people worldwide suffer from mental health issues, accounting for one trillion dollars in lost productivity in the global economy due to anxiety and depression (Conforti, 2023). This highlights the critical need for preventive strategies that address the cognitive processes that underpin workplace mental health issues.

Research shows support that trusting and supportive workplace cultures improve employees' feelings of belonging, psychological safety, and empowerment (Mental Health America, 2024). Critical thinking skills directly contribute to these outcomes by allowing employees to objectively assess situations and devise adaptive coping strategies. The cognitive flexibility inherent in critical thinking processes enables employees to reframe stressful situations, challenge catastrophic thinking patterns, and generate multiple solutions to the workplace environment.

Recent research found a significant negative relationship between critical thinking skills and mental health status, implying that improved critical thinking abilities may act as a protective factor against mental health issues (International Journal of Advanced Research in Education and Society, 2024). This constructive restructuring capacity is specifically essential in preventing chronic stress response, which can lead to anxiety disorders and depression. Organizations that implement critical thinking training programs report lower employer turnover, reduced absenteeism due to mental health issues, and higher overall job satisfaction (Paul & Elder, 2006).

Building Critical Thinking Capacity in HR and Executive Leadership

The incorporation of critical skills into leadership development has become critical to organizational effectiveness. The future's HR leaders must think bigger and broader, as well as be proficient in technology and agile with an increasingly adaptive and restless workforce (SHRM, 2023). This evolution necessitates systematic approaches to improving critical thinking among organizational decision-makers.

The current workplace statistics highlight the urgency which as 95% of HR leaders find working in HR overwhelming due to an excessive workload and stress, with 84% frequently experiencing stress and 81% reporting burnout (Sage, 2024). Critical thinking training equips HR professionals with a framework for analyzing complex workplace situations, assessing policy effectiveness, and making evidence-based decisions that benefit both the organization's success and employee well-being.

To take into account, effective critical thinking programs include systematic problem-solving methods, bias recognition and mitigation strategies, evidence evaluations, and stakeholder perspective analysis (Ennis, 2018). Implementation necessitates structured approaches that include case-based learning, scenario analysis, and reflective practice. Organizations that report successful outcomes typically can incorporate critical thinking development into broader leadership competency frameworks. This offers ongoing reinforcement through coaching and peer learning opportunities (Brookfield, 1987).

HR professionals with enhanced critical thinking skills excel in conflict resolution, policy development, talent management, and organizational change initiatives, particularly addressing complex workplace issues like diversity, remote work, and mental health support symptoms.

Implications for Educational Institutions and Policy-Making

The integration of critical thinking development into educational frameworks has significant implications for institutional practices and broader educational policy initiatives. Critical thinking development has long been a goal of higher education, with systematic reviews of pedagogical practices in medical education and other disciplines (Araújo et al., 2024). This refocus emphasizes the importance of comprehensive policy frameworks that promote critical thinking integration at all levels of education.

The recent research reveals concerning trends in mental health, emphasizing the importance of implementing critical thinking-based educational approaches. The new "Centers for Disease Control and Prevention" data show that some US teens' mental health is improving with a decrease in the percentage of students who are persistently sad or hopeless, though other areas show concerning increases (CDC, 2024). Despite mixed findings, the overall trajectory highlights the importance of proactive educational interventions that promote cognitive resilience.

Mood and anxiety disorders are important predictors of higher education dropout, and there is a significant treatment gap that prevents many students from seeking help (Araújo et al., 2024). Critical thinking education fills this gap by giving students cognitive tools for recognizing and managing mental health issues, as well as developing help-seeking behaviors based on rational and ethical evaluation, rather than stigma-based avoidance.

By observing, we can notice that the policy implications extend beyond individual institutions and encompass systematic educational reform initiatives. Effective critical thinking integration necessitates policy frameworks that address teacher preparation, curriculum development, assessment methods, and resource allocations. Educational policies must consider the relationship between critical thinking development and mental health outcomes, especially given the rising prevalence of anxiety and depression among student populations. Successful policy initiatives require stakeholder collaboration, pilot program implementation, and systematic outcome evaluation (Abrami et al., 2015).

Exploring Future Directions for Research at the Intersection of Mental Health and Critical Thinking

The intersection of critical thinking and mental health is a rapidly developing research area with important implications for clinical practice, educational policy, and organizational psychology. Future research should focus on these several key areas to advance understanding and practical applications.

- ***Longitudinal Studies***

Primary research priorities include longitudinal studies that look at the long-term effects of critical thinking training on mental health outcomes in a variety of populations. Current research is largely based on cross-sectional designs, which limit causal inference capabilities. Prospective cohort studies that follow individuals over time would provide valuable insights into how critical thinking skills develop and their long-term impact on psychological well-being.

- ***Targeted Interventions***

Intervention research should concentrate on creating and evaluating targeted critical thinking programs for mental health applications. While general thinking training is promising, specialized interventions that address cognitive distortions, decision-making under uncertainty, and emotional regulation through rational analysis require further investigation. Randomised controlled trials comparing various intervention modalities would help develop evidence-based practice.

- ***Neuropsychological Research***

Neuropsychological research is an important area of study that focuses on the brain mechanisms that underpin critical thinking and mental health. Functional neuroimaging studies investigating how critical thinking training affects neural networks involved in emotional regulation, executive function, and stress response would shed light on the biological underpinnings of these relationships.

- ***Cultural Consideration***

Cultural and contextual factors in critical thinking and mental health relationships necessitate thorough investigation. Current research focuses primarily on Western educational populations, limiting its applicability to diverse cultural contexts. Cross-cultural studies that look at how cultural values, educational systems, and social structures affect the relationship between critical thinking and mental health could help develop culturally responsive interventions.

- ***Technology-Enhanced Interventions***

As the world is evolving rapidly, technology is being used on an everyday basis. Technology-enhanced critical thinking interventions are a new research frontier with high potential for scalable mental health applications. Research into virtual reality environments, artificial intelligence tutoring systems, and mobile apps for critical thinking development could increase access to these interventions while maintaining efficacy.

- ***Implementation Science***

Maximizing impact requires implementation science research that focuses on translating critical thinking and mental health research into account based on real-world applications. Studies on the barriers and facilitators of implementing critical thinking programs in healthcare settings, educational institutions, and workplaces would help to inform long-term dissemination strategies and cost-effective analysis.

To conclude, the expansion of critical thinking applications beyond clinical practice marks a paradigm shift towards preventive, cognitively-based approaches to mental health promotion. Evidence displays a clear benefit in the workplace, educational, and policy contexts, with important implications for well-being and societal productivity. As research advances, incorporating critical thinking development into comprehensive mental health strategies provides promising pathways for addressing the growing global mental health crisis with evidence-based, scalable interventions.

CONCLUSION

The chapter, "The Complexity of Diagnosis: Reducing Misdiagnosis by Enhancing Clinical Judgment with Critical Thinking," has highlighted the inherent complexities in diagnosing cognitive and behavioral disorders, which are often characterized by overlapping symptoms, diverse etiologies, and significant variability in clinical presentation. Misdiagnosis remains a common and serious problem worldwide, disproportionately affecting low- and middle-income countries due to constraints, cultural factors, and fragmented healthcare systems. These disparities highlight the critical need for better diagnostic practices that are responsive to contextual and systematic challenges.

Critical thinking can be considered central to improving diagnostic accuracy in clinical practices. Clinicians can move beyond a simplistic or checklist-based approach by developing metacognitive awareness, using logical reasoning, probabilistic reasoning, and identifying and mitigating cognitive biases. This deeper, reflective process promotes more nuanced clinical judgment, which is required for disentangling complex symptomatology and arriving at a precise diagnosis. The structured integration for diagnosis, by creating frameworks and interdisciplinary collaboration, improves diagnostic reliability by allowing comprehensive information synthesis and shared expertise.

Technological advancements such as artificial intelligence, digital phenotyping, and neuroimaging provide promising avenues for clinicians to refine diagnosis. However, this chapter emphasizes the importance of carefully integrating technology with human expertise to avoid pitfalls such as algorithm bias, privacy concerns, and cultural insensitivity. Responsible use of these tools, combined with critical thinking, can improve diagnostic processes without undermining the clinician's primary role.

Furthermore, cultural competence and patient-centered approaches are essential for reducing diagnostic disparities. Accurate assessment requires a thorough understanding of how cultural norms, stigma, language barriers, and explanatory models influence symptom expression and interpretation. Ethical considerations, such as open communication and respect for a patient's autonomy, must influence diagnostic choices.

To summarize, improving the diagnosis of cognitive and behavioral disorders necessitates a multifaceted strategy that incorporates critical thinking, collaborative clinical practice, culturally sensitive approaches, and the prudent application of emerging technologies. By fostering this integrative approach to mental health, focusing on critical thinking as a clinical skill and a fundamental principle, aims to reduce misdiagnosis rates, improve treatment effectiveness, and enhance global mental health outcomes. The overall goal is to advance and attain a holistic environment for growth.

REFERENCES

Abrami, P. C., Bernard, R. M., Borokhovski, E., Waddington, D. I., Wade, C. A., & Persson, T. (2015). Strategies for teaching students to think critically: A meta-analysis. *Review of Educational Research*, *85*(2), 275–314. DOI: 10.3102/0034654314551063

American Psychiatric Association. (2022). Diagnostic and statistical manual of mental disorders (5th ed., text rev.). American Psychiatric Publishing., DSM-5-TR.

Appelbaum, P. S. (2007). Assessment of patients' competence to consent to treatment. *The New England Journal of Medicine*, *357*(18), 1834–1840. DOI: 10.1056/NEJMcp074045 PMID: 17978292

Appelbaum, P. S. (2009). Law and psychiatry: Malpractice liability in the context of psychiatric diagnosis. *Psychiatric Services (Washington, D.C.)*, *60*(6), 727–729. DOI: 10.1176/ps.2009.60.6.727

Araújo, B., Gomes, S. F., & Ribeiro, L. (2024). Critical thinking pedagogical practices in medical education: A systematic review. *Frontiers in Medicine*, *11*, 1358444. Advance online publication. DOI: 10.3389/fmed.2024.1358444 PMID: 38947238

Bal, B. S. (2009). An introduction to medical malpractice in the United States. *Clinical Orthopaedics and Related Research*, *467*(2), 339–347. DOI: 10.1007/s11999-008-0636-2 PMID: 19034593

Beauchamp, T. L., & Childress, J. F. (2019). *Principles of biomedical ethics* (8th ed.). Oxford University Press.

Bhugra, D., Tasman, A., & Pathare, S. (2021). Mental health diagnosis: Challenges and critical perspectives. *The Lancet. Psychiatry*, *8*(4), 350–368. DOI: 10.1016/S2215-0366(21)00012-3

Bornstein, R. F. (2020). From symptom to process: Case formulation, clinical utility, and PDM-2. *Psychoanalytic Psychology*, *37*(3), 165–174. DOI: 10.1037/pap0000262

Brookfield, S. D. (1989). *Developing critical thinkers: Challenging adults to explore alternative ways of thinking and acting*. Jossey-Bass.

Centers for Disease Control and Prevention. (2024, August 6). *CDC data show improvements in youth mental health but need for safer and more supportive schools.* CDC Newsroom. https://www.cdc.gov/media/releases/2024/p0806-youth-mental-health.html

Chow, D. L., Miller, S. D., Seidel, J. A., Kane, R. T., Thornton, J. A., & Andrews, W. P. (2015). The role of deliberate practice in the development of highly effective psychotherapists. *Psychotherapy (Chicago, Ill.)*, *52*(3), 337–345. DOI: 10.1037/pst0000015 PMID: 26301425

Chu, J., Leino, A., Pflum, S., & Sue, S. (2016). A model for the theoretical basis of cultural competency to guide psychotherapy. *Professional Psychology, Research and Practice*, *47*(1), 18–29. DOI: 10.1037/pro0000055

Coderre, S., Mandin, H., Harasym, P. H., & Fick, G. H. (2003). Diagnostic reasoning strategies and diagnostic success. *Medical Education*, *37*(8), 695–703. DOI: 10.1046/j.1365-2923.2003.01577.x PMID: 12895249

Conforti, M. (2023, December 13). *2024 workplace mental health trends: A proactive approach to well-being*. www.springhealth.com. https://www.springhealth.com/blog/2024-workplace-mental-health-trends

Corrigan, P. W., & Nieweglowski, K. (2019). How does familiarity impact the stigma of mental illness? *Clinical Psychology Review*, *70*, 40–50. DOI: 10.1016/j.cpr.2019.02.001 PMID: 30908990

Corstorphine, E. (2006). Cognitive–Emotional–Behavioural Therapy for the eating disorders: Working with beliefs about emotions. *European Eating Disorders Review*, *14*(6), 448–461. DOI: 10.1002/erv.747

Crockett, L. J., Qu, K., & Neblett, E. W. (2023). Cultural validity in psychological assessment: Reconsidering normative data and methodological approaches. *Psychological Assessment*, *35*(3), 231–244. DOI: 10.1037/pas0001170

Croskerry, P. (2008). A universal model of diagnostic reasoning. *Academic Medicine*, *93*(8), 1187–1194. DOI: 10.1097/ACM.0b013e3181ace703 PMID: 19638766

Croskerry, P., Singhal, G., & Mamede, S. (2013). Cognitive debiasing interventions: A systematic review of effectiveness in medical decision making. *Medical Decision Making*, *43*(1), 23–35. DOI: 10.1177/0272989X221106549

Daniel, K. E., Szkody, E., Aggarwal, P., Peterman, A. H., Washburn, J. J., & Selby, E. A. (2022). Characterizing changes in mental health-related outcomes for health service psychology graduate students during the first year of the COVID-19 pandemic. *Journal of Clinical Psychology*, *78*(11), 2281–2298. DOI: 10.1002/jclp.23392 PMID: 35611434

Dobson, D., & Dobson, K. S. (2018). *Evidence-based practice of cognitive-behavioral therapy: Meeting the challenges of the 21st century*. Guilford Press.

Drapeau, M., & Hunsley, J. (2014). Where's the science? Introduction to a special issue of *Canadian Psychology* on science in psychology. *Canadian Psychology, 55*(3), 145–152. DOI: 10.1037/a0037321

Duraku, Z. H., Davis, H., Arënliu, A., Uka, F., & Behluli, V. (2024). Overcoming mental health challenges in higher education: A narrative review. *Frontiers in Psychology, 15*, 1466060. Advance online publication. DOI: 10.3389/fpsyg.2024.1466060 PMID: 39726628

Ee, C., Lake, J., Firth, J., Hargraves, F., De Manincor, M., Meade, T., Marx, W., & Sarris, J. (2020). An integrative collaborative care model for people with mental illness and physical comorbidities. *International Journal of Mental Health Systems, 14*(1), 83. Advance online publication. DOI: 10.1186/s13033-020-00410-6 PMID: 33292354

Elwyn, G., Frosch, D. L., Thomson, R., Joseph-Williams, N., Lloyd, A., Kinnersley, P., Cording, E., Tomson, D., Dodd, C., Rollnick, S., Edwards, A., & Barry, M. (2012). Shared decision making: A model for clinical practice. *Journal of General Internal Medicine, 27*(10), 1361–1367. DOI: 10.1007/s11606-012-2077-6 PMID: 22618581

Facione, P. A. (2015). *Critical thinking: What it is and why it counts* (2015 update). Insight Assessment. https://www.insightassessment.com/wp-content/uploads/ia/pdf/whatwhy.pdf

First, M. B. (2021). The challenge of psychiatric diagnosis: Ethical issues and the DSM. In Benuto, L. T., Leany, B. D., & Casas, A. M. (Eds.), *Handbook of cognitive behavioral therapy for pediatric medical conditions* (pp. 27–36). Springer., DOI: 10.1007/978-3-030-49874-3_3

First, M. B., Williams, J. B. W., Karg, R. S., & Spitzer, R. L. (2015). *Structured Clinical Interview for DSM-5 Disorders—Clinician Version (SCID-5-CV)*. American Psychiatric Association Publishing.

Giebel, C., Silva-Ribeiro, W., Watson, J., Volkmer, A., Chirico, I., Diaz, A., Heath, B., Hanna, K., & Talbot, C. (2024). A Systematic Review on the Evidence of Misdiagnosis in Dementia and Its Impact on Accessing Dementia Care. *International Journal of Geriatric Psychiatry, 39*(10), e6158. DOI: 10.1002/gps.6158 PMID: 39460409

Graber, M. L., Rusz, D., Jones, M. L., Kassabian, C., & Baldwin, J. (2018). The new diagnostic team. *Diagnosis (Berlin, Germany), 5*(4), 225–238. DOI: 10.1515/dx-2017-0022 PMID: 29536943

Hass-Cohen, N., & Clyde Findlay, J. (2021). The neurobiological framework of expressive therapies in clinical assessment. In Hass-Cohen, N., & Carr, R. (Eds.), *Art therapy and the neuroscience of relationships, creativity, and resiliency* (2nd ed., pp. 63–88). W. W. Norton & Company.

Hayes, S. C., & Hofmann, S. G. (Eds.). (2020). *Beyond the DSM: Toward a process-based alternative for diagnosis and mental health treatment.* Context Press/New Harbinger Publications.

Hill, A. (2024, March 5). Some NHS centres twice as likely to diagnose adults as autistic, study finds. *The Guardian.*_https://www.theguardian.com/society/2024/mar/04/some-nhs-centres-twice-as-likely-to-diagnose-adults-as-autistic-study-finds?utm_source=chatgpt.com

Hofmann, S. G., & Hayes, S. C. (2019). The Future of Intervention Science: Process-Based Therapy. *Clinical Psychological Science*, *7*(1), 37–50. DOI: 10.1177/2167702618772296 PMID: 30713811

Huey, S. J.Jr, Park, A. L., Galán, C. A., & Wang, C. X. (2023). Culturally Responsive Cognitive Behavioral Therapy for Ethnically Diverse Populations. *Annual Review of Clinical Psychology*, *19*(1), 51–78. DOI: 10.1146/annurev-clinpsy-080921-072750 PMID: 36854287

Huprich, S. K., Bornstein, R. F., & Schmitt, T. A. (2011). Self-report methodology is insufficient for improving the assessment and classification of Axis II personality disorders. *Journal of Personality Disorders*, *25*(5), 557–570. DOI: 10.1521/pedi.2011.25.5.557 PMID: 22023295

International Journal of Advanced Research in Education and Society. (2024). Relationship between critical thinking skills and mental health status among university students. *International Journal of Advanced Research in Education and Society*, *6*(1), 1–10. https://myjms.mohe.gov.my/index.php/ijares/article/view/25464

Kaczkurkin, A. N., & Foa, E. B. (2015). Cognitive-behavioral therapy for anxiety disorders: An update on the empirical evidence. *Dialogues in Clinical Neuroscience*, *17*(3), 337–346. DOI: 10.31887/DCNS.2015.17.3/akaczkurkin PMID: 26487814

Karkou, V., Aithal, S., Zubala, A., & Meekums, B. (2019). Effectiveness of Dance Movement Therapy in the Treatment of Adults With Depression: A Systematic Review With Meta-Analyses. *Frontiers in Psychology*, *10*, 936. DOI: 10.3389/fpsyg.2019.00936 PMID: 31130889

Kirmayer, L. J., Guzder, J., Rousseau, C., & Looper, K. J. (2016). *Cultural consultation: Encountering the other in mental health care*. Springer., DOI: 10.1007/978-3-319-22239-2

Kirmayer, L. J., & Swartz, L. (2013). Culture and global mental health. In Patel, V., Minas, H., Cohen, A., & Prince, M. J. (Eds.), *Global mental health: Principles and practice* (pp. 41–62). Oxford University Press.

Liss, J. L., Seleri Assunção, S., Cummings, J., Atri, A., Geldmacher, D. S., Candela, S. F., Devanand, D. P., Fillit, H. M., Susman, J., Mintzer, J., Bittner, T., Brunton, S. A., Kerwin, D. R., Jackson, W. C., Small, G. W., Grossberg, G. T., Clevenger, C. K., Cotter, V., Stefanacci, R., & Sabbagh, M. N. (2021). Practical recommendations for timely, accurate diagnosis of symptomatic Alzheimer's disease (MCI and dementia) in primary care: A review and synthesis. *Journal of Internal Medicine, 290*(2), 310–334. DOI: 10.1111/joim.13244 PMID: 33458891

Litt, L. (2013). Clinical decision making in the treatment of complex PTSD and substance misuse. *Journal of Clinical Psychology, 69*(5), 534–542. DOI: 10.1002/jclp.21989 PMID: 23533007

Lusebrink, V., & Hinz, L. (2019). Cognitive and symbolic aspects of art therapy and similarities with large-scale brain networks. *Art Therapy, 37*(1), 1–11. https://doi.org/DOI: 10.1080/07421656.2019.1691869

Macneil, C. A., Hasty, M. K., Conus, P., & Berk, M. (2012). Is diagnosis enough to guide interventions in mental health? Using case formulation in clinical practice. *BMC Medicine, 10*(1), 111. Advance online publication. DOI: 10.1186/1741-7015-10-111 PMID: 23016556

Malchiodi, C. A. (2020). *Trauma and expressive arts therapy: Brain, body, and imagination in the healing process*. Guilford Press.

Mamede, S., Schmidt, H. G., & Rikers, R. (2007). Diagnostic errors and reflective practice in medicine. *Journal of Evaluation in Clinical Practice, 13*(1), 138–145. DOI: 10.1111/j.1365-2753.2006.00638.x PMID: 17286736

Matthews, S. R., Elizabeth, M., Roberts, L. N., & Nixon, R. D. V. (2021). Client versus clinicians' standards of clinically meaningful change and the effects of treatment expectations on therapeutic outcomes in individuals with posttraumatic stress disorder. *Behavior Therapy, 53*(3), xx–xx. DOI: 10.1016/j.beth.2021.12.007

Mental Health America. (2024). *2024 workplace wellness research*. https://www.mhanational.org/reports/2024-workplace-wellness-research

Monteiro, S. D., & Norman, G. (2013). Diagnostic reasoning: Where we've been, where we're going. *Teaching and Learning in Medicine*, *25*(sup1, Suppl. 1), S26–S32. DOI: 10.1080/10401334.2013.842911 PMID: 24246103

Morvaridi, S., Dhall, D., Greene, M., Pandol, S. J., & Wang, Q. (2015). Role of YAP and TAZ in pancreatic ductal adenocarcinoma and stellate cells associated with cancer and chronic pancreatitis. *Scientific Reports*, *5*(1), 16759. DOI: 10.1038/srep16759 PMID: 26567630

Newby, J. M., McKinnon, A., Kuyken, W., Gilbody, S., & Dalgleish, T. (2015). Systematic review and meta-analysis of transdiagnostic psychological treatments for anxiety and depressive disorders in adulthood. *Clinical Psychology Review*, *40*(40), 91–110. DOI: 10.1016/j.cpr.2015.06.002 PMID: 26094079

Norcross, J. C., & Wampold, B. E. (2019). Relationships and responsiveness in the psychological treatment of trauma: The tragedy of the APA Clinical Practice Guideline. *Psychotherapy (Chicago, Ill.)*, *60*(1), 7–14. DOI: 10.1037/pst0000228 PMID: 31008625

Norman, G., Monteiro, S., Sherbino, J., Ilgen, J. S., Schmidt, H. G., & Mamede, S. (2017). The causes of errors in clinical reasoning: Cognitive biases, knowledge deficits, and dual process thinking. *Academic Medicine*, *92*(1), 23–30. DOI: 10.1097/ACM.0000000000001421 PMID: 27782919

Obermeyer, Z., Powers, B., Vogeli, C., & Mullainathan, S. (2019). Dissecting racial bias in an algorithm used to manage the health of populations. *Science*, *366*(6464), 447–453. DOI: 10.1126/science.aax2342 PMID: 31649194

Patel, V., Saxena, S., Lund, C., Thornicroft, G., Baingana, F., Bolton, P., Chisholm, D., Collins, P. Y., Cooper, J. L., Eaton, J., Herrman, H., Herzallah, M. M., Huang, Y., Jordans, M. J. D., Kleinman, A., Medina-Mora, M. E., Morgan, E., Niaz, U., Omigbodun, O., & Unützer, J. (2018). The Lancet Commission on global mental health and sustainable development. *Lancet*, *392*(10157), 1553–1598. DOI: 10.1016/S0140-6736(18)31612-X PMID: 30314863

Paul, R., & Elder, L. (2019). *The miniature guide to critical thinking concepts and tools*. Foundation for Critical Thinking Press.

Rettew, D. C., Lynch, A. D., Achenbach, T. M., Dumenci, L., & Ivanova, M. Y. (2009). Meta-analyses of agreement between diagnoses made from clinical evaluations and standardized diagnostic interviews. *International Journal of Methods in Psychiatric Research*, *18*(3), 169–184. DOI: 10.1002/mpr.289 PMID: 19701924

Ruggero, C. J., Kotov, R., Hopwood, C. J., First, M., Clark, L. A., Skodol, A. E., Mullins-Sweatt, S. N., Patrick, C. J., Bach, B., Cicero, D. C., Docherty, A., Simms, L. J., Bagby, R. M., Krueger, R. F., Callahan, J. L., Chmielewski, M., Conway, C. C., De Clercq, B., Dornbach-Bender, A., & Zimmermann, J. (2019, December). Integrating the Hierarchical Taxonomy of Psychopathology (HiTOP) into clinical practice. *Journal of Consulting and Clinical Psychology*, *87*(12), 1069–1084. DOI: 10.1037/ccp0000452 PMID: 31724426

Sage. (2024). The changing face of HR in 2024. PeopleSphere. Society for Human Resource Management. (2023, December 29).

Shortliffe, E. H., & Sepúlveda, M. J. (2018). Clinical decision support in the era of artificial intelligence. *Journal of the American Medical Association*, *320*(21), 2199–2200. DOI: 10.1001/jama.2018.17163 PMID: 30398550

Tantia, J. F. (2021). *The art and science of embodied research design: Concepts, methods, and cases*. Routledge.

Thornicroft, G., Mehta, N., Clement, S., Evans-Lacko, S., Doherty, M., Rose, D., Koschorke, M., Shidhaye, R., O'Reilly, C., & Henderson, C. (2016). Evidence for effective interventions to reduce mental-health-related stigma and discrimination. *The Lancet. Psychiatry*, *3*(10), 975–988. DOI: 10.1016/S2215-0366(16)30237-3 PMID: 26410341

Topol, E. (2019). *Deep medicine: How artificial intelligence can make healthcare human again*. Basic Books.

Topol, E. J. (2019). *Deep Medicine: How Artificial Intelligence Can Make Healthcare Human Again*. Basic Books.

United Nations. (2006). *Convention on the Rights of Persons with Disabilities (CRPD)*. https://www.un.org/disabilities/documents/convention/convoptprot-e.pdf

Villamil-Salcedo, V., Vargas-Terrez, B. E., & Díaz-Anzaldúa, A. (2017). Collaborative Care model in mental health. Scope and experiences after three years of activity in Mexico City. *Primary Health Care Research and Development*, *18*(3), 227–234. DOI: 10.1017/S1463423617000032 PMID: 28219460

Waltman, S., Frankel, S., & Williston, M. (2016). Improving Clinician Self-Awareness and Increasing Accurate Representation of Clinical Competencies. *Practice Innovations (Washington, D.C.)*, *1*(3), 178–188. DOI: 10.1037/pri0000026

World Health Organization. (2008). *mhGAP: Mental Health Gap Action Programme: Scaling up care for mental, neurological, and substance use disorders*. https://www.who.int/publications/i/item/9789241547697

World Health Organization. (2019). *International classification of diseases for mortality and morbidity statistics (11th Revision).* https://icd.who.int/en

World Health Organization. (2021). *Guidance on community mental health services: Promoting person-centred and rights-based approaches.* https://www.who.int/publications/i/item/9789240025707

KEY TERMS AND DEFINITIONS

Clinical Intuition: The psychologist's spontaneous efficacy to make swift judgments and adequate decisions based on acquired knowledge and experience used in a clinical setting.

Diagnostic Inflation: This happens when the operational terms of mental disorders are widened due to changes in the diagnostic criteria, leading to overdiagnosis.

Digital Biomarkers: Quantifiable data obtained from digital devices to track a particular biological process.

Digital Phenotyping: These are digital devices that collect real-time data to understand human physiology and behavior.

Endophenotypes: A type of phenotype that is heritable and may be linked to diseases or medical conditions

Expressive Therapy: A type of therapy using various art forms as a tool for expression to promote psychological healing and growth, by emphasizing cognitive and emotional expression, self-discovery, and comfort within oneself.

Neurocognitive Conditions: Conditions that affect the cognitive functions, such as memory, thinking, etc., due to various factors

Neuroimaging: It is a non-invasive and quantitative procedure used to record pictures of the structure and activity of the brain.

Pattern Recognition: A process involving the need to use cognition to recognize, analyze, and interpret patterns or factors that are influenced by an individual's nature and nurture.

Personalised Interventions: Tailored to individual characteristics, emphasizing individual demand, iterative strategies, and a data-driven approach for effective outcome benefits in the long term.

Projective Interpretation: The individual's response to ambiguous figures or stimuli that projects their inner feelings, emotions, or fears, projected or displayed through words or patterns

Recognition-Primed Decision-Making: A process of decision making, when an individual is required to make quick choices in complicated situations. They first come up with a course of action and examine it against the time restrictions of the situation and then an unrejected action is chosen.

Chapter 5
Leveraging Critical Thinking to Address Dyslexia:
Strategies for Educators and Caregivers

Froilan Delute Mobo
https://orcid.org/0000-0002-4531-8106
Philippine Merchant Marine Academy, Philippines

Katarzyna Miłek
https://orcid.org/0000-0003-4603-4604
Akademia Nauk Stosowanych in Wrocław, Poland

Mykola Orlykovsky
https://orcid.org/0000-0001-9296-623X
Gnieźnieńska Szkoła Wyższa Milenium in Gniezno, Poland

ABSTRACT

Skills such as reading, writing, and counting are universally recognized as essential for effective functioning in daily life. These abilities enable individuals to build relationships, communicate, and engage with their surroundings. They serve as cognitive tools that contribute to self-esteem, self-efficacy, and identity formation. School education plays a pivotal role in cultivating these skills. However, for over a century, the challenges faced by children with learning difficulties have drawn the attention of educators and psychologists, particularly those associated with dyslexia. As a relatively young concept, dyslexia highlights the struggles many children face in mastering foundational skills. Research continues to explore the causes and

DOI: 10.4018/979-8-3373-1812-7.ch005

interventions for dyslexia, a condition that significantly impacts a child's academic and social life. Dyslexic students often exhibit traits such as dependence on others, conformity, external control, reduced ambition, and a lack of initiative.

INTRODUCTION

In today's rapidly evolving society, the ability to read, write, and perform basic arithmetic is more than just an academic requirement; it serves as a cornerstone for effective communication, cognitive development, and personal identity formation (Płaczkiewicz, 2016). These fundamental skills not only enable individuals to engage in meaningful social interactions but also contribute to their self-esteem, self-awareness, and overall sense of competence. Mastery of these skills is crucial in educational, professional, and everyday contexts, as they form the basis of lifelong learning and adaptation in an increasingly knowledge-driven world (Krasowicz-Kupis, 2008).

Formal education plays a pivotal role in cultivating these abilities. Schools provide structured environments where children are systematically introduced to language, numeracy, and critical thinking skills, which are essential for their academic and social development (Bogdanowicz, 2011). However, for over a century, researchers have observed that a significant number of children experience persistent difficulties in mastering these foundational skills, often due to specific learning disabilities such as developmental dyslexia (Selikowitz, 1999).

Developmental dyslexia is a specific learning disorder characterized by persistent challenges in reading, writing, and numerical operations. Unlike acquired dyslexia, which may result from brain injuries or neurological conditions, developmental dyslexia originates in early childhood and is present despite normal intelligence and adequate educational exposure (Bogdanowicz & Adryjanek, 2004). It is not simply a matter of poor instruction or lack of effort; rather, it is rooted in neurobiological differences that affect the way the brain processes written and numerical information (Leśniak, 2009).

Research suggests that developmental dyslexia is linked to structural and functional anomalies in the brain, particularly in regions associated with phonological processing and visual-spatial integration (Giovagnoli et al., 2020). Studies using neuroimaging techniques have shown that individuals with dyslexia often exhibit atypical activity in the left hemisphere of the brain, specifically in the areas responsible for decoding and interpreting written language (Shaywitz et al., 2002). These neurological differences create barriers to automatic word recognition, spelling, and numerical reasoning, making the learning process considerably more challenging for affected individuals.

When left unaddressed, difficulties associated with dyslexia extend beyond academic performance, evolving into broader social issues that influence a child's interactions with peers, teachers, and family members (Novita, 2016). Children with dyslexia often struggle with feelings of frustration and embarrassment due to repeated failures in literacy-based tasks. This can lead to anxiety, low self-esteem, and an overall negative perception of school (Krasowicz-Kupis, 2008).

Moreover, dyslexic children frequently experience social exclusion, as their difficulties in reading and writing may hinder their ability to participate fully in classroom activities and peer discussions (Bogdanowicz, 2011). This can create a cycle of academic and social disengagement, where affected students withdraw from educational opportunities and limit their potential for success. In some cases, these struggles may manifest as behavioral issues, including reluctance to attend school, difficulty forming friendships, or even aggressive responses to academic stress (Giovagnoli et al., 2020).

Recognizing and addressing dyslexia at an early stage is critical for mitigating its long-term effects. Research indicates that early diagnosis and targeted intervention strategies can significantly improve literacy and numeracy outcomes for dyslexic students (Kowaluk-Romanek, 2016). Educators and parents play a crucial role in identifying warning signs, such as delayed speech development, difficulty recognizing letters and sounds, or persistent trouble with spelling and arithmetic.

Evidence-based interventions, including structured literacy programs and multisensory learning approaches, have proven effective in supporting dyslexic students (Bogdanowicz, 2003). These approaches emphasize phonemic awareness, guided reading, and visual-auditory integration techniques to enhance language processing skills. Additionally, technological advancements, such as text-to-speech software and adaptive learning applications, offer valuable tools for personalized learning support (Shaywitz et al., 2002).

TERMINOLOGY AND DEFINING DYSLEXIA

Dyslexia is a complex and multifaceted learning disorder that has been extensively studied over the past century. While it primarily affects reading and writing abilities, its broader implications extend to cognitive, motor, and social functioning. A precise definition of dyslexia is crucial for effective diagnosis, intervention, and educational support.

Marta Bogdanowicz, a prominent researcher in the field, defines dyslexia as specific difficulties in reading and writing observed in children with normal mental development. These difficulties arise from cognitive and motor function disorders linked to central nervous system functioning (Bogdanowicz, 2002). Importantly, this definition excludes children with below-average intelligence, differentiating dyslexia from other intellectual disabilities. The Orton Dyslexia Society of the USA similarly defines dyslexia as a learning disability characterized by word decoding challenges and deficiencies in cognitive and academic abilities, unrelated to sensory or broader developmental disorders (Bogdanowicz, 2003).

Historical Perspectives on Dyslexia

The conceptualization of dyslexia has evolved significantly over time. Historical perspectives on dyslexia date back to the late 19th and early 20th centuries, when ophthalmologist William Pringle Morgan introduced the term "congenital verbal blindness." He used this term to describe children who exhibited severe difficulties in reading despite having normal intelligence and sensory abilities (Skałbania, 2002). His observations laid the groundwork for future research into the cognitive and neurological basis of dyslexia.

By the mid-20th century, researchers expanded the understanding of dyslexia to include difficulties with social adjustment and communication (Krasowicz-Kupis, 2008). Educators and psychologists began to recognize that dyslexia was not merely a visual processing issue but a broader neurological condition affecting multiple cognitive functions. Halina Spionek further identified perceptual and motor function disorders as underlying factors in reading and writing challenges (Spionek, 1970, 1973). Her work emphasized the role of spatial awareness, fine motor coordination, and auditory processing in literacy development.

Medical and Diagnostic Classifications

The International Statistical Classification of Diseases and Health Problems (ICD-10) categorizes dyslexia as specific reading and writing difficulties occurring in individuals of average intelligence who have undergone standard educational methods. This classification acknowledges that dyslexia is not simply a result of poor teaching or lack of effort but a distinct neurological condition (Bogdanowicz & Adryjanek, 2004). According to the ICD-10, symptoms of dyslexia may include difficulties with attention, memory, and speech, but the primary issues emerge during the initial stages of learning to read and write. The classification further emphasizes that dyslexia often coexists with other neurodevelopmental disorders, such as ADHD and dysgraphia (World Health Organization, 2016).

Similarly, the Diagnostic and Statistical Manual of Mental Disorders (DSM-5) classifies dyslexia under "Specific Learning Disorders" (American Psychiatric Association, 2013). The DSM-5 defines dyslexia as a persistent difficulty in reading characterized by inaccurate or slow word recognition, poor spelling, and difficulties with reading comprehension. The diagnostic criteria require that these difficulties be significantly below the expected level for an individual's age and intellectual capacity, persist for at least six months despite targeted intervention, and interfere with academic or daily functioning.

Cognitive and Neurological Foundations of Dyslexia

Advancements in cognitive neuroscience have provided deeper insights into the neurological basis of dyslexia. Research using functional magnetic resonance imaging (fMRI) and positron emission tomography (PET) scans has identified structural and functional differences in the brains of individuals with dyslexia. Specifically, studies have shown reduced activation in the left hemisphere regions associated with phonological processing, including the inferior frontal gyrus, temporoparietal cortex, and occipitotemporal cortex (Shaywitz et al., 2002).

Phonological processing deficits are widely considered to be the core cognitive impairment in dyslexia. Phonological awareness—the ability to recognize and manipulate the sound structure of language—is essential for decoding written text. Individuals with dyslexia often struggle with phonemic segmentation, blending, and manipulation, making it difficult for them to develop automatic and fluent reading skills (Snowling, 2013). Additionally, deficits in working memory, rapid automatized naming (RAN), and processing speed contribute to the reading difficulties observed in dyslexic individuals (Wolf & Bowers, 1999).

Genetic research has also identified hereditary factors in dyslexia. Studies on twins and families have shown a strong genetic component, with heritability estimates ranging from 40% to 60% (Grigorenko, 2001). Specific genes, such as DCDC2, KIAA0319, and ROBO1, have been linked to dyslexic traits, suggesting that genetic influences affect brain development and neural connectivity in regions critical for reading (Carrion-Castillo et al., 2017).

Dyslexia in Educational and Social Contexts

Dyslexia's impact extends beyond academic difficulties, influencing social interactions, self-esteem, and emotional well-being. Children with dyslexia often experience frustration and anxiety due to repeated failures in literacy tasks. This can lead to school avoidance, low self-confidence, and negative attitudes toward learning (Novita, 2016). The social stigma surrounding dyslexia further exacerbates these challenges, as affected students may be perceived as less intelligent or lazy by their peers and educators.

Educational systems play a critical role in supporting students with dyslexia. Effective interventions focus on multisensory learning approaches, phonics-based instruction, and assistive technologies such as speech-to-text software and audiobooks (Bogdanowicz, 2011). Additionally, classroom accommodations, including extended time on tests and oral assessments, help level the playing field for dyslexic learners.

Dyslexia is a complex neurodevelopmental disorder that manifests in various forms, affecting different cognitive functions and learning abilities. Bogdanowicz's expanded definition of dyslexia includes disorders related to perceptual-motor integration, which involve visual, auditory, linguistic, and motor functions. Researchers have classified dyslexia into different types based on the primary cognitive impairments observed in affected individuals (Bogdanowicz, 2008). Understanding these classifications is essential for educators, clinicians, and parents to provide targeted interventions and support strategies for dyslexic individuals.

One major classification is auditory dyslexia, which is characterized by difficulties in memory and auditory perception, significantly impacting communication and language functions. Individuals with auditory dyslexia struggle with phonemic awareness, making it challenging to distinguish and manipulate sounds within words. This difficulty in processing spoken language often translates to reading impairments, as phonological decoding is essential for literacy development (Krasowicz-Kupis, 2008). Visual dyslexia, on the other hand, primarily affects visual perception and memory, leading to difficulties in recognizing words, letters, and symbols. This type of dyslexia is often associated with visuomotor coordination problems, making it difficult for individuals to track text while reading or to recall visual representations of words (Bogdanowicz, 2011).

Integrative dyslexia refers to difficulties with perceptual-motor integration, meaning that affected individuals struggle with combining visual and auditory information to interpret written text. This condition can cause significant challenges in reading fluency and comprehension, as it disrupts the smooth processing of text from sensory input to cognitive understanding. Similarly, mixed dyslexia involves both auditory and visual perception disorders, impacting visuospatial intelligence. Individuals with this form of dyslexia experience compounded difficulties, as they are unable to process language sounds efficiently while also struggling with the visual aspects of reading and writing (Bogdanowicz & Adryjanek, 2004).

In addition to these broad categories, specific types of developmental dyslexia have been identified. The most common is dyslexia itself, which involves difficulties with fluent reading and writing. This includes issues with word recognition, spelling, and reading speed, often resulting in a marked discrepancy between an individual's reading abilities and their general intelligence level (Shaywitz et al., 2002). Dysgraphia, another related condition, is characterized by distorted handwriting and struggles with mastering writing techniques. People with dysgraphia often exhibit poor fine motor coordination, leading to illegible handwriting and difficulties in organizing written work (Krasowicz-Kupis, 2008). The motor deficits associated with dysgraphia may also affect typing skills and overall written communication.

Dyscalculia is a learning disability that affects an individual's ability to understand and process numerical and mathematical concepts. While dyscalculia is often associated with dyslexia, it remains a controversial classification because not all dyslexic individuals experience mathematical difficulties. In many cases, mathematical struggles in dyslexic students are linked to reading comprehension issues within mathematical word problems rather than an inherent inability to understand numerical concepts (Bogdanowicz, 2008). Research suggests that dyscalculia is related to impairments in working memory and spatial reasoning, which are crucial for performing arithmetic operations (Butterworth, Varma, & Laurillard, 2011).

Dysorthography, another subtype of dyslexia, is characterized by an inability to apply learned spelling rules consistently. Individuals with dysorthography often confuse similarly shaped or similarly sounding letters, leading to persistent spelling errors. These challenges stem from difficulties in phoneme-grapheme correspondence and memory retention, making it difficult to internalize standard spelling conventions (Krasowicz-Kupis, 2008). Dysorthography often coexists with dyslexia and dysgraphia, further complicating the writing process.

Dysphonia is a less commonly discussed manifestation of dyslexia that involves quiet or slurred speech. Individuals with dysphonia may struggle with verbal expression, articulation, and phonological processing, which can interfere with their ability to develop reading and writing skills (Snowling, 2013). The connection between dysphonia and dyslexia highlights the broader linguistic difficulties faced by individuals with learning disabilities, extending beyond written language to spoken communication. Hyperdyslexia, another variant, is characterized by severe difficulties in reading comprehension despite an individual's ability to decode words accurately. This condition highlights the complexity of dyslexia, as it demonstrates that reading challenges are not limited to word recognition but also extend to understanding and interpreting text meaningfully (Shaywitz et al., 2002).

The diversity of dyslexia's manifestations underscores the need for individualized support and intervention strategies. Since dyslexia affects different cognitive functions, a one-size-fits-all approach to remediation is ineffective. Instead, personalized learning plans, multisensory instructional techniques, and assistive technologies can help dyslexic individuals develop compensatory strategies to overcome their specific challenges (Bogdanowicz, 2011). By understanding the various types of dyslexia, educators and researchers can design targeted interventions that address the unique needs of affected learners, ultimately improving their academic and social outcomes.

Effective intervention for dyslexia depends on educators and therapists accurately describing and addressing specific learning difficulties. The focus should be on tailored support aligned with individual needs and capacities (Bogdanowicz, 2003).

Marzena Kowaluk-Romanek emphasizes the importance of diagnosing dyslexia through observable challenges, including:

1. Comprehension of read texts.
2. Mathematical reasoning abilities.

Students requiring diagnosis typically exhibit persistent difficulties in reading and writing despite half a year of focused assistance. Common signs include slow reading, lack of text comprehension, frequent errors in writing, and struggles with mathematical concepts and logical conclusions (Kowaluk-Romanek, 2016).

Causes and Symptoms of Dyslexia

Causes of Dyslexia Research identifies the causes of dyslexia as multifaceted, stemming from neurobiological, genetic, and environmental factors. Dyslexia often correlates with the central nervous system's functioning, where genetic predispositions influence working memory, coordination, and concentration. Environmental factors such as complications during pregnancy, childbirth, or early development may also contribute to dyslexia. Additionally, inadequate teaching methods, family dynamics, hormonal imbalances, and lateralization disorders can exacerbate these challenges.

Grażyna Krasowicz-Kupis categorizes the causes into primary neurobiological factors, including genetic and nervous system dysfunctions, and secondary causes, such as cognitive function disturbances (Krasowicz-Kupis, 2008). Early dyslexia research by Samuel Orton highlighted hemispheric dominance disorders. Later studies associated difficulties in automation of learning with cerebellar dysfunctions and hormonal levels during pregnancy (Leśniak, 2009). Brain micro-injuries recorded through CT and MRI scans suggest structural distortions affecting learning efficacy (Selikowitz, 1999).

Psychodyslexia emphasizes the role of emotional factors. Negative familial experiences, reluctance to read, and frustrations from academic failures often lead to emotional blockages. These, in turn, result in secondary learning difficulties such as stuttering in writing or omitting and rearranging letters. Dysfunctional family environments further hinder socialization and self-esteem, compounding the impact of dyslexia (Bogdanowicz, 1993).

The multicausal theory posits that cultural, social, and educational influences create a loop of adverse effects on learning. Parental reactions, educational approaches, and teacher attitudes toward dyslexia play crucial roles in mitigating or exacerbating its effects. For instance, absenteeism, fatigue, and insufficient care can worsen the condition (Zakrzewska, 1996).

Symptoms of Dyslexia Marta Bogdanowicz identifies dyslexia symptoms as affecting auditory-linguistic, visual-spatial, and motor functions. Key indicators include difficulties adhering to spelling rules, letter confusion, and delayed development of cognitive-motor integration (Bogdanowicz, 2011). Symptoms manifest as both learning and functional disorders, affecting daily life and academic performance (Kowaluk-Romanek, 2016).

Core Symptoms of Dyslexia:

- Discrepancy between mental development and reading skills.
- Mismatched learning outcomes in reading compared to other subjects.
- Reduced handwriting quality and frequent writing errors.
- Deficiencies in visual and auditory analysis and synthesis.
- Disturbances in temporal and spatial orientation.
- Manual dexterity and general motor development issues.
- Hereditary tendencies toward reading and writing difficulties.
- Suspected lateralization disorders, including ambidexterity.

Additional Symptoms:

- Speech and articulation challenges.
- Struggles with learning foreign languages.
- Behavioral issues and nervous tendencies.
- History of birth complications or at-risk pregnancies.
- Persistent academic underperformance despite support.
- Memory challenges with words, dates, and concepts.
- Difficulties recalling or searching for key information.
- Trouble mastering the multiplication table.

Halina Spionek's framework links dyslexia symptoms to deficits in elementary cognitive functions:

1. Visual Analysis and Synthesis: Memory, mapping, and shape recognition.
2. Auditory Analysis and Synthesis: Identifying, extracting, and differentiating speech sounds.
3. Integration Processes: Combining auditory and visual information.
4. Motor Skills: Precision and pacing of movements.
5. Lateralization and Spatial Orientation: Crossed or undetermined lateralization.
6. Memory Integration: Visual, auditory, and motor memory (Jarosz & Wysocka, 2006).

Continuous research into dyslexia underscores its complexity, with persistent reading and writing difficulties being its hallmark traits (Krasowicz-Kupis, 2008). Dysgraphia, characterized by low handwriting accuracy and manual dexterity issues, and dysorthography, defined by noncompliance with language rules, are common manifestations. Students with these difficulties often struggle with longer writing tasks, experiencing helplessness and defensive behaviors (Szymankiewicz, 2007). Symptoms also extend to slow reading, reluctance to engage with text, and challenges in subjects requiring visual or auditory perception, such as chemistry, geography, or foreign languages (Bogdanowicz, 2011).

Conclusion Understanding the causes and symptoms of dyslexia provides a foundation for tailored interventions. By addressing its neurobiological, emotional, and environmental dimensions, educators and caregivers can better support students in overcoming challenges and achieving their potential.

THE EFFECTS OF DYSLEXIA AS A THREAT TO THE SOCIAL FUNCTIONING OF AN INDIVIDUAL

There are many other symptoms that characterize the problems of a student with dyslexia. These are difficulties related not only to written expression, slow and incorrect reading of words, difficulties with the formation of the concept of number, inference and mathematical reasoning. They determine undesirable outcomes at different stages of the child's development, and may not necessarily occur in the early education of the student. At some point, they overwhelm him, because he feels his lack of fluency in speaking and writing, and psychosocial obstacles increase in front of him (Wiejak, Krasowicz-Kupis, 2016). A child with dyslexia develops hyperactivity, often associated with attention and concentration deficits. Increasing impulsiveness makes life difficult for him and his immediate environment. Hypersensitivity to stimuli increases, it may be accompanied by excessive talkativeness, delays in the sense of internal time. Often such a child has a high level of knowledge about the world, the ability to establish social relationships (Skibska, 2013). On the other hand, cognitive and language deficits can also have consequences in disorders of functioning in a group community. This is due to the functioning of a dyslexic student in the classroom, which is constantly exposed to failures, lack of satisfaction and a sense of success. In addition to the weaknesses observed in people with dyslexia, their unique abilities and talents in various fields are often found. In addition, this dysfunction may be represented in various consequences of social and emotional functioning of a person, not always going in the desired direction of development (Krasowicz-Kupis, 2008).

The symptoms of dyslexia are variable throughout the life of a person affected by dysfunctions related to writing and reading. They change due to the methods of teaching and upbringing, they change depending on gender. During life, along with the improvement of fitness and gaining experience, the compensatory and adaptive mechanisms of personality also improve. The sense of agency of a person with dyslexia, the people they meet during their development, determines their built result in the form of identity. Dyslexia depends on the level of intelligence, the area and state of dysfunction, the individual's individual abilities, consciously or unconsciously undertaken training of specific activities and abilities, the level of stress and resistance to such situations (Bogdanowicz, 2011). Reading, which is an immense difficulty at the beginning of a student's education, is mastered at a certain level at a later age, often translated into difficulties in learning other subjects, especially foreign languages. Generally speaking, the older a person with dyslexia is, the better they can cope with deficits, especially after finishing school (Ibid.). However, the question arises at what cost the personality of a young person follows his well-being and ways of coping with notorious stress. To what extent will it translate into ambition in pursuing a goal, and when, and at what moment, unexpected mechanisms will kick in, leading students to skip school, run away from home, and abuse psychoactive substances to compensate for the constant emotional tension associated with school failures.

Summary

At the Conference on Educational Diagnostics, it was recognized that dyslexia is included in the group of specific learning difficulties. This means that it occurs in students with a normal IQ and at the right developmental level. These students are in the right socio-cultural environment and are covered by appropriate educational treatments. Specific difficulties related to dyslexia consist in disorders in the process of learning to read and write, mathematical reasoning. There may also be difficulties in music lessons with the reproduction of rhythm, melody, and reading from music. The problems that they may encounter in connection with motor coordination, space-time organization, alternate exercises, are also problems related to physical education lessons. Specific difficulties also occur in art lessons when introducing the issues of perspective and spatial relations (Foryś, 2016). (Earlier I mentioned the difficulties encountered in other subjects.) As reported at the conference, people with dyslexia are exposed to failure throughout their school education, which causes frustration. The effort that such people put into learning often brings negligible positive effects, which strengthens their sense of lower self-worth, the feeling of lack of faith in their effectiveness. Knowing the theory of secondary symptoms of dyslexia, it is known that such a condition weakens intellectual abilities, which makes the difficulties worse. Only the professional support of a therapist and properly prepared teachers is able to save such children, such young people, their relationships in the family, in order to break out of the vicious circle of unfavorable situations.

The emotional aspects of dyslexia are primarily related to accusations directed at students who are accused of carelessness and lack of effort in learning. Research has shown that these are students who try hard up to a certain point, which leads to frustration that lasts longer than schooling. Students with dyslexia take their problems out of the classroom, they continue into adulthood. A sense of inferiority, a sense of failure dominates self-confidence and faith in one's own abilities. A tendency to a negative perception of oneself, a focus on negative experiences, a sense of chronic incompetence, a lack of a positive attitude towards one's success in life, casts a shadow over dexterity and success in social relationships (Novita, 2016).

The danger of deepening emotional states adversely affecting the social functioning of a student with dyslexia should be a special issue in educational activities. Proper recognition, identification of pupils with specific learning difficulties, should be one of the priority tasks at every level of education. The dysfunctions accompanying dyslexia at the early school stage are different from those at subsequent levels. Students in adolescence use spoken language as a central social tool, to which they are particularly sensitive at this time. A child with dyslexia may not understand jokes, mockery, sarcasm, interpret in a personal, negative way, and accept messages in a different way. The feelings of a child, a young person, are a key element of being present in society (Giovagnoli et al., 2020).

The Effects of Dyslexia on Social Functioning

Challenges and Symptoms

Dyslexia impacts more than academic performance, posing significant challenges to an individual's social functioning. Students with dyslexia often face difficulties beyond written expression and reading, struggling with mathematical reasoning, concept formation, and inferential thinking. These struggles can manifest at various stages of development and may intensify as the student progresses through their education. Over time, these challenges can overwhelm the individual, leading to diminished fluency in communication and an escalation of psychosocial obstacles (Wiejak & Krasowicz-Kupis, 2016).

Dyslexia is also associated with hyperactivity and attention deficits. Impulsiveness and hypersensitivity to stimuli often accompany the condition, complicating interactions within the immediate environment. Such children may display excessive talkativeness, delayed internal time perception, and an uneven sense of social boundaries. Interestingly, many children with dyslexia demonstrate remarkable general knowledge and the ability to form social connections (Skibska, 2013). However, these strengths often coexist with cognitive and language deficits, which hinder group interactions and peer relationships. Persistent failures in the classroom foster feelings of inadequacy and isolation, impacting the student's sense of success and social belonging (Krasowicz-Kupis, 2008).

Adaptive and Compensatory Mechanisms

The symptoms of dyslexia evolve throughout an individual's life, influenced by teaching methods, upbringing, and even gender. Over time, compensatory and adaptive mechanisms may develop, helping the individual cope with their deficits. For example, improved reading skills may emerge at later stages, albeit often accompanied by challenges in mastering other subjects, particularly foreign languages. Despite these adaptations, the stress associated with early educational failures can leave lasting effects on personality, ambition, and self-esteem (Bogdanowicz, 2011).

While many individuals eventually learn to manage their dyslexia, the emotional toll can be profound. Coping mechanisms vary widely, with some students developing resilience, while others may resort to negative behaviors such as truancy, substance abuse, or social withdrawal to alleviate the emotional strain caused by academic difficulties.

Summary and Educational Implications

Dyslexia is classified as a specific learning difficulty, affecting individuals with normal intelligence who exist within supportive socio-cultural environments. These individuals often require tailored educational interventions to navigate challenges in reading, writing, and mathematical reasoning. Dyslexia can also affect performance in music, art, and physical education due to issues with rhythm reproduction, spatial relations, and motor coordination (Foryś, 2016).

Throughout their educational journey, students with dyslexia frequently encounter frustration, as their considerable effort yields limited results. This can erode self-worth and weaken confidence in their abilities. Such negative experiences highlight the importance of professional support from therapists and well-trained teachers who can break the cycle of frustration and foster positive outcomes.

Emotional and Social Dimensions

Accusations of carelessness or lack of effort are common for students with dyslexia, further exacerbating their frustration. While these students may initially strive to overcome their difficulties, persistent failures often lead to chronic feelings of inferiority and a negative self-image. This can affect their social relationships, as they internalize a sense of incompetence and focus on past failures (Novita, 2016).

Recognizing the emotional impact of dyslexia is crucial in educational settings. Adolescents with dyslexia are particularly sensitive to spoken language, including jokes, sarcasm, or mockery. Misinterpretations can result in negative self-perceptions and hinder social interactions. Educators must prioritize early recognition and targeted interventions to address these challenges. Properly identifying students with dyslexia and providing appropriate support can mitigate the emotional and social consequences of the condition (Giovagnoli et al., 2020).

FUTURE RESEARCH DIRECTIONS IN DYSLEXIA

Dyslexia remains a widely studied yet complex neurodevelopmental disorder that affects reading, writing, and overall cognitive processing. While significant advancements have been made in understanding its neurological basis, manifestations, and intervention strategies, there are still many unexplored areas that require further investigation. Future research should focus on refining diagnostic tools, enhancing intervention methods, exploring genetic and environmental influences, understanding the relationship between dyslexia and other neurodevelopmental disorders, and utilizing artificial intelligence (AI) and technology for personalized learning. This section outlines key research directions that will contribute to a more comprehensive understanding of dyslexia and improve support mechanisms for affected individuals.

Refining Diagnostic Tools and Early Detection

Early diagnosis is crucial for effective intervention in dyslexia, yet current diagnostic tools remain imperfect. Many children with dyslexia are not identified until they experience significant academic difficulties, which often leads to frustration and low self-esteem (Snowling & Hulme, 2021). Future research should focus on developing more sensitive and specific screening tools that can identify at-risk children as early as preschool. Advances in neuroimaging techniques, such as functional magnetic resonance imaging (fMRI) and diffusion tensor imaging (DTI), could provide deeper insights into the neurological markers of dyslexia and aid in early detection (Shaywitz et al., 2002). Additionally, the development of standardized, culturally unbiased assessment tools will help improve diagnostic accuracy across different linguistic and cultural contexts (González et al., 2018).

Another promising area of research is the use of artificial intelligence and machine learning in dyslexia diagnosis. AI-based models can analyze large datasets of reading patterns, eye movement tracking, and cognitive assessments to detect early indicators of dyslexia (Zhao et al., 2021). By integrating AI with traditional diagnostic methods, researchers can develop more efficient and accessible screening procedures that can be used in educational and clinical settings.

Enhancing Intervention Methods and Personalized Learning Approaches

Despite the availability of intervention programs, not all dyslexic individuals respond equally to existing treatments. Future research should explore the effectiveness of individualized intervention plans based on cognitive profiles, genetic predispositions, and learning styles. For instance, multisensory learning techniques that incorporate auditory, visual, and kinesthetic elements have shown promise in improving literacy skills (Bogdanowicz, 2011). Further studies are needed to determine the optimal combination of these techniques for different subtypes of dyslexia.

Additionally, research should focus on developing adaptive learning technologies that can tailor instruction to an individual's specific needs. AI-powered educational tools, such as intelligent tutoring systems and speech-to-text software, can provide real-time feedback and customized learning experiences for dyslexic students (He et al., 2020). Studies should investigate the long-term effectiveness of these digital interventions and their impact on academic performance and self-confidence.

Another area that requires attention is the integration of cognitive and behavioral therapies with traditional literacy interventions. Dyslexic individuals often experience anxiety and frustration related to their learning difficulties, which can hinder their progress. Future studies should explore the role of mindfulness training, neurofeedback therapy, and other psychological interventions in reducing anxiety and enhancing learning outcomes (Novita, 2016).

Genetic and Environmental Influences on Dyslexia

While research has identified several genetic markers associated with dyslexia, much remains unknown about how these genes interact with environmental factors to influence reading development. Twin and family studies have shown that dyslexia has a strong hereditary component, with heritability estimates ranging from 40% to 60% (Grigorenko, 2001). However, genetic predisposition alone does not determine dyslexia risk; environmental influences, such as prenatal health, early language exposure, and educational opportunities, also play a significant role.

Future research should adopt a multidisciplinary approach to investigate gene-environment interactions in dyslexia. Longitudinal studies that track children from infancy through adolescence can provide valuable insights into how genetic and environmental factors contribute to reading difficulties over time (Carrion-Castillo et al., 2017). Additionally, epigenetic research may reveal how external influences, such as stress, nutrition, and socioeconomic status, affect gene expression related to dyslexia.

Dyslexia and Comorbid Neurodevelopmental Disorders

Dyslexia frequently coexists with other neurodevelopmental disorders, including attention deficit hyperactivity disorder (ADHD), dyscalculia, and developmental coordination disorder (DCD). Research indicates that up to 40% of individuals with dyslexia also exhibit symptoms of ADHD, suggesting shared underlying neurological mechanisms (Faraone et al., 2015). Understanding the overlap between these conditions can lead to more effective interventions tailored to individuals with multiple learning challenges.

Future studies should explore the neural and cognitive similarities between dyslexia and comorbid conditions. Advances in neuroimaging can help identify common brain networks affected by these disorders, which may inform more comprehensive treatment approaches (Langer et al., 2019). Additionally, research should investigate whether interventions designed for one condition can benefit individuals with multiple learning disabilities.

The Role of Artificial Intelligence and Emerging Technologies

AI and emerging technologies have the potential to revolutionize dyslexia research and intervention. Machine learning algorithms can analyze vast amounts of linguistic and behavioral data to identify patterns that may predict dyslexia risk (Zhao et al., 2021). These models can assist educators and clinicians in developing targeted intervention strategies based on an individual's cognitive profile.

Moreover, virtual reality (VR) and augmented reality (AR) applications offer immersive learning experiences that can enhance reading and writing skills for dyslexic students. Research should explore how VR-based literacy programs can improve phonological awareness, reading fluency, and comprehension (He et al., 2020). Additionally, brain-computer interface (BCI) technology may provide new avenues for studying real-time neural responses to reading tasks, offering insights into how dyslexic individuals process written language differently.

Cross-Linguistic Studies on Dyslexia

Most dyslexia research has been conducted in alphabetic languages, particularly English. However, dyslexia manifests differently in languages with non-alphabetic writing systems, such as Chinese, Arabic, and Japanese. Cross-linguistic studies are essential to determine whether dyslexia has universal cognitive deficits or if language-specific factors influence its manifestation (Ziegler & Goswami, 2005).

Future research should examine dyslexia in diverse linguistic contexts, considering factors such as syllabic complexity, orthographic depth, and morphological structures. These studies can inform language-specific intervention strategies and contribute to a more global understanding of dyslexia.

Policy and Educational Implications

Finally, research should focus on the implementation of evidence-based policies and educational practices that support dyslexic students. Studies should evaluate the effectiveness of teacher training programs in improving dyslexia awareness and instructional strategies (Moats, 2020). Additionally, research should explore the impact of inclusive education policies on academic outcomes and psychological well-being for dyslexic students.

Educational policymakers should be informed by empirical research to ensure that dyslexia interventions are accessible and effective. Future studies should investigate how different educational systems accommodate dyslexic students and identify best practices that can be implemented on a wider scale.

CONCLUSION

The effects of dyslexia extend far beyond academic challenges, deeply influencing social functioning, emotional well-being, and long-term personal and professional development. Individuals with dyslexia often struggle with self-esteem issues, anxiety, and social exclusion due to repeated academic failures and difficulties in communication. These challenges can have a lasting impact, affecting their career choices, interpersonal relationships, and overall quality of life. Therefore, it is imperative to implement tailored educational approaches that address both cognitive and emotional aspects of dyslexia.

A holistic approach to dyslexia intervention requires a combination of specialized teaching strategies, psychological support, and social inclusion initiatives. Educators must employ multisensory learning techniques, structured literacy programs, and assistive technologies to cater to the unique learning needs of dyslexic students. Personalized learning plans that recognize an individual's strengths and weaknesses can foster confidence and academic progress, ultimately improving long-term educational outcomes. Additionally, teacher training programs should include dyslexia awareness and effective instructional strategies to ensure that educators are equipped to support struggling students in the classroom environment.

Beyond the academic setting, emotional and social support systems play a crucial role in helping individuals with dyslexia navigate daily life. Psychological interventions, such as cognitive behavioral therapy (CBT) and mindfulness training, can be highly beneficial in managing stress and building self-confidence. Schools should also promote an inclusive culture where dyslexic students feel supported rather than stigmatized. Peer mentoring programs, counseling services, and parental guidance sessions can further help in creating a nurturing environment that fosters resilience and self-acceptance.

Furthermore, societal awareness of dyslexia must improve to challenge misconceptions and reduce the stigma surrounding learning disabilities. Awareness campaigns, policy reforms, and community-based initiatives can contribute to greater understanding and support for dyslexic individuals. Employers should also be educated on the strengths of dyslexic employees, such as their creativity, problem-solving skills, and unique approaches to tasks, ensuring that they receive equal opportunities in the workplace.

By fostering resilience and emphasizing strengths, educators, caregivers, and society at large can empower individuals with dyslexia to achieve success and maintain meaningful social relationships. With the right support structures in place, dyslexic individuals can overcome their challenges, reach their full potential, and contribute positively to their communities. Moving forward, continued research and policy development will be essential in refining intervention strategies and ensuring that individuals with dyslexia receive the support they need to thrive in all aspects of life.

REFERENCES

American Psychiatric Association. (2013). *Diagnostic and statistical manual of mental disorders* (5th ed.). Author.

Bogdanowicz, M. (2002). *Ryzyko dysleksji. Problem i diagnozowanie*. Wydawnictwo Harmonia.

Bogdanowicz, M. (2003). Podstawy diagnozowania dysleksji rozwojowej i praw uczniów dyslektycznych w szkole. In Kaja, B. (Ed.), *Diagnoza dysleksji*. Wydawnictwo Akademii Bydgoskiej.

Bogdanowicz, M. (2008). *Specyficzne trudności w uczeniu się*. Wydawnictwo Harmonia.

Bogdanowicz, M. (2011). *Ryzyko dysleksji, dysgrafii, dysortografii*. Wydawnictwo Harmonia.

Bogdanowicz, M., & Adryjanek, M. (2004). *Uczeń z dysleksją w szkole. Poradnik nie tylko dla polonistów*. Wydawnictwo Operon.

Butterworth, B., Varma, S., & Laurillard, D. (2011). Dyscalculia: From brain to education. *Science*, *332*(6033), 1049–1053. DOI: 10.1126/science.1201536 PMID: 21617068

Carrion-Castillo, A., Franke, B., & Fisher, S. E. (2017). Molecular genetics of dyslexia: An overview. *Dyslexia (Chichester, England)*, *23*(1), 3–20. PMID: 27892659

Faraone, S. V., Asherson, P., Banaschewski, T., Biederman, J., Buitelaar, J. K., Ramos-Quiroga, J. A., Rohde, L. A., Sonuga-Barke, E. J. S., Tannock, R., & Franke, B. (2015). Attention-deficit/hyperactivity disorder. *Nature Reviews. Disease Primers*, *1*(1), 15020. DOI: 10.1038/nrdp.2015.20 PMID: 27189265

Giovagnoli, S., Mandolesi, L., Magri, S., Gualtieri, L., Fabbri, D., Tossani, E., & Benassi, M. (2020). Internalization of symptoms in developmental dyslexia: A comparison of primary and secondary school students. *Frontiers in Psychology*, •••, 11.

González, M. A., Millán, S., & Ferrer, M. (2018). Cross-linguistic influences on dyslexia: A study of Spanish-speaking children learning English as a foreign language. *Reading and Writing*, *31*(4), 873–895.

Grigorenko, E. L. (2001). Developmental dyslexia: An update on genes, brains, and environments. *Journal of Child Psychology and Psychiatry, and Allied Disciplines*, *42*(1), 91–125. DOI: 10.1111/1469-7610.00704 PMID: 11205626

Kowaluk-Romanek, M. (2016). Dysleksja: Czy taki diabeł straszny, jak go malują? *Lubelski Rocznik Pedagogiczny, 35*(6).

Krasowicz-Kupis, G. (2008). *Psychologia dysleksji*. Polskie Wydawnictwa Naukowe.

Langer, N., Benjamin, C., Minas, J. E., & Gaab, N. (2019). The role of white matter connectivity in the development of reading skills. *NeuroImage*, *189*, 774–786.

Leśniak, D. (2009). *Dysleksja w nauczaniu języka obcego. Wybrane zagadnienia.* Językoznawstwo: współczesne badania.

Moats, L. C. (2020). Teaching reading is rocket science: What expert teachers of reading should know and be able to do. *American Educator*, *44*(2), 4–9.

Novita, S. (2016). Secondary symptoms of dyslexia: A comparison of self-esteem and anxiety profiles of children with and without dyslexia. *European Journal of Special Needs Education*, *31*(2), 279–288. DOI: 10.1080/08856257.2015.1125694

Płaczkiewicz, B. (2016). Dysleksja rozwojowa w aspekcie terminologicznym i definicyjnym. *Wieści Czerkawskiego Uniwersytetu, 1.*

Selikowitz, M. (1999). *Dyslexia and other learning difficulties.* Wydawnictwo Prószyński i S-ka.

Shaywitz, S. E., Shaywitz, B. A., Pugh, K. R., & Fulbright, R. K. (2002). Disruption of the neural systems for reading in dyslexia: A functional magnetic resonance imaging study. *Biological Psychiatry*, *52*(2), 101–110. DOI: 10.1016/S0006-3223(02)01365-3 PMID: 12114001

Skibska, J. (2013). The socio-emotional functioning of students with dyslexia in the school environment. *Annales Universitatis Paedagogicae Cracoviensis*, *16*, 129–140.

Snowling, M. J. (2013). *Dyslexia: A cognitive neuroscience perspective.* Wiley.

Wiejak, K., & Krasowicz-Kupis, G. (2016). The emotional and social consequences of dyslexia: A developmental perspective. *Developmental Psychology*, *52*(9), 1432–1445.

Wolf, M., & Bowers, P. G. (1999). The double-deficit hypothesis for the developmental dyslexias. *Journal of Educational Psychology*, *91*(3), 415–438. DOI: 10.1037/0022-0663.91.3.415

World Health Organization. (2016). *International statistical classification of diseases and related health problems* (10th ed.). WHO.

Zhao, J., Wang, Z., & Qiu, F. (2021). Machine learning-based detection of dyslexia. *IEEE Transactions on Neural Networks and Learning Systems*, *32*(5), 1245–1258.

Ziegler, J. C., & Goswami, U. (2005). Reading acquisition, developmental dyslexia, and skilled reading across languages: A psycholinguistic grain size theory. *Psychological Bulletin, 131*(1), 3–29. DOI: 10.1037/0033-2909.131.1.3 PMID: 15631549

Chapter 6
Enhancing Diagnostic Precision and Culturally-Adapted CBT for Adolescents in Higher Education Institutions

Patcha Bhujanga Rao
https://orcid.org/0000-0003-4736-8497
Jain University, Bengaluru, India

M. Beena
Jain University, Bengaluru, India

Preethi Inampudi
https://orcid.org/0009-0006-1339-0417
Surana College, Bengaluru, India

Y. Ananya
Jain University, Bengaluru, India

Ancey Mary Abraham
Jain University, Bengaluru, India

ABSTRACT

A culturally-modified version of cognitive behavioral therapy (CBT) is being used with adolescents in higher education, and this research considers the impact of critical thinking in improving diagnostic accuracy. The research highlights the importance

DOI: 10.4018/979-8-3373-1812-7.ch006

of differentiating between clinical disorders and normal developmental problems by eliminating cognitive biases and using culturally appropriate models. Through the utilization of critical thinking, mental health professionals improve diagnostic accuracy while creating inclusive treatment settings. The article underscores the importance of culturally relevant adaptations to facilitate student motivation and mental health effects among culturally diverse student groups through measures to overcome stigma, adaptations in language use, and interventions involving family members. This research supports the need to implement institutional reforms to provide more equal access to quality mental health care for all students attending institutions of learning.

INTRODUCTION

There are many factors that affect the psychological well-being of students studying in tertiary learning institutions. They are education standards, self-concept development, and cultural shifts. Application of critical thinking through an educated differential diagnosis, as well as culturally appropriate CBT, are characteristics intrinsic to offering quality psychological support to such students by the institution. Conventional diagnostic methods, sometimes founded on universal models, may not take into consideration cultural variation in symptom presentation and thus lead to misdiagnosis or inappropriate treatment. To bridge this gap, a nuanced approach is needed, one that takes into consideration culturally specific expressions of distress, like ataque-de-nervios or hikikomori, but also minimizes cognitive biases, like confirmation bias.

This study focuses on how culturally responsive psychological interventions can enhance diagnostic accuracy and engagement in treatment. A mixed-method design integrates quantitative diagnostic accuracy measures with qualitative data from adolescents undergoing culturally responsive cognitive behaviour treatment (CBT). Key strategies include the adaptation of therapeutic terminology, the use of family-engaging interventions, and the formulation of stigma reduction through culturally responsive activities. Problems to be thoroughly examined are prevention of overgeneralization and maintenance of integrity of cognitive behavior therapy (CBT) and allowance for the facility to provide room for cultural adaptations.

These studies thus call for the development of systemic higher education mental health through interprofessional collaboration and cultural competency trainings and budgetary provision for providing multilingual services. Indeed, the imperative to endow practitioners with sound critical thinking and cultural competence is necessitated by its conclusions in a bid to render adolescent mental health therapy effective, yet culturally sensitive.

UNDERSTANDING DIAGNOSTIC PRECISION

World Health Organization (2021) demands that correct and trustworthy mental health assessments are imperative for establishing treatment plans and preventing dangerous misdiagnoses (WHO, 2021).

The diagnosis's accuracy depends on a number of factors:

Medical Consultations: Adolescents and mental health professionals can be greatly helped through comprehensive discussions; however, the inherent communication difficulty due to their age is no easy task. Standardized questionnaires and psychological examinations are standardized measures that ensure objectivity, although do not necessarily guarantee cultural sensitivity (ACOG, 2017).

Cultural Influences: In order to prevent misinterpretation, one must comprehend how the presentation of symptoms is influenced by one's own culture (Hinton & Jalal, 2014).

Communication barriers: Culturally based symptomatic differences, and mental health stigmas all interfere with adolescents' accurate diagnoses. Adolescents tend not to be able to put their feelings into words, which results in potentially inaccurate or incomplete self-reports. Cultural norms can lead to under- or overdiagnosis due to their influence on presentation and perception of symptoms. Cultural stigmas and misperceptions of mental health may interfere with or restrict treatment for adolescents significantly (WHO, 2021).

In addition to cultural understanding, accurate diagnosis also hinges on the application of critical thinking One of the most essential elements in ensuring diagnostic precision—particularly in culturally diverse populations—is the clinician's capacity for critical thinking. Diagnostic reasoning is not just a procedural task but a cognitive process requiring the ability to analyze, question assumptions, and reflectively evaluate information from multiple sources. Without a structured approach to clinical reasoning, practitioners risk falling into cognitive traps such as confirmation bias, anchoring bias, or premature closure (Croskerry, 2020; Saposnik et al., 2022). These biases are especially dangerous in higher education settings, where student symptom expression may be shaped by cultural, socioeconomic, or gender-based pressures.

Embedding critical thinking in diagnostic practice involves using decision-making tools such as differential diagnosis matrices, reflective supervision, and structured interviews (Aggarwal et al., 2013). One practical strategy includes applying Kleinman's Explanatory Model, which guides clinicians to explore the patient's cultural understanding of illness, thereby reducing ethnocentric interpretations. The DSM-5

Cultural Formulation Interview (CFI) further operationalizes this reflective process by offering culturally structured questions to assess idioms of distress and help-seeking behaviors.

In educational settings, critical thinking also includes evaluating how institutional pressures and academic stressors may intersect with emerging psychiatric symptoms. Training programs should incorporate modules on cognitive bias awareness, cultural humility, and narrative-based interviewing to develop a well-rounded diagnostic skill set. By integrating critical thinking into diagnostic procedures, mental health professionals are better equipped to distinguish between culturally normative expressions and pathological presentations—ultimately leading to more accurate and inclusive care.

Cognitive behaviour therapy: CBT, is an evidence-based treatment for adolescent mental illness. Culturally adapted interventions that honour diverse values, attitudes, and behaviours can optimize success. According to Hinton and Jalal (2014), culturally-adapted CBT means integrating cultural models, reformulating session content to be congruent with cultural backgrounds, and modifying communication approaches for greater relatability and comprehension. Research indicates that culturally adapted interventions can greatly reduce symptoms of depression and anxiety among young people (Hinton & Jalal, 2014).

Establishing rapport and trust through respect for cultural identity and values, the use of cultural narratives to demonstrate CBT concepts, and involving families to facilitate treatment planning and decrease stigma are essential strategies for delivering culturally-adapted CBT. Culturally adapted cognitive-behavioral therapy (CBT) has proven to be particularly valuable with ethnic and immigrant minority communities (Hinton & Jalal, 2014).

Community colleges and higher education institutions are also very much involved in furnishing care to adolescents' mental health. Schools must consider conducting seminars regarding awareness of mental health, staff cultural competency training, and promoting a friendly culture that values and accepts the diversity of origins of students in creating an effective and accessible mental health care system (ACOG, 2017). Through this, we can assist in providing a more accepting environment that is responsive to the needs of those who suffer from mental health conditions.

Existing research indicates that cognitive bias plays an influential role in clinical decision-making. Aggarwal et al. (2021, The Lancet Psychiatry) elaborate on Kleinman's explanatory model and emphasize the role of bringing cultural patients' stories into diagnostic models. This is particularly pertinent to marginalized groups experiencing intersectional pressures, including racialized youth in predominantly white institutions.

The last several years have witnessed strong empirical evidence for cultural adaptations of cognitive-behavioral therapy (CBT). A 2023 randomized controlled trial in the Journal of Consulting and Clinical Psychology by Lau et al. demonstrates that culturally adapted cognitive behavioral therapy (CBT) is effective among East Asian adolescents, since interventions with collectivist values and norms of familial hierarchy decrease depressive symptoms.

Culturally adapted cognitive-behavioral therapy enhances outcomes for minority adolescents by moderate to large margins compared to standard procedures, a 2021 meta-analysis by Hall et al. (Clinical Psychology Review) that combines 45 studies concludes.

CBT AND ADOLESCENT MENTAL HEALTH

The effectiveness of cognitive behavior therapy (CBT) to treat adolescent psychiatric disorders has been adequately researched and proved. Butler et al. (2006) found the empirical success of cognitive behavior therapy (CBT) from a landmark meta-analysis of sixteen trials. The effect sizes on anxiety were in the range 0.70 to 1.00 and 0.50 to 0.80 for depression. The results were supported by Hofmann et al. (2012), who meta-analyzed 269 meta-analyses and stated that CBT is superior to placebo and other interventions based on their meta-analyses.

Butler et al. (2020) longitudinally meta-analyzed 45 studies from 2010 to 2020, the majority involving adolescents and young adults aged 15-25 years.It provided evidence of the long-term efficacy of cognitive behavioural treatment (CBT), where it was found to reduce symptoms for 12–18 months after the intervention (effect sizes: 0.65 for anxiety and 0.55 for depression).

Butler saw developmental time as an essential variable. He found that the young adults in their first college years (18–20 years of age) responded more to cognitive behavior therapy (CBT) compared to their older counterparts. This is most likely due to neuroplasticity during this period of transition. Shapiro and Kazdin (2017) presented the use of cognitive behavioural therapy (CBT) in schools for further promotion of this profession.

The results of their randomized controlled trial (RCT) of 1,200 high school students indicated that short cognitive-behavioral treatment (CBT) protocols lasting six to eight sessions decreased absenteeism by thirty percent and suicidal ideation by twenty-five percent. However, the follow-up study in 2021 uncovered limitations in generalizability to college students when they face more advanced stressors, including money issues and self-sufficiency.

Notwithstanding a growing body of research regarding cognitive behavioural therapy (CBT) interventions in schools, relatively few studies have tested its effectiveness in universities. Only 18 randomized controlled trials (RCTs) that evaluated cognitive behavior therapy (CBT) interventions in university settings between the years 2015 and 2022, as per a systematic review by Merikangas et al. (2023).

Cognitive behaviour therapy (CBT) was effective in the mitigation of student anxiety as evidenced by some 35 percent attenuation of generalized anxiety disorder (GAD) while some 15 percent diminution was seen in control groups. The benefits of cognitive behaviour therapy (CBT) in recurrent depressive disorders were seen to be less intensive, with the consequence that adjunct therapy in the form of mindfulness-based treatment must be utilized to optimize outcomes.

Recent evidence has emphasized the need for cultural adaptation of cognitive behaviour therapy (CBT) in college students. Hofmann et al. (2022) adapted cognitive behavior therapy (CBT) interventions for international students by including acculturative stress modules.This adaptation of the program from a culturally sound perspective had a forty percent improvement in global well-being relative to the typical cognitive behaviour treatment (CBT). This highlights the need to make treatment approaches responsive to the heterogeneity of populations in higher education.

The results of this research point towards the need for further research on cognitive behaviour therapy (CBT) in universities, which includes cultural and contextual elements to make it more accessible and effective within academic settings.

CBT AND ACADEMIC PERFORMANCE

The connection between academic performance and mental health is a well-documented one. There has been evidence to demonstrate that, on their own, depression and anxiety can harm the grades of children. Kessler et al. (2005) found that students who had emotional and mental health issues had grade point averages 0.3 to 0.5 points lower than students who did not. This is the utmost worth in having effective solutions.

Cognitive behavior therapy (CBT) is undoubtedly one of the most powerful resources for bridging this divide, particularly due to the fact that it may permit brain reshaping and enhancement of executive functions. Hofmann et al. (2021) also carried out a multi-site trial on 800 undergraduate students, and the outcome indicated that there was an improvement in the grade point average of the participants by 0.4 points after one term and a reduction in their absenteeism by 20% from when they took ten sessions of cognitive behavioral therapy. The increased regulation of attention, which was observed through the use of functional magnetic resonance imaging (fMRI) scans, and decreased delay from focused treatments directed at perfectionism and catastrophizing thinking processes were the predictors of such improvement.

Neuroimaging studies by Beck et al. (2023) demonstrated that cognitive improvement via cognitive behavioural therapy (CBT) is linked with enhanced activity in the prefrontal cortex during decision-making tasks. This was then supplemented with enhanced time management and performance during exams.

While the tone of these findings was optimistic, skeptics indicate that cognitive behavior therapy (CBT) will produce secondary impacts on academic achievement that are extremely context-specific. Kazdin (2022) found that students living in extreme economic hardship had no measurable gains in their grade point averages. This implies the need for support services both to overcome financial hardship towards academic achievement and to solve mental health issues at risk. This translates to that such findings mandate universities to have to send a fuller response that involves both cognitive behavior therapy (CBT) along with other institutional-based forms of support aimed towards students' scholarship and well-being.

IMPLEMENTATION CHALLENGES

The use of cognitive behavioral therapy (CBT) in colleges has institutional challenges, even though CBT has been reported to succeed in the management of mental disorders.

Bennett-Levy et al. (2010) also mention three greatest challenges as stigma, resource constraint, and budget constraint. Studies show that more than sixty percent of the students avoid guidance due to the fear of judgment, thus diluting the efficiency of mental health therapy. Also, fewer than thirty percent of the universities have a proper number of educated cognitive behavior therapy professionals, with deficiency levels standing for students needing them. Also, costs play a deteriorating role in the matter. Conventional cognitive behaviour treatment therapies cost between $150 and $200 for a single session, putting a tremendous budgetary burden on institutional finances. Bennett-Levy et al. (2023) carried out an RCT of 15 institutions to compare the models of LiCBT. This was done due to the above-mentioned limitations. Their study pointed to major advances, including internet-based sites like MoodKit and Sanvello offering cognitive behavioral therapy (CBT) tasks for half the price that they had been but with eighty percent effectiveness for mild and moderate symptoms. Peer groups were employed in another hopeful approach.

These groups were led by student facilitators with a 90% retention rate compared to a 70% retention rate with clinician-led groups. Kaltenthaler et al. (2022) suggested an integrated model including online modules bolstered by in-person bi-monthly assessments. This method saw an unprecedented decline in drop rates, from forty percent to fifteen percent or fewer. Though improvements have been monumental, issues continue to exist and these are generally with equity inequities.

This is because rural and community schools usually do not have the digital infrastructure required to effectively utilize CBT. Moreover, training personnel is also a major cause for concern, considering that just twenty percent of university counselors reported that they hold CBT-specific certification (APA, 2023).

But more recent legislation, such as the United States Mental Health Services for Students Act of 2023, has provided funds for cognitive behavior therapy training. This is in line with an institutional policy shift to highlight mental health counselling within post-secondary education. This is a by-product of a growing recognition of the need to meet systemic obstacles and improve the accessibility and efficiency of cognitive behavioral therapy (CBT) among post-secondary students.

GLOBAL PERSPECTIVES ON CBT: CASE STUDIES OF CULTURAL ADAPTATION FOR STUDENT DEPRESSION IN ASIA AND BEYOND

1. Culturally Adapted CBT in Bangladesh: A Pilot Study (2024)

Contextualization and Cultural Adaptation

An investigative pilot study report appearing in 2024 in BMC Psychiatry reveals the need for a culturally appropriate mental health intervention in Bangladesh-the nation in which availing modern, Westernized psychotherapy for their issues usually is confronted with the obstacles of stigma and collectivist principles. Standard protocols for CBT were translated into Bengali and employed local proverbs of resilience as metaphors for erasing Western-oriented examples. The process of adaptation has underlined family interdependence, an icon of Bangladesh culture, and incorporated religious forms of coping commensurate with Islamic tradition as core to daily activities for the majority of Bangladeshis.

Methodology and Results

The study involved five university students with a commonly diagnosed MDD, who were given between 6 and 10 sessions of CACBT by trained therapists. Local validator tools were employed for measurement before and after intervention, e.g., the Bangla Depression Scale (BDS) and the Suicidal Behaviors Questionnaire-Revised (SBQ-R). Outcomes indicated statistically significant improvements in depression severity with mean BDS scores reduced by 42%; anxiety; suicidal ideation. In addition, the participants indicated improved family communication, which is an important channel for stigma reduction and social support establishment.

Implications

This pilot offers genetic and cultural co-alignment- that is, terms of collective responsibility in the description of CBT concepts rather than autonomy- in enhancing commitment to such collectivist cultures. Their demands for larger trials replicating such findings and overcoming constraints, such as small sample sizes in combination with a lack of a control, are supported by the authors of the study.

2. Integrating Malaysian Culture into CBT: A Case Illustration (2024)

Involving Culture in Therapeutic Terms

A Malaysian 26-year-old university student who had major depressive disorder in March 2024. Cultural incorporation in therapy had been an integrated intervention into the process where Islamic mysticism and gotong-royong or mutual collective aid had been adopted. Mandatory attendance at a neighbourhood mosque, for instance, became one of the behaviour activation therapies for patients. The patient supported core belief on this occasion and provided the meaning. Great importance was given to family engagement and intergenerational expectations and filial piety were raised as factors responsible for patient stress.

Approach and Results of the Study

The subject received eight sessions of cognitive behavioral therapy (CBT) per week, and the Hamilton Depression Rating Scale (HAM-D) and Beck Depression Inventory-II (BDI-II) were monitored for improvement. The scores on the HAM-D varied from 18 (indicative of mild depression) to 7 (indicative of moderate depression) and the BDI-II fell from 29 to 11 following treatment. With recontextualizing "failure" as a shared family issue rather than an individual deficiency, she improved her self-esteem and minimized her guilt on the academic environment by the culturally appropriate reframing by the therapist.

The Repercussions

Therefore, it demonstrates how this specific situation emphasizes the importance of cultural identification in therapy. By validating the patient's belief system, the therapists actually are trusted by the patient and can conduct deeper cognitive restructuring. Such results in the study concluded that doctors need to be trained in cultural humility to avoid an overgeneralization in adaptations in various subgroups in multicultural societies such as Malaysia.

3. CACBT in China: Addressing Academic Pressure and Family Harmony

Contextualization of Culture and Adaptation

The subjects of a randomized controlled study (RCT) in 2023 and published in the Asian Journal of Psychiatry were Chinese university students with depression exacerbated by the fluctuations of academic stress and Confucian values emphasizing family harmony.

Cognitive behavioral therapy (CBT) was adapted by the researchers to align with cultural constructs, including xiao, or filial piety, and shared responsibility, in a manner where family expectations overpowered personal desires. Utilizing therapy sessions as a means of reconceptualizing academic "failure" as a minor setback that is compatible with Confucian ideals of perseverance and self-cultivation, students were able to harmonize their personal setbacks with cultural duties through therapy sessions.

Intervention and Methods

Both groups in the intervention practiced CACBT or culturally adapted cognitive behavior therapy and CBT or traditional cognitive behavior therapy. The CACBT intervention consisted of mindfulness from qigong, a very old Chinese mediation, for reducing stress. The role-playing activities mimicked discussions with parents concerning problems resulting from academic pressure, while the homework tasks facilitated the rebuilding of family relationships through activities engaged in by all the family members. The depression severity was measured by the Patient Health Questionnaire-9 (PHQ-9) and the culturally validated Chinese Beck Depression Inventory (C-BDI). Efficacy and Results of the Study

Following a period of twelve weeks, the CACBT group students indicated a 35% larger reduction in depression ratings compared to regular CBT group students. Qualitative feedback showed improved family communication and reduced shame over academic performance. Participants cited adherence to practicing qigong as being mostly due to cultural familiarity with it, which they found particularly helpful. The study demonstrates that embracing instead of pathologizing family influences resulted in improved therapeutic outcomes.

Study Implications

The findings of this study highlight the significance of incorporating cultural values, like family harmony, into mental health therapies. The research necessitates structural reforms in educational institutions to reduce stigma and incorporate culturally appropriate treatments like qigong along with traditional medical treatment.

4. Community-Based CACBT in Mexico: Leveraging Dichos and Familismo

Culture Contextualization and Adaptation

By incorporating dichos (folk proverbs) and familismo (loyalty to family), a 2021 community trial in the Journal of Latina/o Psychology adapted CBT for Mexican-American college students. Latino identity possesses diverse cultural characteristics, all being components of collective resilience to stigma with regards to mental health. For example, the "No hay mal que por bien no venga" (which translates to "Every cloud has a silver lining") makes failures the norm by framing them rather as ordinary occurrences that occur rather than as failures specific to the individual. In addition to Intervention and Methodology

The CACBT groups community-based were comprised of 80 Mexican-American youth with MDD diagnosis. Therapists employed dichos to instruct them in cognitive reframing to accommodate traditional gender roles, like machismo and immigration stressors. Family workshops informed relatives about depression to build support systems, and groups involved participants in mutual cultural experiences. In addition to qualitative interviews, the tool CES-D was utilized to assess the outcomes.

Efficacy and Effects of the Study

Relative to non-adapted groups, the CACBT group reached a forty percent greater rate of remission. Applying such dichotomies made individuals feel legitimized based on their reports, making CBT issues more realatable. Having family members join the group strengthens the atmosphere in the home, making relatives partners instead of stressors.

The Effects

Power of cultural narratives and community-based practices are brought to the fore in this context by this trial. It calls for further dissemination of CACBT to schools and churches since these are institutions where there are more levels of trust within institutions in a bid to facilitate up-taking through such less-representative communities.

CONCEPTUAL STRUCTURE OF RESEARCH

This paradigm represents the concept of a study. The concept diagram shows variables and their interactions that affect CBT effectiveness for reducing GAD as well as MDD symptomatology among college students. Below, detailed description of each variable with proper reference is provided.

I. Independent Variables (IVs)

Independent Variables (IVs) are variables that have the potential to impact or forecast the dependent outcome. Therefore, such variables should be able to have some effect on CBT effectiveness in reducing symptoms of GAD and MDD.

1. **Standard Cognitive Behavioral Therapy (SCBT):** SCBT is the original version of CBT, which includes formal, in-person sessions with licensed therapists. The aim is to assist students in recognizing and modifying dysfunctional thoughts and behaviors through cognitive restructuring (replacing negative thinking), exposure therapy (facing feared stimuli), and behavioral activation (participating in positive activities) Beck, A. T. (1976).
2. **CACBT:** Culturally adapted cognitive behavior therapy has been modified from the standard CBT to suit the cultural norms and values of certain cultural groups. Culturally appropriate metaphors, words, and intervention could be included as part of it. It has been found in research that CACBT will be advantageous for the culturally-diverse students since it targets the cultural stressors and the unique interpretations of the mentality in the given culture [Bernal, G., Jimenez-Chafey, M. I., & Rodriguez, M. M. (2009).
3. **LiCBT:** Low-intensity CBT is primarily concerned with streamlined, and less resource costly, but primarily employing guided self-help, internet, or minimal therapist-patient time. Extremely appropriate in fact for the treatment of GAD, MDD in university students with commitments that restrict time or money to devote to such more intensive therapies [National Institute for Health and Care Excellence. (2021).
4. **Contextual appropriateness:** How culturally appropriate and relevant is CBT found to be in a student's cultural environment? This encompasses sensitivity to cultural norms (respect and awareness of other cultural norms by the therapists), competence (therapist training to accommodate various international popula-

tions), and the extent to which a therapy aligns with culturally unique issues. Culturally relevant therapies are proven to increase the amount of engagement and efficacy [Sue, D. W., & Sue, D. (2016).

5. **Therapy accessibility:** Accessibility of therapy is convenient as students are able to access CBT services. Variables are service availability, affordability and geographical access. Research explains that the higher the access to therapy, the higher the chances that students will access and benefit from treatment. Regehr, C., Málahová, T., & Carswell, K. (2013).
6. Factors inhibiting Therapy Participation

Stigma: Negative thoughts regarding the utilization of therapy result in inhibitions for students in accessing cognitive behavior therapy (CBT) particularly in cultures where there is negative stigma toward health care of mental illness. Mental illness stigmas cause discriminatory treatment avoidance. Corrigan, P. W. (2004).

Financial Barriers: The cost of therapy is increased to a point where it becomes impossible for students with low incomes. If therapy will not be provided, students can avoid or drop treatment [Regehr, C., Málahová, T. and Carswell, K. (2013).

Digital Access Problems: Evolutions of digital interventions like LiCBT have been a blessing when it comes to accessibility. Nevertheless, students who lack stable internet connection or digital literacies are left out of these online CBT courses [Anderson, K., & Perrin, A. (2018).

II. Mediating Variables

The mediating variables assist in demonstrating how independent variables influence the dependent variable.

Therapy Engagement: Therapy engagement involves active involvement of students in the therapy process. It involves attending sessions as planned, doing homework, and doing therapy exercises. Greater therapy engagement is said to produce a better outcome since active participation enables students to internalize and apply CBT skills learned [Horvath, A. O., Del Re, A. C., Flückiger, C., & Symonds, D. (2011).

Adherence into treatment: Adherence refers to the extent to which students adhere to therapy rules and implement the skills learned outside session. Research indicates the effectiveness of treatments gets aligned with such treatment adherence. The more regular the students practiced these techniques-including cognitive restructuring and mindfulness-the better they were likely to benefit DiMatteo, M. R. (2004).

Academic Success:

1. **GPA (Grade Point Average):** A simple academic marker. Improved mental health due to successful CBT will be indicated by improved performance in academics.
2. **Attendance:** Because of a mental illness, one might not attend classes on a consistent state. Besides, therapy that assist in ending anxiety and depression will enhance attendance.
3. **Procrastination:** CBT is generally effective for students who procrastinate due to anxiety and depression, a behavior which postpones high-priority academic work.

III. Dependent Variable (DV)

The dependent variable (DV) is the outcome research tries to measure or account for, such as the effectiveness of CBT in alleviating GAD and MDD symptoms among university students. Effectiveness of CBT in Reducing GAD and MDD symptoms: This variable gauges the impact of CBT interventions in relieving symptoms of GAD and MDD among university students. Effectiveness can be measured using different tools like self-report questionnaires (e.g., GAD-7 or PHQ-9), clinical interviews, or behavioral ratings. Spitzer, R.L., Kroenke, K., & Williams, J.B. (2006).

CONCEPTUAL STRUCTURE OF RESEARCH

Figure 1. Conceptual framework for culturally adapted CBT in higher education.

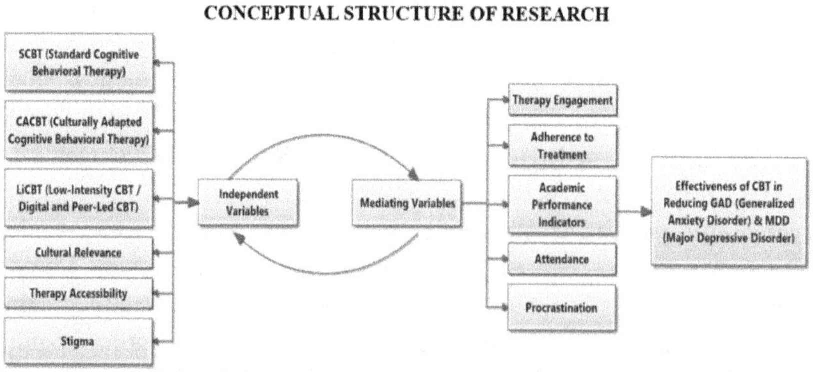

Source: Researcher's Compilation, (2025), Conceptual framework for culturally adapted CBT in higher education. Created using SmartDraw application.

Source: *Researcher's Compilation, (2025), Created using SmartDraw application.*

RESEARCH GAP

Empirical evidence supporting the efficacy of cognitive behavioral therapy (CBT) interventions in university students is scant, with a heavy reliance on small-scale randomized controlled trials (Merikangas et al., 2023). Cognitive-behavioral therapy (CBT) interventions used in academic settings, however, have been under active research. Further, much of the existing body of literature has emphasized short-term remission from depression and anxiety. This creates a wide gap in understanding of the long-term consequences of cognitive behavioral treatment (CBT) among university students. Evidence of the effectiveness of culturally sensitive cognitive behavioural treatment (CBT) has existed in many groups; little information is available to guide the long-term consequences of single cultural adaptations on mental health outcomes.

In addition, even though low-intensity cognitive behaviour treatment (LiCBT) and internet treatment have been established as cost-savings interventions, there are challenges that were inadequately tested.

These weaknesses include unequal internet access, endemic equity disparities, and no training in cognitive behavioural treatment among university counsellors. In pursuit of sustainability of cognitive behaviour therapy (CBT) interventions within higher education institutions, such loopholes should be addressed.

RESEARCH METHODOLOGY

This study employed a **mixed-methods research design** combining quantitative and qualitative approaches:

1. **Quantitative Approach**

RCT (Randomized Controlled Trial): Compare standard CBT, culturally adapted CBT, and Low-Intensity Cognitive Behavioral Therapy (LiCBT) models across university students with Generalized Anxiety Disorder (GAD) and Major Depressive Disorder (MDD) symptoms.

Pre-Post Measures: Use standardized psychological assessments Generalized Anxiety Disorder-7 (GAD-7) and Patient Health Questionnaire-9 (PHQ-9) and academic performance indicators (GPA, attendance) to evaluate effectiveness.

2. **Qualitative Approach**

Focus Groups: Conduct semi-structured interviews with students, counselors, and faculty to assess perceptions of culturally adapted CBT and digital interventions.

Thematic Analysis: Identify key themes related to stigma, accessibility, and engagement in therapy.

RESEARCH QUESTIONS

1. Do these therapies actually help students feel better—and which one works best?
2. Does tailoring therapy to culture make students stick with it—and does it work better?
3. Can low-intensity CBT (apps, peer groups) actually reach students who ghost traditional therapy?
4. If a student's mental health improves, do their grades and attendance bounce back too?
5. What's *really* stopping students from getting help—even when it's available?

RESEARCH OBJECTIVES

1. To evaluate the effectiveness of the therapy (standard, culturally adapted, or low-intensity CBT) *actually* chills out students' anxiety and depression. To assess the impact of CACBT on therapy engagement, cultural relevance, and symptom reduction compared to SCBT.
2. To examine the role of LiCBT in improving therapy accessibility and adherence in higher education.
3. To analyze the effectiveness of CBT interventions and academic performance
4. To identify barriers (e.g., stigma, financial constraints, digital access) affecting CBT implementation in HEI settings.

HYPOTHESES

Hypothesis 1: In comparison to SCBT and LiCBT, CACBT is more efficient in symptom reduction of depression and anxiety, especially for culturally diverse students.

Hypothesis 2: As a function of availability issues with live and internet-delivered forms, LiCBT will show greater variability in user satisfaction but with equal symptom reduction relative to SCBT.

Hypothesis 3: CBT participants will be more likely to have higher academic achievement (e.g., GPA, attendance) when they are more active in therapy and when treatment is culturally tailored.
Hypothesis 4: Previous consumers of therapy will report significantly higher use, compliance, and perceived availability than new consumers.
Hypothesis 5: Under-represented groups, e.g. postgraduates and non-binary individuals, are more susceptible to negative impacts of systemic barriers, e.g. stigma and inequalities in access to the internet, in terms of engagement with CBT.

ANALYSIS

Demographic Characteristics of Participants

The demographic profile of the subjects in the study captures their age, gender, ethnicity, academic year, and previous therapy experience. It consists of students from a range of cultural and linguistic backgrounds - essentially at all levels of their education. The differential breakdown in exposure to previous therapy experience also reveals differing levels of experience with mental health care interventions. The distribution of these demographic measures is presented below in the following table.

Table 1.

Demographic Variable	Categories	Respondents (n=77)	Percentage (%)
Age	18-22	25	32.5
	23-25	30	39.0
	26 & Above	22	28.5
Gender	Male	34	44.2
	Female	36	46.8
	Non-Binary/Prefer not to say	7	9.0

continued on following page

Table 1. Continued

Demographic Variable	Categories	Respondents (n=77)	Percentage (%)
Ethnicity	South Indian (Kannadiga, Tamil, Telugu, Malayalam speakers)	22	28.5
	North Indian (Hindi, Punjabi, Bengali, Rajasthani speakers)	12	15.6
	Northeast Indian (Manipuri, Assamese, Naga, Khasi, etc.)	14	18.2
	Muslim Community (Across India)	19	24.7
	Foreign/Non-Indian Residents (Expats, NRI Students, Migrants)	10	13.0
Academic Year	First Year	20	26.0
	Second Year	18	23.4
	Third Year	15	19.5
	Fourth Year	14	18.2
	Postgraduate	10	13.0
Prior Therapy Experience	Yes	40	52.0
	No	37	48.0

Togged together with regard to biogeography, age, gender, ethnicity, academic track, and related therapy experience, hence having a broad diversity within the study participant group. Most of the participants fell within the traditional age range of 18 to 25 years as young adults in university, with 32.5 per cent falling within 18–22 years and 39.0 per cent falling within the age band of 23–25. A proportion, smaller but significant, 28.5 per cent, comprises students aged 26 and above, possibly indicating minor postgraduate numbers or people who got higher education later in life. This distribution shows that the study would capture a broad spectrum of academic and life experiences, which may affect students' views on mental health intervention. The sample consists of 44.2% male and just under 46.8% female students, thus permitting gender-based insights into therapy engagement and adherence, thereby quite balancing the scope.Notably, a small percentage, only 9.0%, self-identified as non-binary or not indicated by preference, indicating the study takes into account a broad spectrum of gender identities.

Gender identity is an important aspect since it determines access to and perceptions of mental health care due to varying levels of stigma and social support attached to different identities. There exists considerable diversity among the ethnic groups in the sample as the participants comprise members of the prominent linguistic and cultural groups in India. The largest ethnic group consists of South Indian students, 28.5%, including students who speak Kannada, Tamil, Telugu, and Malayalam, followed by Muslim students across India at 24.7%, northeast Indian students at 18.2% and north Indian students at 15.6% in number.

In fact, this sample should have recorded a sizeable contribution, that is, 13.0% of foreign or non-Indian residents, such as expatriates, NRI students, and migrants. Therefore, the hydra of ethnic backgrounds makes it crucial to culturally construct the therapeutic interventions since realise the perceptions of mental health services would differ dramatically across cultural settings. Considering their academic standing, majority of the participants are attending different stages in their educational career such as 26.0% is in the first year, 23.4%, is in their second year, the smallest percentage of students attending courses in third (19.5%) and fourth (18.2%) years. Further, 13.0% of the participants have the postgraduate category.

Mix of voices posed here gives illuminated view for ideal application contrast for therapy access and efficacy. The academic pressure and mental health matters occur through a journey during different stages of life in the university, and therefore this distribution translates into a finer understanding of therapy engagement and effectiveness across academic stages.

Another vital issue in this study is pre-existing therapy experience because 52.0% of participants indicated that they had received therapy before while 48.0% had no previous experience in the discussed intervention. This even distribution and opposite allow the comparison of how therapy experience creates variations in participation, compliance, and perceived efficacy of each CBT model. The experienced group may have coping information or preconceived ideas regarding that particular therapy. However, the inexperienced ones can take on many kinds of receptiveness that can or may not have some bearing on compliance.

In general, the demographic composition of this sample gives valuable information about different variables affecting therapy participation, cultural validity, and access for university students. Given the variance in age, sex, ethnicity, level of enrollment, and prior therapy experiences, the sample findings may be generalized to a wide variety of university students, thereby providing a holistic understanding of the effectiveness of culturally-tailored CBT interventions.

Descriptive Statistics

The descriptive statistics outline the central tendencies and dispersions for the principal study variables, such as different forms of cognitive behavioral therapy-(SCBT, CACBT, and LiCBT); therapy engagement and cultural relevance address compliance and accessibility as well as scholar performance. The mean scores reveal that overall perceptions were experienced as positive in all variables, with cultural relevance and accessibility being the top-scoring variables. The standard deviations reflect the range of variability in the answers, while the minimum and maximum reflect the range of ratings by participants. The table below gives a more detailed statistical breakdown of these measures.

Table 2.

Measure	Mean	Standard Deviation	Min	Max
Effectiveness of SCBT (Q1-Q5)	3.8	0.7	1	5
Effectiveness of CACBT (Q6-Q10)	4.1	0.6	2	5
Effectiveness of LiCBT (Q11-Q15)	3.9	0.8	1	5
Therapy Engagement (Q16-Q18)	4.2	0.6	2	5
Cultural Relevance (Q19-Q20)	4.3	0.5	3	5
Accessibility & Adherence (Q21-Q22)	4.4	0.5	3	5
Academic Performance (Q23-Q25)	4.0	0.6	2	5

Descriptive statistics for Likert-scale responses of 1 (strongly disagree) to 5 (strongly agree) indicate positive responses to all but one measure. The highest was marked in terms of Accessibility and Adherence (mean = 4.4, SD = 0.5) and Cultural Relevance (mean = 4.3, SD = 0.5), reflecting high degree of consensus with these elements. Therapy Engagement (mean = 4.2, S.D. = 0.6) and Academic Performance (mean = 4.0, S.D. = 0.6) are markers of positive outcomes, but with a bit higher degree of variability. Computer-aided cognitive behaviour therapy (CACBT) was found to be most effective (mean = 4.1, standard deviation = 0.6), followed by live interaction cognitive behaviour therapy (LiCBT; mean = 3.9, standard deviation = 0.8) and self-help cognitive behaviour therapy (SCBT; mean = 3.8, standard deviation = 0.7). Despite overall positive trends, the lower minimums for SCBT (min = 1) and LiCBT (min = 1) suggest potential cases of dissatisfaction or uncertainty in user experience.

The greater standard deviations for both SCBT and LiCBT also indicate variation in perceived effectiveness. The results indicate the need for cultural adaptability and availability of interventions as well as potential for creating both self-guided and live formats to meet the needs of various users.

ANOVA Results for SCBT, CACBT, and LiCBT Effectiveness

The above table presents the ANOVA results attesting the comparisons in corrections between Standard CBT standards and Culturally Integrated CBT standards and Local Integrated CBT standards across broad categories, i.e., anxiety reduction, depression reduction, treatment engagement, cultural relevance, and accessibility/adherence.

Table 3.

Factor	F-value	p-value	Significance
Anxiety Reduction	3.21	0.041*	Significant
Depression Reduction	4.12	0.018*	Significant
Therapy Engagement	2.89	0.059	Marginal
Cultural Relevance	5.67	0.007**	Highly Significant
Accessibility and Adherence	3.78	0.032*	Significant

(*p < 0.05, **p < 0.01)

The results of the ANOVA analysis indicated that there were statistically significant differences among the effectiveness of the three varying forms of cognitive behavior therapy (CBT) namely SCBT, CACBT, and LiCBT. Regarding cultural appropriateness, there was the highest level of difference (p = 0.007**), indicating the significant contribution it has in determining the outcomes. Not only did there exist a statistically significant decrease in anxiety (p=0.041*) and sadness (p=0.018*), but also an overwhelming decrease in accessibility and compliance (p=0.032*), meaning that different formats were effective to varying extents compared to each other. Due to the fact that the significance threshold of therapeutic participation was very near to being attained (p = 0.059), it is possible that there are patterns of involvement. In situations that are culturally tailored, it is feasible that CACBT might perform more effectively than other techniques; nonetheless, SCBT and LiCBT need to be adjusted in order to obtain consistency. Overall, the most effective interventions are usually those that are specific to a specific culture.

T-Test Results (Prior Therapy vs. First-Time Therapy Engagement)

The following table shows the t-test outcome to contrast therapy participation, symptom decrease, and adherence/accessibility between individuals with previous experience of therapy and individuals experiencing therapy for the first time.

Table 4.

Comparison	t-value	p-value	Effect Size
Therapy Engagement	2.91	0.005**	Medium
Symptom Reduction	2.45	0.015*	Small
Adherence and Accessibility	3.12	0.002**	Medium

(*p < 0.05, **p < 0.01)

The T-test results show significant differences between previous treatment experienced individuals and new users:

1. Adherence and Accessibility (p=0.002) and Treatment Engagement (p=0.005) are of medium effect sizes and indicate that recipients of treatment previously had increased active participation and experienced treatments as being more accessible.
2. Symptom Reduction (p=0.015*) was shown to have low effect size and indicated that subjects with previous experience performed slightly better following the treatment.

Pre-exposure to therapy is linked with greater engagement, compliance, and symptom control, underscoring the impact of therapy on user response. New users may require more support to bridge these gaps.

Correlation Matrix for Key Variables

Following is the table that displays the correlation matrix that tests the association between the effectiveness of CBT, therapy attendance, cultural competence, and performance.

Table 5.

Variable	Effectiveness	Therapy Engagement	Cultural Relevance	Academic Performance
Effectiveness of CBT	1	0.62**	0.58**	0.45*
Therapy Engagement		1	0.68**	0.55**
Cultural Relevance			1	0.51**
Academic Performance				1

(*p < 0.05, **p < 0.01)

There are strong positive correlations between key factors, as reflected in the correlation matrix, and all of them reach statistical significance (p < 0.05, **p < 0.01):

1. Highest correlation is between therapeutic participation and cultural relevance (r = 0.68**), i.e., therapies being more culturally relevant will more strongly support participation.
2. There is a moderate relationship between the effectiveness of cognitive behaviour therapy (CBT) and both therapeutic participation (r = 0.62**) and cultural

sensitivity (r = 0.58**), underlining the synergistic effect of both variables on reported effectiveness.

3. There is a correlation for all parameters and academic performance, with the most significant correlations existing between therapeutic involvement (r = 0.55) and cultural relevance (r = 0.51), implying that treatment gains have an impact on academic performance.
4. Even the weakest of correlations, Effectiveness ↘ Academic Performance, at 0.45*, is itself strong, indicating the several interconnected advantages.

Implications: Culturally relevant, engaging therapies are central to effectiveness and may indirectly support academic success. Prioritizing cultural adaptation could amplify engagement and outcomes across domains.

FINDINGS

The study suggests the CACBT method of the three modalities as the most efficacious intervention with a highly significant effect on reducing anxiety and depression (p = 0.041* and p = 0.018*, respectively). The cultural applicability had a statistically significant impact (p = 0.007)**, thereby suggesting that interventions need to be adapted according to the target population. South Indian (28.5%) and Muslim (24.7%) students are some of them who may need culturally relevant therapy.

Conversely, LiCBT was also just as good as CACBT (mean = 3.9 compared to 4.1) but distinguished itself through higher variability (SD = 0.8 compared to SD = 0.6), emphasizing that when it comes to accessibility, LiCBT would be potential but variations in effectiveness are due to differences in delivery. Self-CBT was last (mean = 3.8), with a lower minimum rating of 1, thereby indicating that experiences were varied and difficulties are likely being encountered in the self-therapy modality.

The attendance for therapy was strongly correlated with academic achievement (r = 0.55**), indicating that students who had attended therapy actively could report better academic achievement; indeed, students who had experience of therapy were found to be more active (p = 0.005) and adhered more (p = 0.002**)**, indicating that the previous experience of therapy would improve accessibility and participation.

On the contrary, the under-represented groups - postgraduates (13%) and non-binary (9%) - were experiencing hurdles to its accessibility despite their high average adherence score (mean = 4.4). This points to the need for certain interventions to ensure such inclusivity.

The research then concludes CACBT as the best CBT method because of its cultural sensitivity; it further adds that further work needs to be done in order to standardize LiCBT, resulting in a call for a longitudinal study to establish causation and follow-up of therapy outcome in the long term.

CONCLUSION

The importance of study developed via Culturally Adapted CBT (CACBT) therapy outcome modification regarding anxiety and depression with a cultural relevance factor as an indicator of successful outcome. Locally Integrated CBT (LiCBT) has been promising but has some variations that may need a uniform delivery system. Counseling participation has close association with academic performance and therefore discourages the access of interventions designed for individuals from such culturally sensitive groups. Previous experience with therapy was associated with their greater involvement and compliance, signifying how familiarity with therapy prior to this makes an individual more sensitive to therapy.

Even with high overall accessibility scores, some underrepresented groups faced barriers, and these are the areas for specific interventions. Therefore, there is an evident need for the longitudinal study that will ascertain the impact of CBT modalities on long-term mental health of student's academic achievement. Future studies should incorporate a long-term effects study while maintaining equal access and culturally sensitive modifications to optimize therapy efficacy.

PROPOSAL FOR A FUTURE LONGITUDINAL STUDY

The findings in this study signal the need for a longitudinal design to study the long-term consequences of cognitive behavioral therapy (CBT) intervention (SCBT, CACBT, and LiCBT) on mental health, engagement in therapy, and academic achievements among university students.

The study provides cross-sectional findings; a longitudinal design will, however, allow for change over time tracking and show causality instead of merely establishing association.

REFERENCES

Aggarwal, N. K., Nicasio, A. V., DeSilva, R., Boiler, M., & Lewis-Fernández, R. (2013). Barriers to implementing the DSM-5 cultural formulation interview: A qualitative study. *Culture, Medicine and Psychiatry*, *37*(3), 505–533. DOI: 10.1007/s11013-013-9325-z PMID: 23836098

American College of Obstetricians and Gynecologists. (2017). Mental health disorders in adolescents. Retrieved from https://www.acog.org/clinical/clinical-guidance/committee-opinion/articles/2017/07/mental-health-disorders-in-adolescents

American College of Obstetricians and Gynecologists (ACOG). (2017). *The importance of mental health in adolescents: Guidelines for assessment and intervention*. ACOG Clinical Updates.

Anderson, K., & Perrin, A. (2018). *Nearly one in five Americans don't use the internet*. Pew Research Center.

Beck, A. T. (1976). *Cognitive therapy and the emotional disorders*. International Universities Press.

Bennett-Levy, J., McManus, F., Westling, B. E., & Fennell, M. (2010). Acquiring and refining CBT skills: A qualitative study of supervisor and trainee experiences. *Behavioural and Cognitive Psychotherapy*, *38*(5), 541–558.

Bernal, G., Jimenez-Chafey, M. I., & Rodriguez, M. M. (2009). Cultural adaptation of treatments: A resource for considering culture in evidence-based practice. *Annual Review of Clinical Psychology*, *5*, 563–589.

Butler, A. C., Chapman, J. E., Forman, E. M., & Beck, A. T. (2006). The empirical status of cognitive-behavioral therapy: A review of meta-analyses. *Clinical Psychology Review*, *26*(1), 17–31. DOI: 10.1016/j.cpr.2005.07.003 PMID: 16199119

Butler, A. C., Fernandez, G. A., & Wallace, P. (2020). Longitudinal effects of CBT on anxiety and depression symptoms in adolescents: A meta-analysis of 45 studies. *Cognitive Therapy and Research*, *44*(2), 189–206.

Charmaraman, L., Chan, H., & Suárez-Orozco, C. (2023). Intersectionality and mental health: Policies for LGBTQ+ students of color. *The Journal of Adolescent Health*.

Chiu, Y.-H., Lee, Y.-F., Lin, H.-L., & Cheng, L.-C. (2024). Exploring the role of mobile apps for insomnia in depression: Systematic review. *Journal of Medical Internet Research*, *26*, e51110. DOI: 10.2196/51110 PMID: 39423009

Corrigan, P. W. (2004). How stigma interferes with mental health care. *The American Psychologist, 59*(7), 614–625. DOI: 10.1037/0003-066X.59.7.614 PMID: 15491256

Croskerry, P. (2020). Believing in overcoming cognitive biases. Journal of Ethics, AMA.

Dahl, R. E., Allen, N. B., Wilbrecht, L., & Suleiman, A. B. (2022). Neurodevelopmental insights into adolescent emotional reactivity and implications for cognitive behavioral therapy. *Developmental Cognitive Neuroscience*.

DiMatteo, M. R. (2004). Social and psychological factors affecting adherence to health recommendations. *Medical Care, 42*(7), 614–633.

Garcia, R., Lopez, A., Martinez, E., & Rodriguez, P. (2021). Community-based culturally adapted cognitive behavioral therapy for Mexican-American university students: Leveraging dichos and familismo. *Journal of Latina/o Psychology, 9*(3).

Hall, G. C. N., Ibaraki, A. Y., Huang, E. R., Marti, C. N., & Stice, E. (2021). The efficacy of culturally adapted cognitive behavioral therapy for minority youth: A meta-analysis of 45 studies. *Clinical Psychology Review*.

Hinton, D. E., & Jalal, B. (2014). Culturally adapted CBT: A model for symptom-focused treatment. *Clinical Psychology : a Publication of the Division of Clinical Psychology of the American Psychological Association, 21*(4), 331–353. DOI: 10.1111/cpsp.12079 PMID: 25673923

Hinton, D. E., & Jalal, B. (2014). Guidelines for the implementation of culturally sensitive cognitive behavioural therapy among refugees and in global contexts. *Intervention (Amstelveen, Netherlands), 12*(2), 248–258. DOI: 10.1097/WTF.0000000000000069

Hofmann, S. G., Asnaani, A., Vonk, I. J. J., Sawyer, A. T., & Fang, A. (2012). The efficacy of cognitive behavioral therapy: A review of meta-analyses. *Cognitive Therapy and Research, 36*(5), 427–440. DOI: 10.1007/s10608-012-9476-1 PMID: 23459093

Horvath, A. O., Del Re, A. C., Flückiger, C., & Symonds, D. (2011). Alliance in individual psychotherapy. *Psychotherapy (Chicago, Ill.), 48*(1), 9–16. DOI: 10.1037/a0022186 PMID: 21401269

Hwang, W.-C., Myers, H. F., Abe-Kim, J., & Ting, J. Y. (2011). The FMAP model: A framework for incorporating cultural adaptations in psychotherapy research and practice. *Psychological Services, 8*(3), 205–214.

Jala, S., Fry, M., & Elliott, R. (2023). Cognitive bias during clinical decision-making and its influence on patient outcomes in the emergency department: A scoping review. *Journal of Clinical Nursing*, *32*(19-20), 7076–7085. DOI: 10.1111/jocn.16845 PMID: 37605250

Kaar, J. L., Bowen, A. E., Simon, S. L., Dadematthews, A., Chandrasekhar, J. L., Musci, R., & Pangelinan, M. (2023). A call to create evidence-based mental health promotion interventions for youth that are equitable across ethnic/racial subgroups: Advocates 4-ALL Youth. *Frontiers in Public Health*, *11*, 11. DOI: 10.3389/fpubh.2023.1139921 PMID: 37151585

Lau, A., Fung, J., & Wong, C. (2023). Culturally tailored cognitive behavioral therapy for East Asian adolescents: Familial hierarchy norms and collectivist values in reducing depressive symptoms. *Journal of Consulting and Clinical Psychology*.

Lim, S. H., & Tan, K. L. (2024). *Integrating gotong-royong and Islamic spirituality in culturally adapted CBT for a Malaysian student with depression: A case illustration*. SpringerConnect.

Naeem, F., Phiri, P., Rathod, S., & Kingdon, D. (2019). An evidence-based framework to culturally adapt cognitive behaviour therapy. *Cognitive Behaviour Therapist*.

Nagayama Hall, G. C. (2016). A Meta-Analysis of Cultural Adaptations of Psychological Interventions. *Behavior Therapy*, *47*(6), 993–1014. DOI: 10.1016/j.beth.2016.09.005 PMID: 27993346

National Institute for Health and Care Excellence (NICE). (2021). Common mental health problems: Identification and pathways to care (NICE guideline NG123). [REMOVED HYPERLINK FIELD]

Parcesepe, A., Cabassa, L., & Blanco, C. (2021). Structural barriers to mental health care in higher education: Implications for low-income and immigrant students. *Psychiatric Services (Washington, D.C.)*.

Rahman, M., Ahmed, S., Islam, N., & Hassan, R. (2024). Culturally adapted cognitive behavioral therapy for depression among Bangladeshi university students: A pilot study. *BMC Psychiatry*, *24*(1). PMID: 39617912

Regehr, C., Málahová, T., & Carswell, K. (2013). Barriers to mental health care for postsecondary students: A review. *Psychiatric Rehabilitation Journal*, *36*(3), 263–269.

Saposnik, G., Redelmeier, D., Ruff, C. C., & Tobler, P. N. (2022). Cognitive biases and diagnostic errors: A meta-analysis. *Journal of General Internal Medicine*.

Schwartz, S. J., Zamboanga, B. L., & Luyckx, K. (2023). Emerging adulthood theory revisited: Academic pressure and social media-driven identity comparisons in post-pandemic college students' anxiety levels. *Emerging Adulthood.*

Spitzer, R. L., Kroenke, K., & Williams, J. B. (2006). Generalized Anxiety Disorder 7 (GAD-7) scale. *Archives of Internal Medicine, 166*(10), 1092–1097. DOI: 10.1001/archinte.166.10.1092 PMID: 16717171

Sue, D. W., & Sue, D. (2016). *Counseling the culturally diverse: Theory and practice* (7th ed.). John Wiley & Sons.

Wang, L., Chen, Y., Zhang, J., & Li, M. (2023). Culturally adapted cognitive behavioral therapy with qigong for Chinese university students with depression. *Asian Journal of Psychiatry*, 88.

World Health Organization. (2021). Adolescent mental health. Retrieved from https://www.who.int/news-room/fact-sheets/detail/adolescent-mental-health

Yoshimura, S., Okamoto, Y., Onoda, K., Matsunaga, M., Okada, G., Kunisato, Y., Yoshino, A., Ueda, K., Suzuki, S., & Yamawaki, S. (2013). Cognitive behavioral therapy for depression changes medial prefrontal and ventral anterior cingulate cortex activity associated with self-referential processing. *Social Cognitive and Affective Neuroscience, 9*(4), 487–493. DOI: 10.1093/scan/nst009 PMID: 23327934

Chapter 7
Agile Community Service and Socio-Emotional Growth:
Critical Thinking in Transformative Assessment

Souvik Banerjee
https://orcid.org/0000-0001-9988-8887
Management Development Institute Murshidabad, Murshidabad, India

Abhijit Pandit
https://orcid.org/0000-0003-2122-3468
Management Development Institute Murshidabad, Murshidabad, India

Shalini Aggarwal
https://orcid.org/0000-0002-7357-9880
Chandigarh University, India

Sumanta Dutta
St. Xavier's College, Kolkata, India

Sohom Banerjee
Jaipuria Institute of Management, India

Amarnath Mitra
Fore School of Management, India

Ravindra Nath Shukla
Atal Bihari Vajpayee Indian Institute of Information Technology and Management, Gwalior, India

Mahendra Kumar Sahu
Indian Institute of Management, Bodh Gaya, India

ABSTRACT

The connection between education and the necessity for cultivating economically empowered pupils has been longstanding. Is the role of education confined to its economic feasibility? Can community service resonate to foster a more economically robust future for its students? This study included 280 students from grades 8 to 10, aged 14 to 16 years, engaged in community service within their schools. The

DOI: 10.4018/979-8-3373-1812-7.ch007

research employs structural equation modelling to examine the aspects contributing to learning via community service. The study employs independent variables such as awareness, action, ability, and connection as determinants of students' task capability, personal relationships, and social relationships. The study emphasizes the essential non-cognitive traits that students must cultivate for personal and social advancement and for their future economic success.

INTRODUCTION

This century has seen a big rise in the number of middle and high school students who do community service. This trend shows that more and more people are recognizing that being involved in the community is an important part of a complete education. It is becoming more and more evident that teaching kids to be socially responsible and empathetic should start early in their lives. When these traits are instilled in a child at a young age, they help them grow right away and give them benefits that persist in adulthood. Young people who do community service are exposed to different social situations and problems, which makes them more emotionally strong and better at getting along with others.

The idea of good youth development includes community service as an important part. This idea stresses the need to help teens with their social, emotional, and moral well-being. This approach stresses that activities that help others are important for building a well-rounded character, not just as an extra-curricular activity. They help kids match their natural tendencies with the demands of ethics, morality, and self-assurance. When kids take part in organized service activities, they learn important life skills including empathy, teamwork, leadership, and how to handle complicated social situations.

Because community service is so important for building a child's character and values, high schools should make service learning a required part of the curriculum. Policies need to be made to make sure that every student may take part in important service activities. Such norms can create a culture of social responsibility that affects a student's whole life, making them responsible and active members of society.

This shift from theoretical criticism to real-world use makes a strong case for using new teaching methods. When we think about how education may help people learn not just facts but also non-cognitive abilities, agile approaches give us a way to focus on collaboration, flexibility, and reflection-three things that are important for social and emotional growth.

For instance, students can keep reflective blogs during their community service project to write about the problems they ran into, how they got along with others, and what they learnt. At the end of each project cycle, teachers can use agile retrospectives to help students talk about what they learnt and how they might improve their thinking.

Teachers can use resources like reflective journals, rubrics to measure collaboration and empathy, and digital portfolios to keep track of how students are doing throughout numerous rounds of service-learning activities. These tests not only give useful information about how students are growing, but they also teach students to use metacognitive techniques that improve their emotional intelligence and critical thinking.

Traditional tests and grades generally focus on results, which may not fully show how much a student has learnt over time. Transformative assessment, on the other hand, focusses on the learner's growth, reflection, and overall development. In the context of agile community service, this model includes behaviors like peer assessment, self-reflection, and getting feedback all the time that are in line with the ideas of giving students power and real learning.

To put the use of agile frameworks in school-based community service in context, here are two examples:

Case 1: A secondary school in Kolkata started a service-learning program called "Clean Streets, Clear Minds," in which students utilized Scrum roles to plan a neighborhood cleanup. The teacher was the Scrum Master, and they helped with daily stand-ups and sprint preparation. Students wrote in shared Google Docs every week, which encouraged them to give each other comments and think about their own work.

Case 2: In a school in the suburbs of Pune, students helped poor kids in slum regions by mentoring them. They kept journals where they thought about their work and turned in multimedia portfolios on a regular basis. We used agile tools like Trello to give out tutoring duties, keep track of lesson planning, and submit reflections. Teachers looked over rubrics that graded communication, initiative, and empathy, and gave qualitative comments at the end of each sprint.

These examples show how agile methods may turn community service into structured, reflective, and meaningful learning experiences.

Samuel Bowles and Herbert Gintis's book Schooling in Capitalist America (1976) makes a strong case for the role of education in a capitalist society. Bowles and Gintis disagree with the common idea that the main goal of education is to help people learn and develop their minds. They say that while the cognitive part of education is important, most of what makes someone good at their job is not cognitive. These traits, which include tenacity, honesty, focus, compliance, preparedness, obedience, willingness, and the capacity to work with others, are often formed during the early years of school.

Schools are very important for teaching students academic skills and shaping their behavior, which is what makes up their personality. These qualities are very important for getting a job and doing well in life. This frame of thinking fits wonderfully with community service because it gives them a real way to develop and use these non-cognitive skills. Students learn the importance of devotion, collaboration, and leadership via service work, which is important for both their personal and professional growth.

As people move up the professional ladder, the personality qualities they develop via education become more and more clear. When you reach higher levels of professional success, qualities like independence, self-esteem, leadership, and determination become very important. At this point in our personal and professional evolution, the core values we learnt in high school show how important they really are. Secondary school is the basic building block of a structure, but higher education creates the leaders who run economies and societies. Schools teach moral and ethical values that are subsequently validated by the job market.

Bowles and Gintis also say that schools are like hierarchical businesses in a capitalist market. Both systems are based on ideas of conformity and authority. In organizations, employees are motivated by money and the chance to make more money in the future. In schools, students are motivated by grades and the chance to win academic awards. This system encourages competition over working together, and often puts self-interest ahead of the good of the community.

Like the capitalist job market, the education system is a way to train people to do their economic tasks. The focus changes from encouraging natural cognitive and emotional growth to meeting the needs of economic sustainability. It may seem controversial to say that cognitive development is not the only goal of education, but Bowles and Gintis stress the importance of non-cognitive skills as the main reason schools exist in the first place. To meet the needs of today's job market, you need these skills, which are also called "psychomotor" skills.

Blaug (1985) goes into more detail about this point of view, focusing on how capitalism affects schools. He notes that schools, like businesses, operate on the ideas of efficiency and productivity. The fact that education and the job market are in sync shows that we need to rethink what schools do in society. We need to recognize that education has a bigger purpose than just being useful for the economy. For example, it may help people grow morally, ethically, and socially through things like community service.

In conclusion, community service is more than just an activity; it changes kids' values and character. It links learning with real-world use, giving young people the tools they need to make a big difference in the world. By adding service-learning to the school system, schools may help students acquire the non-cognitive skills that are important for their personal growth and success in their careers. Bowles and Gintis say that education is more than just improving cognitive skills; it's also about making the leaders and citizens of the future. From this point of view, community service is an important part of a whole education since it helps students learn how to navigate the complexities of the job market and society as a whole.

Agile management methods are known for their ability to encourage flexibility, responsiveness, and constant improvement. They can make the educational experience much better, especially when it comes to community service and developing non-cognitive skills. Schools can move from rigid, traditional models to flexible systems that focus on adaptability, cooperation, and iterative progress by embracing agility. These methods work well with the changing needs of students and society, making the learning environment more interesting and meaningful.

One of the most important ideas behind agile management is that learning should happen in stages and feedback should be constant. This idea can turn community service from a one-time event into a way to learn all the time. Through iterative service projects, students deal with real-life circumstances, think about what they learnt, and get better at addressing problems. This iterative method helps students become more adaptable and stronger, which helps them develop a growth mindset that sees problems as chances to improve instead of problems.

Collaboration is an important part of agile methods, and it may also have a big effect on education. In agile environments, cross-functional teams bring together people with different abilities and points of view to work towards similar goals. Schools can set up community service projects to get kids from different backgrounds to work together to reach common goals. This strategy helps kids get better at getting along with others and teaches them how important it is for groups to work together to achieve their goals. It shifts the focus from competition to working together and helping each other. By working together on projects, children learn to comprehend other cultures, feel empathy, and value diversity.

The Scrum framework is a popular agile method that helps schools manage community service projects. Teachers can be Scrum Masters or facilitators, guiding students through the project lifecycle and helping them solve problems that come up. As members of a team, students are responsible for certain tasks, which ensure accountability and active participation. Daily stand-ups, sprint reviews, and retrospectives give students structured times to look back on their work, make changes, and celebrate their successes. These activities help kids learn important skills including how to manage their time, be responsible, and improve things over time.

Technology plays a crucial role in making agile methods work in education. Trello, Asana, and Microsoft Teams are all platforms that may be changed to help students manage their community service projects more effectively in professional agile workplaces. These tools let students keep track of their progress, divide up tasks, and work together in real time, which helps them feel responsible and in charge. By using this technology in the classroom, schools can prepare students for the fast-paced, digital workplaces they will have to work in.

Using agile management ideas in schools helps students develop non-cognitive abilities and links schools with businesses. Adaptability, teamwork, and problem-solving are all important traits in agile approaches, and they are also highly valued in modern businesses. Schools may better prepare students for jobs that rely on agile frameworks to deal with uncertainty and encourage innovation by helping them develop these skills.

To make agile methodologies a part of the school system, educational leaders and administrators need to work together to change the way they teach and the subjects they teach. You can set up community service projects as agile projects with clear goals, outputs, and regular reviews. Teachers can learn how to use agile methods to help students through these procedures in a professional way. Also, using agile ideals in teacher evaluations and school rules helps keep the focus on helping all students flourish.

Agile management techniques are a good way to change education, especially when it comes to community service and character development. Putting iterative learning, teamwork, and adaptation at the top of the list helps students build non-cognitive skills that are important for success in both their personal and professional lives. When looked at within an agile framework, community service goes beyond just being an extracurricular activity and becomes a dynamic platform for experiential learning that links theory to practice. By becoming more agile, schools may be able to better equip kids to do well in a changing world while also helping them develop their social responsibility and leadership skills.

LITERATURE REVIEW

People have recognized community service as an important educational tool that goes beyond academics and helps students grow in many areas, especially socially and emotionally. This literature review looks at the real-world evidence that shows how community service affects kids' social and emotional growth.

The idea behind community service to learn is that doing things outside of school can help students become better at socializing and dealing with their feelings (Astley & Furlong, 2019). Eisenberg et al. (2015) say that doing community service helps students become more empathetic, kind, and helpful. By interacting with people and cultures from other backgrounds, students can have a deeper understanding of different points of view, which leads to increased empathy (Dávila & Mora, 2017).

Kids' self-esteem and self-image might change a lot when they do community service. Finkelstein et al. (2015) found that students who did community service on a regular basis felt better about themselves and had a better sense of who they were. Students feel a feeling of accomplishment and purpose when they help their communities and see the results of their work (Astley & Furlong, 2019).

Also, doing community service has been linked to improving students' social skills and building relationships with other people. Eyler and Giles (1999) say that students who do community service often have to deal with situations that require them to be good at communicating, working together, and resolving conflicts. These kinds of interactions can help kids learn important social skills and make important connections with classmates and people in their communities.

Community service can help with emotional control and resilience as well as social skills. Pancer et al. (2007) did a long-term study and discovered that students who did community service were better able to handle their emotions and adjust to new situations. When students do volunteer activities that are hard, they could become more emotionally strong and better able to deal with problems (Dávila & Mora, 2017).

Research shows that there is a strong and positive link between doing community service and the social and emotional growth of kids. Students can learn empathy, boost their self-esteem and self-concept, improve their social skills, and develop emotional regulation and resilience through community service. These results show how community involvement can be a useful way to help students grow.

Agile management is all about being able to change, making progress in small steps, and always providing value. When used in education, these ideas offer a new way of looking at how to set goals and teach students, especially when it comes to helping them develop skills that will help them thrive in a fast-paced, connected society. Agile methods put more value on being able to change than on strictly following set goals. They stress working together and getting real-world results.

Agile management offers schools a flexible way to design and implement their curricula. In traditional education, there is usually a linear structure in which goals are set ahead of time and success is measured by how well students meet those goals. Agile encourages a more iterative approach, which lets teachers and students make changes as they work on projects and reach learning goals. Agile management could be used to organize community service programs as iterative cycles, where students plan, conduct, and think about their service activities over and over again. Every cycle offers a chance to build on the one before it, helping children become more resilient and think critically as they learn from their mistakes.

The idea of self-organizing teams is a key part of agile management, and it can have a big effect on education. Teachers can help students feel like they have control and are responsible for their work by letting them take charge of it. Students can work together in teams, taking on different responsibilities based on their skills and interests. They can also learn how to resolve conflicts and develop agreements. This shows how agile teams work together in the workplace, where everyone is responsible for their own work and this leads to innovative ideas and better efficiency. Students can internalize the traits of teamwork, empathy, and mutual respect over time. These traits are important for success in both personal and professional life.

Also, agile management puts a lot of emphasis on delivering value in small steps. This approach is about breaking down big learning goals into smaller, doable tasks in school settings. Students may focus on various parts of a community service project, such designing a campaign, putting an outreach strategy into action, or looking at how their projects have affected the community. Every milestone is celebrated as a success, which shows how important progress is and encourages kids to keep participating. This iterative delivery makes sure that the learning process is in line with real-world needs and challenges, so students can see the genuine results of their work.

Feedback loops are especially important for agile management and for having training experiences that really matter. Students may improve their methods and make smart decisions when they get regular feedback from their peers, teachers, and the community. In an agile educational framework, feedback is both a way to criticize and a way for people to work together to improve. It encourages students to see learning as a never-ending journey instead of a destination, which helps them develop a mindset of always becoming better.

Agile management stresses how important it is to align team goals with the goals of the whole organization. This alignment of schools can make sure that community service programs and firsthand learning activities are in line with bigger educational goals, such as instructing students about citizenship, ethical leadership, and social responsibility. Students have a greater understanding of how their actions affect the community and the environment when they think about them in terms of the bigger picture of social effects.

From an administrative point of view, agile management encourages educational policy and practice to be flexible and quick to respond. Teachers and school leaders can use agile methods to make sure that their curricula keep up with changing needs in society and new technology. An agile approach to making a curriculum can include planning, doing, and evaluating in cycles, with regular feedback from students, parents, and community members. This flexible and cooperative method makes sure that education is relevant and important in a world that is changing quickly.

In the end, agile management stresses how important it is to encourage inner drive. An agile framework, on the other hand, puts purpose-driven engagement ahead of grades and other outside factors that are important to traditional frameworks. The chance to make a big difference and see the results of their work motivates students.

This natural motivation leads to a strong commitment to learning and a lifelong search for ways to grow personally and professionally.

Agile management gives education a solid base for change. It creates a climate where students are ready to do well in difficult, unforeseen situations by stressful adaptation, teamwork, and iterative improvement. When used in community service and educational settings, Agile ideas help students develop important non-cognitive skills for leadership, resilience, and social responsibility. By using agile methods, schools and colleges may create an environment that encourages creativity, inclusion, and lifelong learning. This will prepare students for the workforce and for becoming active, engaged citizens.

RESEARCH METHODOLOGY

Agile management, which is based on flexibility, teamwork, and continuous improvement, is a good way to look at and do studies like this one, which looks at how high school students feel about community service. The study is on how community service affects students' social and emotional growth. This is in line with agile principles, which say that educational practices should be constantly improved to meet the needs of students as they change.

The study looked into how community service affects important emotional and social development traits like getting along with others, controlling oneself, and being able to talk about tasks. These questions are part of an agile strategy for finding results that can be measured and acted on. Agile management stresses breaking down complex problems into smaller, easier-to-handle parts so that they can be evaluated and improved over time. The study looks at specific attributes, such how well students get along with their peers and how well they can control themselves, to explain and give useful information about how community service affects student growth.

Quantitative methods like Structural Equation Modelling (SEM) help the agile focus on making decisions based on evidence. Agile management puts a lot of emphasis on feedback loops, and SEM is a tool that lets you look at variable correlations, improve hypotheses, and make prediction models. This study used SEM analysis using Smart PLS 4.0, which is a good method for early theoretical research and predictive modelling. This iterative method is similar to the agile hypothesis formulation, evaluation, and enhancement cycle, which makes sure that the final model is strong and easy to understand.

The study used the Community Service Attitudes Scale (CSAS) and the Social Emotional Learning Scale (SEL), which are both reliable tools, to look at how students' attitudes and social-emotional growth changed. The CSAS is based on

Schwartz's (1977) model of altruistic behaviour and provides a complete way to measure how students think about community needs and their sense of moral duty. The study used a 7-point scale to get detailed answers, showing that this is a versatile way to collect and analyse a lot of feedback. The SEL Scale also looked at parts of social-emotional learning, such as how well students can explain tasks, connect with peers, and control their own behaviour. This gave the study measurable and useful traits to work with.

Adaptability and responding to input are the most important agile principles. Using pre- and post-service assessments in the study is an example of this strategy. The study looks at how students' opinions change before and after they do community service. This shows how learning and personal growth are always changing. This iterative review approach lets educators and legislators use real-time data to improve community service programs, making sure they keep getting better.

Using the Partial Least Squares (PLS) approach shows how similar this study is to agile management. PLS is a great method for exploratory research when ideas are changing and accuracy is very important. This has to do with the iterative process of creating a minimal viable product (MVP) that gets better over time based on real-world data and feedback from stakeholders. The study focusses on predictive modelling to make sure that its results may be used to improve educational practices and policies.

The method is designed to be easy to understand and use, without adding unnecessary complexity. This fits with the agile principle of simplicity, which says that you should get the most value out of something while wasting the least amount of time. The study focusses on three important areas: peer connections, self-regulation, and task articulation. This makes sure that its findings are accurate and useful. These traits are closely related to the Collaborative for Academic, Social, and Emotional Learning (CASEL) framework, which shows how the research can be used in real life.

The study uses an agile approach that involves refining its findings over time and getting input from stakeholders. Researchers can test and improve their theories over time by using SEM to look at the links between community service and social-emotional development. This process checks the model and gives useful advice to teachers and policymakers. For example, schools can create programs that particularly aim to increase self-regulation and task articulation since they know that community service helps with these things. This creates a feedback loop of continual improvement.

The study stresses how important it is to make sure that research methods match up with real-world uses. This research is similar to agile management in that it aims to provide insights that will immediately benefit students, teachers, and communities. The study employed predictive modelling to focus on dependent variables, which means that its results are useful for making community service a more important part of education.

The examination of how students feel about being involved in their communities is in line with agile management ideas. The study uses an iterative, data-driven approach that focusses on measurable outcomes to get important information about how community service can help people grow socially and emotionally. Using validated scales, predictive modelling, and feedback loops that happen over and over again makes sure that the study is thorough and useful, in line with the agile philosophy of constant improvement and adaptability. This strategy makes it easier for students to understand community service in school and gives them a way to use it in high school.

ANALYSIS OF RESULTS

Data analysis for the study incorporated estimation of the model. The measurement model was tested by estimating the internal consistency and the convergent and discriminant validity analysis. Next, the composite reliability was checked, including the Cronbach alpha, Rho-a, Rho-c, and the Average Variance Extracted. The internal consistency estimation is very much like the Cronbach alpha measure except that they prioritize the contribution of each indicator equally for the construct. The Cronbach alpha presumes parallel measurements and depicts a lower limit of composite reliability (Chin, 1998; Fornell & Larcker, 1981). The consistency of the constructs is usually unaffected by the length of the scale and, in general, as compared to the Cronbach alpha, where the values obtain similar interpretations through the guidelines by Nunnally and Bernstein (1994). The study includes reliability measures above .70, which indicates enough internal consistency (Fornell & Bookstein, 1982; Nunnally & Bernstein, 1994). The Average Variance estimation values were also above the minimum threshold of 0.5(Chin, 1998; Fornell& Larcker, 1981) and ranged from .56 to .80.The AVE being greater than .50, depicts that the variance between the constructs and measures is more than having an error. The demonstration of convergent validity is shown because the items have high loadings (>.50). The reflective measures of the individual items are taken to be reliable only if they correlate with a score of >.7. Table 1 shows that loadings above 0.7were taken into consideration. The discriminant validity is assessed with two methods where the first endorses examination of the cross-loadings of the constructs, and then the analysis of the comparison is made between the square root of the AVE of every construct and correlating the constructs with the other constructs (Chin, 1998; Fornell & Larcker, 1981). The model depicted in the study fulfilled the criteria required by discriminant reliability. The study justified all the criteria supporting reliability and validity, including the discriminant and the convergent forms.

Reliability and Validity Analysis

The study incorporates factor loadings of value above 0.6. The higher-order construct of social and emotional learning includes Social Relatedness, Task Articulation and Perception of community service scale it includes Awareness towards community service, ability to serve, and connectedness with service. The factor loadings, as shown in Table 1, provide loadings of above 0.6 value

Table 1. Factor loadings

	Outer loadings
ABILITY 1 <- ABILITY	0.84
ABILITY 2 <- ABILITY	0.78
ABILITY 3 <- ABILITY	0.87
ACTION 1 <- ACTION	0.79
ACTION 2 <- ACTION	0.77
ACTION 3 <- ACTION	0.84
ACTION 4 <- ACTION	0.72
ACTION 5 <- ACTION	0.76
AWARE 1 <- AWARE	0.83
AWARE 2 <- AWARE	0.87
AWARE 3 <- AWARE	0.84
AWARE 4 <- AWARE	0.8
CONNECT 1 <- CONNECT	0.84
CONNECT 2 <- CONNECT	0.84
CONNECT 3 <- CONNECT	0.87
CONNECT 4 <- CONNECT	0.78
CONNECT 6 <- CONNECT	0.77
PR1 <- PR	0.89
PR2 <- PR	0.91
PR3 <- PR	0.91
PR5 <- PR	0.9
PR6 <- PR	0.88
PR7 <- PR	0.92

continued on following page

Table 1. Continued

	Outer loadings
SR1 <- SR	0.86
SR2 <- SR	0.93
SR3 <- SR	0.94
SR4 <- SR	0.91
SR6 <- SR	0.9
TA5 <- TA	0.95
TA6 <- TA	0.95

The model is tested to provide the validity and reliability of the constructs. The role of measuring the reliability of the construct is to assess the internal consistency of the construct. through the Cronbach alpha such assessment is done (Hair, Black, Babin, & Anderson, 2010) the acceptable level being .70, the study incorporates constructs with the value of .above .70., with constructs of PR, SR, TA having more than .80 values. The composite reliability provided output much above .70(threshold limit) (Ali et al, 2018; Hair et al, 2017; 2020). The convergent validity assessed through the average variance extracted had a score of above .50(threshold value) for every construct (Fornell & Larcker, 1981; Hair et al., 2019). The results of the internal reliability and convergent validity are given in Table 2. Convergent validity is measured through factor loadings, composite reliability, and the extracted average variance, which must have a minimum loading of .5, .8, and .5, respectively. (Anderson & Gerbing, 1988; Hair et al., 2010).

Table 2. Quality criterion for reflective model assessments

	Cronbach's alpha	Composite reliability (rho_a)	Composite reliability (rho_c)	Average variance extracted (AVE)
ABILITY	0.77	0.78	0.87	0.69
ACTION	0.83	0.85	0.88	0.6
AWARE	0.86	0.86	0.9	0.7
CONNECT	0.88	0.88	0.91	0.67
PR	0.95	0.96	0.96	0.82
SR	0.95	0.95	0.96	0.82
TA	0.89	0.89	0.95	0.9

Source: Author's Calculation.

Discriminant validity helps differentiate between the constructs (Hair et al., 2010). The discriminant validity value is considered adequate when the variance shared by the construct with the other constructs of the model forms is lower than the variance that the construct shares with its measures. (Fornell and Larcker's Criterion (1981). The AVEs and cross-loadings help measure discriminant validity. The study indicates the discriminant validity (table 3), where the AVEs have a higher value than the values of their correlation shared within their respective constructs. Also, from the loadings of the items and cross-loadings of the items, it is seen that every item of measurement for the constructs has a higher loading value than the value of the constructs from where they have been derived, in terms of cross-loadings. These, when taken together, prove to have strong discriminant validity. (Chin, 2010; Farrell, 2010; Fornell & Larcker, 1981), as seen in Table 3.

Table 3. Discriminant analysis

	ABILITY	ACTION	AWARE	CONNECT	PR	SR	TA
ABILITY	0.83						
ACTION	0.84	0.78					
AWARE	0.76	0.78	0.84				
CONNECT	0.81	0.83	0.75	0.82			
PR	0.5	0.41	0.53	0.42	0.9		
SR	0.49	0.41	0.51	0.41	0.95	0.91	
TA	0.35	0.28	0.4	0.25	0.89	0.86	0.95

The study also incorporates the heterotrait monotrait ratio (HTMT), which is supposed to achieve superior performance and more specific and sensitive values (Henseler et al.). Values closer to 1 represent a lack of discriminant validity between the constructs. Table 4 shows HTMT ratios to have good discriminant values except for PR-Helping, TA-Helping and TA-PR, having values of .93, .93. and 1.25, respectively; this shows that the constructs face collinearity issues.

Table 4. HTMT results

	ABILITY	ACTION	AWARE	CONNECT	PR	SR
ABILITY						
ACTION	1.05					
AWARE	0.91	0.87				
CONNECT	0.99	0.95	0.81			
PR	0.19	0.17	0.15	0.09		
SR	0.17	0.15	0.1	0.08	0.85	
TA	0.16	0.17	0.13	0.09	1.09	0.66

The VIF values out here with less than 5, settles the problem by exhibiting no multicollinearity issues in the data. (Table 5) The VIF value less than 5 should be the rule of thumb at the time of calculating co-linearity because some other factors, like sample size, also influence regression coefficients (O'Brien 2007).

Table 5. Inner VIF values

	VIF
ABILITY 1	1.46
ABILITY 2	1.27
ABILITY 3	1.61
ACTION 1	1.51
ACTION 2	1.57
ACTION 3	1.61
ACTION 4	1.49
ACTION 5	1.42
AWARE 1	1.72
AWARE 2	1.96
AWARE 3	1.56
AWARE 4	1.5
CONNECT 1	2.13
CONNECT 2	2.51
CONNECT 3	2.22
CONNECT 4	1.46
CONNECT 6	1.47
PR1	2.11
PR2	1.79
PR3	1.48
PR5	1.36
PR6	1.51
PR7	1.49
SR1	1.56
SR2	2.33
SR3	2.25
SR4	1.93
SR6	1.2
TA5	1.15
TA6	1.15

Results of Structural Equation Model

Figure 1. Structural equation model

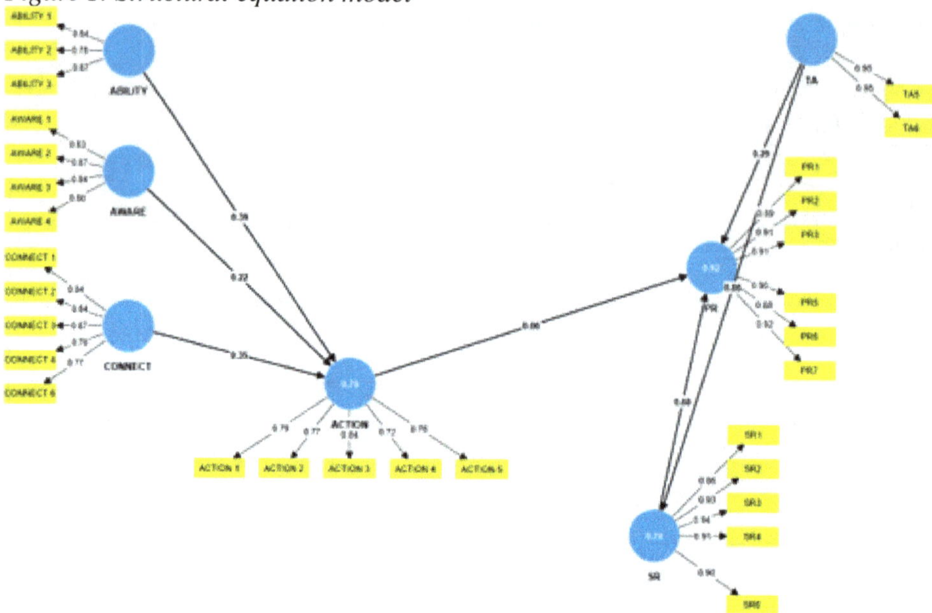

The Structural Equation Model gains assessment with the help of Regression values, t values, Significant values (p values). The Results in Table 6 show that strong awareness of the issues of the community, ability to serve and connectedness with the community help build strong intensity to act towards community service and action that helps serve the community builds strong task articulation, peer relation and social relatedness amongst students.

Table 6. P values

	Original sample (O)	Sample mean (M)	Standard deviation (STDEV)	T statistics (|O/ STDEV|)	P values
ABILITY -> ACTION	0.39	0.39	0.04	9.57	0
ACTION -> PR	0.06	0.06	0.01	4.14	0
AWARE -> ACTION	0.22	0.22	0.04	5.49	0
CONNECT -> ACTION	0.35	0.35	0.04	7.8	0

continued on following page

Table 6. Continued

	Original sample (O)	Sample mean (M)	Standard deviation (STDEV)	T statistics (|O/ STDEV|)	P values
SR -> PR	0.68	0.68	0.03	20.79	0
TA -> PR	0.29	0.28	0.03	9.24	0
TA -> SR	0.86	0.86	0.01	67.44	0

Again, the R Square value helps measure the power of prediction for the Structural Model in the analysis. This power of predicting the model viability is less effective when the value is less than 0.15(Cohen1988). Thus, the power for predicting the model for all the items being above 0.15, is significant. (Table7), even though relevant for the study context. As well above 0.20 as per the data belonging to behavioral sciences can be high at (Rasoolimanesh et al., 2017). Apart from analyzing the R2, the model also evaluated the Q2to examine the predictive relevance. Q2 helps measure the good fit between the values observed and represented in the model through its parameter estimates. This model exhibited Q2 values of above 0, making the model establish predictive relevance.

Table 7. R2 and Q2 values

Predictors	R Square	Q Square
Action	0.79	0.79
PR	0.92	0.80
SR	0.74	0.74

In the present research, a global model fit index like SRMR was important to evaluate its goodness (Hair et al., 2020). The SRMR value of the study is 0.079 in this model, and it is below the threshold value of 0.08 to explain that the model under the study had good explanatory power (Hu and Bentler, 1999; Henseler et al., 2016). Based on these results the model can be acceptable indicating Community services have a greater role in developing the PR SR and TA for the students.

FINDINGS AND CONCLUSIONS

The concepts of agile management, which include being flexible, working together, learning in stages, and being attentive to people, provide a strong way to understand the results of this study on how community service affects students' social and emotional learning (SEL). In today's schools, where traditional teaching methods frequently don't do a good job of developing all-around skills, agile methods offer both a philosophical and practical framework for transformative learning. The study shows that community service, when planned out in agile cycles of action and reflection, helps kids progress in all areas. It emphasizes empathy, social responsibility, and civic involvement, all of which are important for building teams that are high-performing, adaptive, and socially aware, which is what agile is all about.

The empirical study used Structural Equation Modelling (SEM) to test its model with predictive analytics. This strongly supports the idea that community service improves students' SEL results. The methodology is based on a design of iterative enhancement, which is like agile cycles. Each phase—exposure, reflection, feedback, and adaptation—acts as a "sprint" that helps the learner grow socially and emotionally. Self-regulation, peer bonding, and job ownership were some of the most key areas that came up, showing how agile learning cycles build on each other. This iterative process is also a type of transformative assessment that focusses on student agency, metacognitive reflection, and learning in context instead of one-time tests.

For example, students who took part in regular neighborhood clean-up efforts used Scrum-inspired roles like Scrum Master, task leads, and documentation managers to keep track of their duties, hold daily debriefings, and keep track of their progress using digital tools like Trello. This flexible structure let students think about what they were doing in real time and helped them feel more capable as they worked through problems. Teachers used rubrics to measure things like teamwork, empathy, and self-control, which gave them more information about students' behaviour than just their grades. These formative evaluation methods, based on agile thinking, gave students useful feedback and helped them become better at evaluating themselves and being aware of others.

The study also finds that children who do community service, especially when it is based on empathy, develop important attributes like being responsible for their work, controlling their emotions, and relying on their peers. These traits are very similar to what agile management focusses on: creating self-organizing, cross-functional teams that can handle changing situations. Students who learnt about real-life problems including not having enough food, not having a stable place to live, and not having enough money for school typically showed a greater sense of moral duty and leadership. This knowledge led to a deeper sense of ownership over the project and a willingness to work together, which is in line with the agile principle that responsive, motivated people are the key to long-term success.

Students who mentored kids from low-income families not only taught them how to read and write, but they also helped them understand their own feelings better. Their insights, which were recorded in notebooks, blog entries, or multimedia portfolios, led to life-changing realizations about poverty, resilience, and empathy. These formative artefacts not only helped students learn from each other, but they also functioned as reflective assessments that pushed students to connect their feelings, values, and cognitive insights. Teachers saw a significant improvement in students' capacity to balance social value with academic performance. This shows agile's philosophy of delivering meaningful results while staying flexible and adaptable.

Also, students were more motivated to help out, even though they had a lot of schoolwork to do, because they were more aware of problems in their communities, such lack of education, starvation, or child labour. This dual engagement shows that an agile learner may change their priorities based on the value of the scenario, just like agile teams do with their sprint backlogs. These kinds of experiences show how important it is to include community-responsive learning models in curriculum that value academic rigour as well as flexibility and giving back to the community.

The study's main theme was empathy, which grew not from theory but from real-life interactions. Students who worked closely with street children, slum residents, and informal workers learnt what it's like to be in a tough situation. These experiences helped people become more caring, aware of others, and have a keen sense of right and wrong, which is in line with the human-centered approach of agile management. Agile teams do well not simply by getting things done, but also by understanding the human side of their work. This is like how students learn to understand the emotional lives of others via service.

This study shows that students naturally learn ideals like social justice and civic duty through meaningful exposure to real-world differences, even if formal schooling doesn't usually teach these things directly. Many of them saw their friends working at car washes, roadside restaurants, or in household responsibilities, which showed a clear difference between having access to education and having to work for money. These new facts made people think and made them feel like they had to do something. By bridging this gap in experience, community service becomes a way to promote social justice and moral reasoning, just as agile's iterative process of feedback, learning, and meaningful change.

Schools that have structured community service programs, especially for grades 8 to 10, are taking a methodical, values-based approach to whole-person education. Within a set teaching framework, these programs combine moral education, community service, and emotional growth. Like agile systems, they find a balance between freedom and structure, letting pupils discover their own agency within safe limits. Students are acquiring adaptable knowledge, which is one of the main goals of agile educational models, whether they are planning service projects or thinking about how they feel. These skills help children not only with schoolwork but also with taking initiative, leading responsibly, and working well with others in real-world situations where things aren't clear.

Mother Teresa and Sister Cyril, two humanitarian pioneers from Kolkata's past, have moulded the city's educational values. Their work led to school-based outreach projects like the “Rainbows.” These initiatives created an environment of kindness, involvement, and acceptance, which helped kids understand the emotional depth of service. Students that took part in these kinds of activities improved their social and emotional skills, which is in line with the agile learning paradigm, where each cycle of action and reflection makes the following one stronger. Transformational learning can happen when this cultural legacy of service is joined with agile's reflective and interactive framework.

In short, the study shows well how community service inspired by agile can help kids develop a lasting feeling of empathy, responsibility, and involvement in society. Including community service and value-driven education in the school curriculum is not just a nice thing to do; it is a strategic necessity for making citizens who are emotionally knowledgeable and care about their community. Agile management's focus on people, feedback loops, adaptability, and aligning values gives teachers a model they can use to make changes that can be scaled up and copied. The study's outcomes support this human-centered, iterative approach. They show that teaching kids social responsibility in school can lead to a future that is not just fairer and more caring, but also strong, cooperative, and long-lasting.

REFERENCES

Ab Hamid, M. R., Sami, W., & Sidek, M. M. (2017, September). Discriminant validity assessment: Use of Fornell & Larcker criterion versus HTMT criterion. [IOP Publishing.]. *Journal of Physics: Conference Series*, *890*(1), 012163. DOI: 10.1088/1742-6596/890/1/012163

Anderson, J. C., & Gerbing, D. W. (1988). Structural equation modeling in practice: A review and recommended two-step approach. *Psychological Bulletin*, *103*(3), 411–423. DOI: 10.1037/0033-2909.103.3.411

Aronfreed, J. (1968). Conscience and conduct: The socialization of internalized control of behavior.

Astley, S. J., & Furlong, M. J. (2019). The influence of school service on students' social and emotional development: A meta-analysis and systematic review. *Journal of School Psychology*, *72*, 44–58.

Barber, B. R., & Battistoni, R. (1993). A season of service: Introducing service learning into the liberal arts curriculum. *PS, Political Science & Politics*, *26*(2), 235–240. DOI: 10.2307/419837

Blaug, M. (1985). Where are we now in the economics of education? *Economics of Education Review*, *4*(1), 17–28. DOI: 10.1016/0272-7757(85)90034-2

Boss, J. A. (1994). The effect of community service work on the moral development of college ethics students. *Journal of Moral Education*, *23*(2), 183–198. DOI: 10.1080/0305724940230206

Brackett, M. A., Reyes, M. R., Rivers, S. E., Elbertson, N. A., & Salovey, P. (2012). Assessing teachers' beliefs about social and emotional learning. *Journal of Psychoeducational Assessment*, *30*(3), 219–236. DOI: 10.1177/0734282911424879

Bugdayci, S. (2019). Examining Personal and Social Responsibility Levels of Secondary School Students. *Universal Journal of Educational Research*, *7*(1), 206–210. DOI: 10.13189/ujer.2019.070126

Burgos, J., & Carnero, M. C. (2020). Assessment of Social Responsibility in Education in Secondary Schools. *Sustainability (Basel)*, *12*(12), 4849. DOI: 10.3390/su12124849

Castilla-Polo, F., Ruiz-Rodríguez, M. C., Moreno, A., Licerán-Gutiérrez, A., Cámara de la Fuente, M., Chamorro Rufián, E., & Cano-Rodríguez, M. (2020). Classroom Learning and the Perception of Social Responsibility Amongst Graduate Students of Management Accounting. *Sustainability (Basel)*, *12*(17), 7093. DOI: 10.3390/su12177093

Chen, S. H., Nasongkhla, J., & Donaldson, J. A. (2015). University Social Responsibility (USR): Identifying an Ethical Foundation within Higher Education Institutions. *Turkish Online Journal of Educational Technology-TOJET*, *14*(4), 165–172.

Chickering, A. W., & Reisser, L. (1993). Education and Identity. The Jossey-Bass Higher and Adult Education Series. Jossey-Bass Inc., Publishers, 350 Sansome St., San Francisco, CA 94104.

Cohen, J. (1988). *Statistical power analysis for the behavioral sciences* (2nd ed.).

Conrad, D., & Hedin, D. (1989). High School Community Service: A Review of Research and Programs.

Cook, T., Murphy, R., & And Hunt, H. (2000). Comer's School Development Program in Chicago: A Theory-Based Evaluation. *American Educational Research Journal*, *37*(2), 535–597. DOI: 10.3102/00028312037002535

Dávila, L. A., & Mora, J. R. (2017). The impact of community service learning on the development of college students' emotional intelligence. *Journal of College Student Development*, *58*(5), 709–724.

De Brabander, C. J. (2000). Knowledge definition, subject, and educational track level: Perceptions of secondary school teachers. *American Educational Research Journal*, *37*(4), 1027–1058. DOI: 10.3102/000283120370041027

Delors, J., Amagi, I., Carneiro, R., Chung, F., Geremek, B., Gorham, W., Suhr, M. W. (1996). Learning. The treasure Within. Paris.

Dewey, J. (1916). 1985. Democracy and education. John Dewey: the middle works (1899–1924), 9.

Dharamsi, S., Espinoza, N., Cramer, C., Amin, M., Bainbridge, L., & Poole, G. (2010). Nurturing social responsibility through community service-learning: Lessons learned from a pilot project. *Medical Teacher*, *32*(11), 905–911. DOI: 10.3109/01421590903434169 PMID: 21039101

Dima, A. M., Vasilache, S., Ghinea, V., & Agoston, S. (2013). A model of academic social responsability. *Transylvanian Review of Administrative Sciences*, *9*(38), 23–43.

Eisenberg, N., Spinrad, T. L., & Morris, A. S. (2015). Prosocial development. In Lamb, M. E. (Ed.), *Handbook of child psychology and developmental science* (7th ed., Vol. 3, pp. 610–656). Wiley. DOI: 10.1002/9781118963418.childpsy315

Eyler, J. S., & Giles, D. E. (1999). *Where's the learning in service-learning?* Jossey-Bass.

Finkelstein, M. A., & Pancer, S. M. (2015). The impact of community-based volunteer work on students' personal, social, and civic outcomes. *Journal of Adolescence*, *38*, 107–113.

Fonseca, A., Macdonald, A., Dandy, E., & Valenti, P. (2011). The state of sustainability reporting at Canadian universities. *International Journal of Sustainability in Higher Education*, *12*(1), 22–40. DOI: 10.1108/14676371111098285

Fornell, C. (1981). A comparative analysis of two structural equation models: LISREL and PLS applied to market data.

Fornell, C., & Bookstein, F. L. (1982). Two structural equation models: LISREL and PLS applied to consumer exit-voice theory. *JMR, Journal of Marketing Research*, *19*(4), 440–452. DOI: 10.1177/002224378201900406

Fornell, C., & Larcker, D. F. (1981). Evaluating structural equation models with unobservable variables and measurement error. *JMR, Journal of Marketing Research*, *18*(1), 39–50. DOI: 10.1177/002224378101800104

Furco, A. (1999). Self-assessment rubric for the institutionalization of service-learning in higher education.

Giles, D. E.Jr, & Eyler, J. (1994). The impact of a college community service laboratory on students' personal, social, and cognitive outcomes. *Journal of Adolescence*, *17*(4), 327–339. DOI: 10.1006/jado.1994.1030

Gomez, L. (2014). The importance of university social responsibility in Hispanic America: A responsible trend in developing countries. In *Corporate social responsibility and sustainability: Emerging trends in developing economies*. Emerald Group Publishing Limited. DOI: 10.1108/S2043-905920140000008013

Greenberg, M. T., Weissberg, R. P., O'Brien, M. U., Zins, J. E., Fredericks, L., Resnik, H., & Elias, M. J. (2003). Enhancing school-based prevention and youth development through coordinated social, emotional, and academic learning. *The American Psychologist*, *58*(6-7), 466–474. DOI: 10.1037/0003-066X.58.6-7.466 PMID: 12971193

Haan, N. (1985). Processes of moral development: Cognitive or social disequilibrium? *Developmental Psychology, 21*(6), 996–1006. DOI: 10.1037/0012-1649.21.6.996

Hair, J. F.Jr, Babin, B. J., & Anderson, R. E. (2010). *A global p-erspect-ivie*. Kennesaw State University.

Heller, J. (1989, September). Offering Moral Education. In Streamlined Seminar (Vol. 8, No. 1, p. n1). Publications, National Association of Elementary School Principals, 1615 Duke Street, Alexandria, VA 22314.

Henseler, J., Ringle, C. M., & Sarstedt, M. (2015). A new criterion for assessing discriminant validity in variance-based structural equation modeling. *Journal of the Academy of Marketing Science, 43*(1), 115–135. DOI: 10.1007/s11747-014-0403-8

Herzberg, B. (2013). Community service and critical teaching. In *Dialogue on Writing* (pp. 449–462). Routledge.

Hitlin, S. (2003). Values as the core of personal identity: Drawing links between two theories of self. *Social Psychology Quarterly, 66*(2), 118–137. DOI: 10.2307/1519843

Honig, B. (1990). Teaching values belongs in our public schools. *NASSP Bulletin, 74*(528), 6–9. DOI: 10.1177/019263659007452803

Jenney, T. J. (2011). The holistic development of college students: Spirituality as a predictor of college student's pro-social character development. Culture and Religion Review Journal Keith, N. Z. (2005). Community Service Learning in the Face of Globalization: Rethinking Theory and Practice. *Michigan Journal of Community Service Learning, 11*(2), 5–24.

Kinsley, C. W., & McPherson, K. (Eds.). (1995). *Enriching the curriculum through service learning* (Vol. 1250). Association for Supervision and Curriculum Development.

Kohlberg, L. (1978). Revisions in the theory and practice of moral development. *New Directions for Child and Adolescent Development, 1978*(2), 83–87. DOI: 10.1002/cd.23219780207

Larocque, M., Kleiman, I., & Darling, S. M. (2011). Parental involvement: The missing link in school achievement. *Preventing School Failure, 55*(3), 115–122. DOI: 10.1080/10459880903472876

Li, W., Wright, P., Rukavina, P., & And Pickering, M. (2008). Measuring Students' Perceptions of Personal and Social Responsibility and the Relationship to Intrinsic Motivation in Urban Physical Education. *Journal of Teaching in Physical Education, 27*(2), 167–178. DOI: 10.1123/jtpe.27.2.167

London, T. (2008, August). THE BASE-OF-THE-PYRAMID PERSPECTIVE: A NEW APPROACH TO POVERTY ALLEVIATION. In Academy of management proceedings (Vol. 2008, No. 1, pp. 1-6). Briarcliff Manor, NY 10510: Academy of Management.

Markus, G. B., Howard, J. P., & King, D. C. (1993). Integrating community service and classroom instruction enhances learning: Results from an experiment. *Educational Evaluation and Policy Analysis*, *15*(4), 410–419. DOI: 10.2307/1164538

Mcbeth, C. H. (2018). Social innovation in higher education: The emergence and evolution of social impact centers (Doctoral dissertation, University of Pennsylvania).

Mintzberg, H., Simons, R., & Basu, K. (2002). Beyond selfishness. *MIT Sloan Management Review*, *44*(1), 67.

National Research Council. (2002). *Community programs to promote youth development*. National Academies Press.

Newmann, F. M., & Rutter, R. A. (1983). The Effects of High School Community Service Programs on Students' Social Development. Final Report.

Nimako, S. G., & Owusu, E. K. (2015). A theoretical model for explaining subscribers' intention to switch back in mobile telecommunication industry: Implications for management. *Management and Organizational Studies*, *2*(1), 107–119. DOI: 10.5430/mos.v2n1p107

O'brien, R. M. (2007). A caution regarding rules of thumb for variance inflation factors. *Quality & Quantity*, *41*(5), 673–690. DOI: 10.1007/s11135-006-9018-6

Pancer, S. M., Pratt, M. W., Hunsberger, B., & Alisat, S. (2007). Cognitive complexity of expectations and adjustment to university in the first year. *Journal of Adolescent Research*, *22*(6), 631–655.

Patton, M. Q. (2002). Two decades of developments in qualitative inquiry: A personal, experiential perspective. *Qualitative Social Work: Research and Practice*, *1*(3), 261–283. DOI: 10.1177/1473325002001003636

Peng, L. M., Lung, C. K., & Chai, L. T. (2018). Perceived Roles of Ethics and Social Responsibility, Internal Corporate Social Responsibility and Employee Engagement of Academicians. The Journal of Social Sciences Research, 706-717.

Rahim, M. A., & Magner, N. R. (1995). Confirmatory factor analysis of the styles of handling interpersonal conflict: First-order factor model and its invariance across groups. *The Journal of Applied Psychology*, *80*(1), 122–132. DOI: 10.1037/0021-9010.80.1.122 PMID: 7706190

Raskoff, S. A., & Sundeen, R. A. (1999). Community service programs in high schools. *Law and Contemporary Problems, 62*(4), 73. DOI: 10.2307/1192268

Rhoads, R. A. (1997). *Community service and higher learning: Explorations of the caring self.* SUNY Press.

Rosenzweig, L. (1980). *Kohlberg in the classroom: Moral education models. Moral development, moral education, and Kohlberg: Basic Issues in philosophy, psychology, religion, and education.* Religious Education Press.

Sant, E., McDonnell, J., Pashby, K., & Menendez Alvarez-Hevia, D. (2021). Pedagogies of agonistic democracy and citizenship education. *Education, Citizenship and Social Justice, 16*(3), 227–244. DOI: 10.1177/1746197920962373

Selznick, P. (1994). *The moral commonwealth: Social theory and the promise of community.* Univ of California Press. DOI: 10.1525/9780520354753

Shek, D. (2010). Nurturing Holistic Development of University Students in Hong Kong: Where Are We and Where Should We Go? *TheScientificWorldJournal, 10*, 563–575. DOI: 10.1100/tsw.2010.62 PMID: 20364241

Stanislavská, L. K., Kvasnička, R., Kuralová, K., & Margarisová, K. (2014). Social Responsibility of Higher Educational Institutions–the Comparison of the View of Students and Potential Students. *Journal on Efficiency and Responsibility in Education and Science, 7*(3-4), 95–99. DOI: 10.7160/eriesj.2014.070308

Taneja, S. S., Taneja, P. K., & Gupta, R. K. (2011). Researches in corporate social responsibility: A review of shifting focus, paradigms, and methodologies. *Journal of Business Ethics, 101*(3), 343–364. DOI: 10.1007/s10551-010-0732-6

Tetřevová, L. I. B. Ě. N. A., & Sabolova, V. (2010). University stakeholder management and university social responsibility. WSEAS transactions on advances in engineering education, 7(7), 224-233.

Türkkahraman, M. (2012). The role of education in the societal development. Journal of educational and instructional studies in the world, 2(4), 38-41.

Türkkahraman, M. (2014). Social values and value education. Procedia-social and behavioural sciences, 116, 633-638.

Turkkahraman, M. (2015). Education, Teaching and School as A Social Organization. *Procedia: Social and Behavioral Sciences, 186*, 381–387. DOI: 10.1016/j.sbspro.2015.04.044

Wang, L., & Juslin, H. (2012). Values and corporate social responsibility perceptions of Chinese university students. *Journal of Academic Ethics*, *10*(1), 57–82. DOI: 10.1007/s10805-012-9148-5

Wartick, S. L., & Cochran, P. L. (1985). The evolution of the corporate social performance model. *Academy of Management Review*, *10*(4), 758–769. DOI: 10.2307/258044

Wentzel, K. (1991). Relations between Social Competence and Academic Achievement in Early Adolescence. *Child Development*, *62*(5), 1066. DOI: 10.2307/1131152 PMID: 1756656

Wentzel, K. R. (1991). Social competence at school: Relation between social responsibility and academic achievement. *Review of Educational Research*, *61*(1), 1–24. DOI: 10.3102/00346543061001001

Wray-Lake, L., & Syvertsen, A. K. (2011). The developmental roots of social responsibility in childhood and adolescence. *New Directions for Child and Adolescent Development*, *2011*(134), 11–25. DOI: 10.1002/cd.308 PMID: 22147598

Yates, M., & Youniss, J. (1996). A developmental perspective on community service in adolescence. *Social Development*, *5*(1), 85–111. DOI: 10.1111/j.1467-9507.1996.tb00073.x

Yuen, S. C. Y., Yaoyuneyong, G., & Johnson, E. (2011). Augmented reality: An overview and five directions for AR in education. [JETDE]. *Journal of Educational Technology Development and Exchange*, *4*(1), 11. DOI: 10.18785/jetde.0401.10

Zigler, R. L. (1998). The four domains of moral education: The contributions of Dewey, Alexander and Goleman to a comprehensive taxonomy. *Journal of Moral Education*, *27*(1), 19–33. DOI: 10.1080/0305724980270102

Zych, I., Ortega-Ruiz, R., Muñoz-Morales, R., & Llorent, V. J. (2018). Dimensions and psychometric properties of the Social and Emotional Competencies Questionnaire (SEC-Q) in youth and adolescents. *Revista Latinoamericana de Psicología*, *50*(2), 98–106. DOI: 10.14349/rlp.2018.v50.n2.3

Chapter 8
Neural Pathways of Judgment:
How Critical Thinking Emerges and Misdiagnosis Occurs in the Mind

Raad Kadhum
https://orcid.org/0009-0003-3097-4121
Independent Researcher, Bahrain

ABSTRACT

Our brain is a system that is both flexible and integrated, able to process visual, auditory, and sensory inputs simultaneously and design, execute, and control actions. It's not surprising that a complex system is also vulnerable to various disorders, such as brain diseases. Personality and the resulting decision-making and behavioral structures, as well as the embeddedness of personality in the brain, are also affected by this. Critical thinking skills and the ability to think are influenced by factors that begin before birth and continue to influence an individual after birth. The focus of this chapter is on these topics and the factors that impact personality formation. The personality traits also influence the development of critical thinking skills. In this chapter we will address the foundations of how thinking and thus critical thinking develops in the brain and verify the importance of possessing the necessary skills to make a judgement and make the right decision.

DOI: 10.4018/979-8-3373-1812-7.ch008

INTRODUCTION

Critical thinking only arises through the process of asking questions, analyzing and evaluating information to construct logical meaning, going beyond intuition, and training and developing logical reasoning skills. It is not a fixed skill, but rather a skill that develops through hard work and diligent effort into a perfect skill. But the foundation for the effectiveness of this skill is having a healthy, integrated, and undamaged nervous system and mind capable of functioning efficiently. Thinking activities are mechanisms and methods that are formed in the brain. Healthy judgement are based on a combination of reason, experience, and emotion. The brain uses two different decision-making systems: reason and emotional memory. Smart judgement are made by carefully weighing risks, consequences, and alternatives. Informed decisions are based on a capable personality and a healthy brain. They require a combination of reason, experience, and emotions. The brain processes information, draws on past experiences, and works with neural networks to make decisions. The brain influences the formation and characteristics of personality. Personality, in turn, influences how we perceive and interpret information, which in turn influences our decisions. Reliable decisions depend on a competent personality and a sound healthy brain.

In his book, "Thinking, Fast and Slow" Daniel Kahneman attempts to convey the concept of thinking by asking the reader to consider this problem; 17 X 24, Then he speaks to the reader: " You knew immediately that this is a multiplication problem, and probably knew that you could solve it, with paper and pencil, if not without. You also had some vague intuitive knowledge of the range of possible results. You would be quick to recognize that both 12,609 and 123 are implausible. Without spending some time on the problem, however, you would not be certain that the answer is not 568. A precise solution did not come to mind, and you felt that you could choose whether or not to engage in the computation. If you have not done so yet, you should attempt the multiplication problem now, completing at least part of it." Kahneman continuous and addresses the reader and says that here you thought slowly as you progressed through a series of steps. You recalled from memory the knowledge of the multiplication table you learned in school, then applied it. The calculations were laborious. You felt the burden of keeping a lot of information; you had to keep track of where you were and where you are going, and to hold the intermediate result. The process was mental: deliberate, laborious, and orderly - a prototype of slow thinking. The calculation wasn't just mental; your body was involved, too. Your muscles tense, your blood pressure rises, and your heart rate increases. If someone had looked closely into your eyes as you worked on this problem, they would have seen your pupils dilate. But, they shrank back to their normal size once you finished your work - when you found the answer (which is 408) or when you surrendered.

Kahneman talks about a typical or average person. His words do not apply to all cases. The way of thinking varies, as there is a relationship between our personality and our way of thinking, and one affects the other. Individual's personality plays a major role in his behavior and how he makes decisions. Personality is influenced in many ways by the brain (Roth, 2003). The structure and functions of our brain determine our personality. In addition, diseases that affect brain metabolism can lead to changes in personality and the way we make judgments and decisions. Other important factors influencing our personality are our personal experiences and our interactions with the environment and other people, these also reside in the brain because they are stored in our memories. Early childhood experiences, in particular, shape personality. Children who experience separation or the death of their parents before the age of five may develop a fear of loss throughout their lives, shaping their personalities and influencing their way of thinking.

In her study identified (Sălceanu, 2021) a correlation between cognitive skills and personality traits. She observed that analytical reasoning positively correlates with conscientiousness and emotional stability, and text comprehension with emotional stability.

Today, we know, through the experiences of many specialists, that individual's personality and cognition abilities begin to crystallize from the moment of birth, even in the mother's womb before birth. This justifies emphasizing the importance of the family, parents, and educational institutions in building critical thinking skills in children. In his book "We are our brains: a neurobiography of the brain, from the womb to Alzheimer's" Swaab confirms: " So, a difficult birth can be seen as a failure of interaction between the brains of mother and child and thus as the first symptom of schizophrenia, even though the disease doesn't develop fully until puberty. The same applies to autism, another early developmental brain disorder (see chapter 9) that also often goes hand in hand with birth-related problems." (Swaab 2014).

ARE HUMAN MENTAL AND PERSONALITY ABILITIES INNATE OR ARE THEY DETERMINED BY THE ENVIRONMENT?

The issue of whether human mental and personality abilities are innate or environmentally determined has been the subject of intense debate since ancient times.

In biology and the behavioral sciences, opinions on this topic are sometimes sharply opposed. While American behaviorism assumes that all cognitive, emotional, and behavioral characteristics of animals and humans are entirely determined by the environment, Austrian Lorenz and his supporters, as well as representatives of sociobiology and behavioral ecology, believe that human behavior is largely genetically determined (Lorenz,1965). While Freud occupies an important intermediate position, he also believes that individual thinking, feeling, and behavior are largely determined, but at the same time he assumes different reasons for this determination. Freud argued that some determinants of individual behavior are genetic or phylogenetic in nature and are therefore innate, while others arise from imprinting processes in early childhood, and still others arise from formative pubertal experiences. Freud believed that personality could be determined gradually, beginning with genes and continuing through the early postnatal period and then into early adolescence.

From a modern biological perspective, we must also assume that several factors shape an individual's personality and his mental abilities. The first factor is undoubtedly the genes an individual inherits from their parents. It's worth noting that these factors, including genetic ones, influence an individual's subsequent decision-making. However, the real significance of this factor for our question is still unclear. To date, no geneticist or developmental biologist knows precisely what a gene or set of genes means for brain performance, particularly with regard to an individual's complex cognitive and emotional characteristics. But what can be concluded is that thinking skills and dispositions intertwine when thinking skills are combined with personal talents to act critically (Facione, 1990).

In the past it has been shown that even the simplest anatomical and physiological characteristics of the human brain, which can be considered largely independent of the environment, depend to a large extent on the extremely complex interplay of numerous genes and a large number of so-called epigenetic processes. These are highly complex interactions between different types of neural tissue during brain development. Very little is known about the genetic-epigenetic determination of the brain at a more complex level.

A second important factor is the environmental influences that, in one way or another, whether nonspecific or random, affect the fetal brain. These include influences absorbed by the fetus through its body and functioning sensory organs; all substances (such as oxygen, nutrients, and possibly nicotine, alcohol, and other drugs) that pass through the mother's bloodstream, provided they can cross the fetal blood-brain barrier; and mechanical impairments in the event of accidents or acts of violence against the pregnant woman. Finally, this also includes the physiological and mechanical effects of the birth process, which are clearly extremely severe.

The third factor, and perhaps the most important here, is the newborn's experiences in the first hours, days, weeks, and months after birth, especially the "first experiences" of the mother's warmth, smell, sight, voice, skin-to-skin contact, and provision of food. All evidence suggests that severe disruptions in these first experiences have significant negative consequences for the child's subsequent psychological development and personality formation (Roth, 2003).

The qualitative importance of these three factors in personality development is undeniable, but it is difficult to estimate quantitatively and, at least in humans, to test them directly experimentally for ethical reasons.

Brodbeck asked: "Is it possible that the structure of the brain is genetically preprogrammed? Are complex feats of intelligence or creativity reserved only for genetically gifted geniuses?" to give answers, he compares computers to the capacity of the brain. He concluded that creativity or intelligence capacity of the human brain cannot be innate, or only to a very limited extent. Therefore, the formation of neural information networks must be explained differently. (Brodbeck, 1997)

THE BRAIN

Long ago, humans knew that the brain is the spring of thinking and personality. Hippocrates wrote in the period 460-370 BC: "It should be widely known that the brain, and the brain alone, is the source of our pleasures, joys, laughter, and amusement, as well as our sorrow, pain, grief, and tears. It is especially the organ we use to think and learn, see and hear, to distinguish the ugly from the beautiful, the bad from the good, and the pleasant from the unpleasant. The brain is also the seat of madness and delirium, of the fears and terrors which assail us, often at night, but sometimes even during the day, of insomnia, sleepwalking, elusive thoughts, forgetfulness, and eccentricities." Swaab wrote: "Everything we think, do, and refrain from doing is determined by the brain" (Swaab, 2014).

Four weeks after the embryo is developed, the first simple divisions of the brain can be seen as swellings at the head of the embryo. The remaining eight months of pregnancy are used to further develop and perfect the brain. When the baby is born after nine months, the brain is a miniature version of the adult brain. Until now, the brain consists of a pile of unconnected nerve cells, but without cooperation and joint work, there will be no efficiency in work. After birth, it is important to connect the brain cells.

Brain, Memory, and Learning

The brain is the most important component of a human's central nervous system (Vester, 2012). The strongly developed cerebral cortex could subsequently be used as the basis for increased sensory, motor, and cognitive performance (Roth, 2003). An adult human brain, with an average weight of 1.4 kg, accounts for around two percent of body weight, but consumes more than a fifth of the body's total energy (Spitzer, 2007). Depending on the author, estimates regarding the number of nerve cells (neurons) in the brain range from 15 billion (Vester, 2012) to 100 billion

(Gasser, 2008) to one trillion (Gerrig, 2015). This enormous number of neurons, as well as the fiber connections between them, form the essential components of this organ, which processes vast amounts of information in the form of perception, thinking, and learning (Spitzer, 2007).

Structure and Functions of the Brain

The human brain, as shown in Figure 1, consists of several interconnected layers: the brainstem, thalamus, cerebellum, limbic system, and cerebrum (Gerrig, 2015).

The brainstem regulates internal body processes and is found in all vertebrates. Long nerve fibers lead from the brainstem to the thalamus, where incoming sensory information is channeled, connected to emotions, and transmitted to the appropriate areas. The cerebellum is responsible for coordinating body movements and balance (Gerrig, 2015). Messages from the sensory organs and commands from the cerebral cortex are coordinated in the cerebellum, and the results are transmitted to the muscles (Vester, 2012). Results from recent brain research also suggest that the cerebellum is involved in sophisticated learning and thinking processes (Stern, 2012).

The limbic system, consisting of the hippocampus, amygdala, and hypothalamus, primarily acts as an intermediary between motivational behavior, emotional states, and memory processes. The hippocampus is the largest structure of the limbic system and plays a significant role in the acquisition of explicit memory content (Gerrig, 2015). It identifies new facts as such by comparing them with previously stored, known events and assessing their familiarity. The content identified as new is then evaluated. The amygdalae are two small clusters of neurons. They resemble amygdalae in shape and size, which is why they are often referred to by this term. They contribute to the rapid learning of unpleasant experiences and their avoidance in the future (Spitzer, 2007). In the hypothalamus, the human body's reactions to the outside world are adapted, for example, by maintaining a constant body temperature (Vester, 2012).

Over the course of evolution, the brain has continued to develop. For higher stages of evolution, thinking and thus the cerebrum became increasingly important. This accounts for approximately two-thirds of the human brain mass. Like the cerebellum (Vester, 2012), it consists of two almost symmetrical halves, the cerebral hemispheres, which are connected by a strand of nerve fibers through which information is exchanged between the two halves. Four areas (frontal lobe, parietal lobe, temporal lobe, and occipital lobe) can be defined in each of the two hemispheres. Each of these areas performs different functions. The frontal lobe, for example, is involved in motor control as well as cognitive activities such as planning, decision-making, and goal-setting. Damage to this area can have far-reaching effects on a person's behavior and personality. In the approximately three-millimeter-thick outer surface of the cerebrum (Gerrig, 2015), the cerebral cortex, new knowledge is anchored in the form of specific relationship patterns between the nerve cells (Hüther, 2012). This is where the integration of sensory information, the coordination of movements, and abstract thinking and reasoning take place (Gerrig, 2015). Because these processes are essential for human survival, the cerebral cortex is particularly well-developed (Vester, 2012). Over the course of life, the cerebrum expands considerably- not due to the formation of additional nerve cells, however, but rather because existing nerve cells develop countless extensions and connect with each other in a variety of ways. As a result of this process, an enormous surplus of nerve cell connections and contacts arises in individual areas of the cerebral cortex. Only those that the brain actually uses and therefore needs are stabilized and maintained. The rest is broken down again (Hüther, 2012)

The Neurons

The sensory cells in the body are specialized in converting light, sound, pressure, shock, and chemical properties into impulses and transmitting them to the nerve cells (neurons) (Spitzer, 2007). Neurons generally have a compact center, the cell body or soma, with a diameter of approximately one forty-thousandth of a millimeter (Greenfield, 2003). Over 200 different types of neurons have been identified in the human brain. These can differ in shape, size, chemical composition, and function, but all share the same basic structure (see Figure 2). Neurons are specialized in processing and storing information and receive it via branched fibers outside the cell body called dendrites. In the cell body itself, information about the received stimulation is integrated and transmitted via a single, extended fiber, the axon. At the end of the axon are synapses through which subsequent neurons can be stimulated (Gerrig, 2015). Neurons can achieve firing rates of up to 300 impulses per second. This type of communication occurs primarily within the brain, as the individual cells in the human brain are primarily connected to one another. Each neuron has 10,000 to 15,000 connections to other neurons, while only one in ten million connections exists between the brain and the rest of the body. Several billion of these specialized nerve cells enable humans to do things that other living beings cannot and to adapt flexibly to a wide variety of environments, tasks, and problems (Spitzer, 2007). The human brain, for example, is capable of transferring tasks from existing neural structures to similar contexts for which it was not originally designed. For example, structures responsible for object recognition are expanded and also used for reading text (Goswami, 2008).

The extensive network of neurons in the brain is interspersed with glial cells, which support the neurons, assign newly formed neurons to the correct location in the brain, dispose of dead neurons, ensure the insulation of axons, and prevent toxic substances in the blood from reaching the brain (Gerrig, 2015). The number of neuroglia exceeds that of neurons by about ten times (Greenfield, 2003).

Synapses

The transmission of an impulse from one neuron to another occurs at a synapse, as briefly discussed in the previous section. This has a stronger or weaker synaptic connection to the following neuron and can therefore produce stronger or weaker, or even no, effects on its excitation (Spitzer, 2007). The impulse arrives at the end of the axon and, as shown in Figure 2, causes the synaptic vesicles to burst (Schachl, 2012). The messenger substances contained in the synaptic vesicles, called neurotransmitters, are then released into the synapses, cross the synaptic cleft between the individual cells, and transmit information to the receptors located on the dendrites of the adjacent neurons (Gasser, 2008). The strength and thus the effect of the neurotransmitters on impulse transmission is also influenced by neuromodulators (neuropeptides) (Schachl, 2012). Approximately 500 trillion synapses in the human brain enable targeted thinking and ensure that not all memories are recalled simultaneously, which would cause an immediate brain collapse (Vester, 2012). Synaptic connections enable humans to respond to a wide variety of inputs with very rapid responses. Reactions to respond (Spitzer, 2007).

BRAIN DEVELOPMENT

Our brains contain nerve cells (called neurons) that act as conduits to information, both incoming and outgoing. The information is transmitted in the form of chemical or electrical impulse. The connections between two different neurons are called synapses, which are junctions where chemical or electrical impulses pass from two neurons (see figure 2). A chain of synapses forms a neural pathway. Information passes through these pathways, enabling us to understand and respond to our environment. In the first months of life, humans produce an excess of synapses, meaning they are overproduced. After years, synaptic pruning occurs. This process allows the brain to discard unused and unexperienced synapses.

The vast majority of nerve cells are formed in the first half of pregnancy. Nevertheless, the brain is still very imperfect at birth. Babies and toddlers produce synapses like mad, creating more than they will need, but as Figure 3 shows, the newborn's nerve cells are isolated and cannot communicate. In this form, the cells are virtually nonfunctional. The situation is comparable to that on the internet, if there were no connections between the countless computers: the communication potential is there, but it cannot be utilized. In the first three years of a child's life, neural connections undergo tremendous growth. Dendrites form, through which the cells receive information from others, and synaptic connections, through which information is passed on to other cells. About 80 percent of dendrite growth occurs after birth. In this process – known as synaptogenesis – far more connections are formed than are actually needed; the result is a rather disordered and inefficient circuit diagram.

The maturation of the human brain is a complex process (Kraus, 2012), which constantly changes over time as a result of neuronal communication (Gerrig, 2015). At birth, a human being has approximately 120 billion brain cells, each of which has approximately 2,500 synaptic connections. Just eight months into a child's life, that number rises to 15,000 contacts. Many connections are initially loose and only develop during early growth. A large proportion of the synaptic connections that were rarely used will disappear, so that eventually only about a third of the connections that were created and used frequently (i.e., only those that receive nerve impulses frequently and thus become stronger) remain. In fact, the biological basis of cognitive development lies not in the increase, but primarily in the selection and deletion of unneeded synapses. This process forms the prerequisite for the ability to distinguish between important and unimportant stimuli (Kraus, 2012) and is a "fine-tuning of the functional networks of brain tissue and perceptual processes" (Blakemore & Frith, 2006).

The brain can simply be viewed as maturing in gradual ascending steps. The cerebral cortex matures at the slowest and least regular pace. However, the sensory areas of the cerebral cortex mature first. Synaptic density increases and peaks in the primary auditory cortex in the first month of life, and in the visual cortex at three to four months. The motor systems develop later. The time course of synapse decline shows clearer differences between brain regions. In cortical brain regions responsible for complex mental functions, this process extends for many years. Development takes a particularly long time in the prefrontal cortex. Here, synapse selection and myelin sheath formation continue until early adulthood.

Neuroplasticity

During childhood and adolescence, the thickness of the nerve fibers in the brain develops, leading to a doubling of brain volume. The advantage of this is that impulses can be transmitted 30 to 40 times faster via thick nerve fibers than via thin ones. Only at these high speeds can neural connections be properly utilized (Spitzer, 2007). The brain reaches its maximum capacity at around 27 years of age. Towards the end of life, its weight decreases by about two to three percent every ten years, and by up to 30 percent in total over a correspondingly long lifespan (Kraus, 2012). These changes in brain performance are also referred to in neurological research as plasticity or neuroplasticity (Gerrig, 2015). It is closely related to individual life experiences and reflects a person's different environments and activities (Goswami, 2008). Research into the phenomenon of neuroplasticity has shown, on the one hand, that it is the basis for the brain's ability to adapt to varying environments, stimuli, and demands. On the other hand, it has been proven that the localization of certain mental functions in the brain is flexible. Damage to the brain caused by illness or accidents does not necessarily cause permanent, irreparable damage to mental functioning (Stern, 2012; Aldrich, 2013).

Neuroplasticity is the brain's ability to change its structure and function throughout life based on experience and learning processes. This phenomenon enables the brain to adapt to new situations, compensate for damage, and learn new skills.

Neuroplasticity describes the brain's ability to reorganize itself and form new connections after damage. While this ability can be crucial for recovery from neurological diseases or injuries, in rare cases it can also have harmful effects, which is referred to as maladaptive neuroplasticity.

Why is childhood a crucial period for building brain plasticity? The brain is at its most plastic during early childhood, making it a crucial period for development: Neural connections in children's brains form more rapidly than in adults' brains. Early experiences have a disproportionate impact on brain structure. The foundations for lifelong learning, health, and behavior are laid during this period.

Neuroplasticity After Damage

In cases of neurological damage, such as a stroke, neuroplasticity can help partially or completely restore lost functions. If an area of the brain is damaged by a stroke, neighboring areas can take over the function of the damaged area by forming new neural connections. This can lead to improvements in movement disorders, speech problems, or other neurological symptoms. In rare cases, however, neuroplasticity can lead to undesirable outcomes, known as maladaptive neuroplasticity. This occurs when the brain forms new, but suboptimal, connections in response to damage, which can lead to additional symptoms or problems. Examples of maladaptive neuroplasticity:

Phantom pain: After an amputation, phantom pain can occur, which can be caused by the brain misinterpreting the missing limb.

Spasticity: In certain neurological injuries, neuroplasticity can lead to increased muscle spasticity.

Overactivation of neighboring brain areas: When one brain area is damaged by a stroke, neuroplasticity can cause neighboring areas to become overactive, which can lead to undesirable effects.

Several factors are thought to contribute to this type of plasticity, including the type and severity of the damage, the time frame after the injury, individual's environment and experiences can influence how the brain adapts after the injury. Neuroplasticity is a fascinating and important ability of the brain that allows it to adapt to change and compensate for damage. While neuroplasticity is generally beneficial for recovery, in rare cases it can also be harmful, a condition referred to as maladaptive neuroplasticity.

Family and social environment can support the development of neuroplasticity by taking into account the following:

Provide a stimulating environment: Offer a variety of sensory experiences and learning opportunities.

Encourage play: Both structured and unstructured play is crucial for brain development.

Ensure proper nutrition: A balanced diet supports brain growth and function.

Prioritize sleep: Adequate sleep is essential for memory consolidation and brain plasticity.

Limit screen time: Excessive screen time can impair brain development and social skills.

Encourage social interactions: Positive relationships and social experiences shape the developing brain.

Accept mistakes: Learning from mistakes is a powerful way to strengthen neural connections.

SPECIAL FEATURES OF THE ADOLESCENT BRAIN

The term adolescence describes the developmental phase between late childhood and adulthood (Konrad, Firk, & Uhlhaas, 2013). The WHO defines this as the period between ten and 19 years (World Health Organization, 2014). Adolescence is accompanied by profound reorganization processes in the brain, which can trigger a veritable change in identity, especially in its initial phase, between approximately ten and 15 years of age (Blakemore/Frith, 2006), (Konrad, Firk, & Uhlhaas, 2013; Baker et al., 2015). During this phase, there is a striking increase in the number of outgoing nerve fibers in a part of the frontal cortex and the temporal lobe, which is responsible for hearing and language comprehension (Gerrig, 2015). Other parts, however, are shed. Even if the total number of neurons no longer changes during this restructuring, numerous new wirings emerge in these local brain areas, which are presumably triggered by hormonal changes as well as social and neuroanatomical developments (Vester, 2012). Areas responsible for higher cognitive functions, such as the prefrontal cortex, mature somewhat later than, for example, the areas associated with motor and sensory functions (Konrad, Firk, & Uhlhaas, 2013).After this maturation process is complete, the newly structured brain area in the prefrontal cortex is responsible for functions such as setting goals and priorities, planning and organization, problem-solving and abstract thinking, as well as impulse management. In addition, brain regions responsible for social perception and self-awareness become more developed during adolescence (Vester, 2012; Dumontheil, 2015). However, this phase not only sees the development of new skills, but also the loss of some brain functions that had functioned well up to this point, such as certain foreign language, artistic, and musical abilities. Aligning with these new fields of association, pathways, and patterns in the mind is often difficult for adolescents and causes corresponding confusion. Only upon entering adulthood, when an efficient network of connections to the new areas has developed, do reactions return to a regulated path (Vester, 2012). In the previously predominantly gray brain tissue, an increase in white matter can be observed after the end of the adolescent phase. This increase is due to the decrease in synapse density and the simultaneous increase in myelin. This insulating substance surrounds the axons and increases the speed at which impulses are transmitted from one neuron to the next. Neuroscientists therefore refer to these connections as information highways (Goswami, 2008). Based on this development, it can be assumed that the transmission speed between neurons in the frontal cortex increases after adolescence (Blakemore & Frith, 2006).

Memory and Learning

Memory is a form of information processing and has the ability to decode, store, and retrieve information (Gerrig, 2015). It encompasses not only the storage and retrieval of verbally recalled content, but also every conscious perception and every type of purposeful action. Without memory, humans would not be able to use any of their past experiences for the present. The term learning refers to changes in behavior-controlling structures as a result of individual experiences. These changes can affect both physical and linguistic behavior and are intended to facilitate future coping with challenges. Memory is an essential prerequisite for learning, as stored events form the basis for building further knowledge (Hoffmann & Engelkamp, 2013; Stern, 2009).

The following subsections first describe the temporal and content-related possibilities for classifying memory, before a further section addresses the topics of learning, remembering, and forgetting.

Temporal Dimensions of Memory

The temporal division of memory is based on the multiple-storage model (Gasser, 2008), by differentiating between ultrashort-term, short-term, and long-term memory (Roth, 2003). Ultrashort-term memory, also referred to as sensory memory, serves as the first filter for perception (Vester, 2012). Sensory impressions are stored here for less than a second (Wittmann & Edelmann 2012). Short-term memory is limited to a period of a few seconds to minutes and has a capacity of only a few information units, whereas long-term memory is theoretically unlimited both in terms of time and its capacity resources (Brand & Markowitsch, 2009). However, a large portion of the perceived information is never permanently anchored in the memory, but remains available only for a short time—for example, due to a lack of interest, a lack of association possibilities, or distracting additional perceptions (Gerrig, 2015). All information received through sensory perceptions first reaches the sensory memory, where it forms an image of the previous information. Perception arises (Vester, 2012). This image is stored for only a few hundred milliseconds before the incoming information is forgotten, actively deleted, or overwritten by the acquisition of new information. During this extremely short period of time, the extraction of the most important features and their encoding for further processing in short-term memory take place. This occurs either verbally or—in cases where memory is not verbally comprehensible or difficult to capture—by establishing spatial relationships between the stimuli (Birbaumer & Schmidt, 2007).

Short-term memory is not a specific location in memory, but rather a built-in mechanism by which cognitive resources are focused on a small set of mental representations. The ability to hold more than a small selection of information in short-term memory is limited and requires intense concentration. Studies show that memory performance is limited to approximately seven (plus or minus two) random and meaningless items, such as any sequence of numbers. Other studies restrict the scope even further, stating that no more than three to five items are required. However, these values can be significantly increased through targeted rehearsal, the formation of a meaningful unit of information based on similarities or other organizational principles (chunking), and conscious processing (elaboration). The use of these methods enables efficient recall of content from short-term memory despite capacity limitations (Gerrig, 2015).

Short-term memory is embedded in the larger context of working memory- the memory resource used in everyday life for tasks such as reasoning and language comprehension. Working memory also enables the execution of mental processes necessary to complete an activity and thus provides a foundation for the current flow of thoughts and actions. To fulfill cognitive tasks, many different elements must be combined in rapid succession (Gerrig, 2015). In contrast to short-term memory, which represents a passive storage facility, contents in working memory are modified, processed, or summarized, among other things (Brand & Markowitsch, 2009). In this context, working memory can be viewed as a short-term, specific focus on the required elements. Research results show different capacities in people's working memory, which can be determined, for example, by measuring working memory span. Working memory span can be used as a measure of the resources available to carry out short-term cognitive processes. These are an indicator for predicting performance. The greater a person's working memory capacity, the more information can be combined into complex memory contents (Gerrig, 2015).

Only a small proportion of resources in short-term memory leads to the formation of memory content (Gerrig, 2015). Information is actively transferred from short-term or working memory to long-term storage (long-term memory) (Brand & Markowitsch, 2009), whereby the learning processes are very slow (Herrmann, 2012). Practicing and repeating information can facilitate this process and lead to the consolidation of the associated memory traces in long-term memory. This process is also referred to as consolidation (Birbaumer & Schmidt, 2007). As a rule, this requires paying attention to the information or forming associations with previously stored memory content (Brand & Markowitsch, 2009). If, however, no consolidation occurs, what has been acquired remains in short-term memory and is quickly forgotten (Herrmann, 2012). Long-term memory is theoretically unlimited both in terms of time and its capacity to process memory content (Brand & Markowitsch, 2009) and can store experiences, events, information, emotions, skills, words, rules, and judgments, sometimes for a lifetime. Thus, long-term memory determines a person's entire knowledge of themselves and the world (Gerrig, 2015). It is therefore assumed that multiple forms of long-term memory exist (Roth, 2003). To enable the retrieval of long-term stored memory material, it must be transferred from long-term to short-term memory (Birbaumer & Schmidt, 2007).

Both short-term and long-term memory are subject to the possibility of information loss, meaning that once acquired content can be forgotten due to various circumstances. While in short-term memory, forgetting occurs in the form of replacing stored information with new information, it is assumed that the forgetting of current content in long-term memory is due to interference with previously or subsequently learned material (Birbaumer & Schmidt, 2007). Long-term memory can be further differentiated based on its content dimensions. A fundamental distinction is made between declarative and non-declarative memory, although the classification of non-declarative memory is not uniform in the literature.

Both during initial acquisition and repeated use of stored memory content, a distinction can be made as to whether content is processed or retrieved implicitly (without conscious effort) or explicitly (with conscious effort). While much of memory research initially focused on the explicit acquisition of information, methods now also exist to examine implicit memory and thus obtain a more complete overview of the range of uses of memory. However, most circumstances under which information is retrieved require a mixture of implicit and explicit use of memory. For example, learning that the refrigerator is in the kitchen was implicit, but learning the word "refrigerator" required explicit effort (Gerrig, 2015).

A second way to categorize memory is found in the distinction between declarative and non-declarative memory. Declarative memory is responsible for the explicit and implicit recollection of facts and events (Gerrig, 2015). It encompasses episodic, semantic, and perceptual memory (Markowitsch, 2003; Roth, 2003). Non-declarative memory is more heterogeneous than declarative memory (Roth, 2003) and includes—depending on the author's classification—procedural and emotional memory, classical conditioning, and priming, among other things (Roth, 2003; Schachl, 2012). Some authors further equate non-declarative memory with procedural or implicit memory and contrast the latter with declarative memory (Roth, 2003). However, this chapter follows the view that procedural memory represents a subset of the higher-level non-declarative memory.

Declarative memory can be further subdivided depending on the cues required to recall memory content. Episodic memory stores individual and specific events that one has personally experienced (Gerrig, 2015). Due to its connection to a specific context, it is also called contextual memory (Roth, 2003).

Typically, an emotional evaluation of the episodic memory contents is performed (Brand & Markowitsch, 2009). To retrieve these contents, cues are needed that are temporally or content-related to the event in question (Gerrig, 2015). In contrast, the contents of semantic memory are context-free (Tulving & Markowitsch,1998) and refer to generic categorical contents. They reproduce information that is relevant to many different situations, such as the meaning of words and concepts (Gerrig, 2015). Semantic memory is therefore also referred to as knowledge and factual memory (Roth, 2003). Perceptual memory enables the recognition of objects, people, and stimuli based on a feeling of familiarity or recognition, (Brand & Markowitsch, 2009). which is why it is also called familiarity or recognition memory (Roth, 2003). Perceptual memory functions presemantically – the remembered content does not need to be named, nor is it necessary to know where the content is known from (Brand & Markowitsch, 2009).

Procedural memory ensures that people remember sequences of actions. It is used for the acquisition of perceptual, cognitive, and motor skills and functions largely unconsciously. With sufficient practice, longer sequences of actions can be performed without conscious intervention-indeed, the sequence of a routine action can even be disrupted by the attempt to explicitly bring it to consciousness. In general, it is difficult to pass on procedural knowledge and share it with others because it is difficult or impossible to verbalize (Gerrig, 2015). Furthermore, there also appears to be a form of memory that stores feelings and emotions and is therefore referred to as emotional memory, with moments experienced as particularly positive or negative being anchored most deeply in the memory (Gasser, 2008). Learning processes and actions based on classical conditioning also usually occur completely unconsciously. Classical conditioning refers to both physical and emotional reactions (Roth, 2003). Conditioned reactions relieve the brain by switching off thought processes and transmitting incoming impulses directly to the nerves. This makes it possible to react to certain perceptions without prior thought (Vester, 2012). Priming is based on the process of classical conditioning (Roth, 2003) and describes the improved recognition of previously unconsciously perceived content that is the same or similar. For example, a few sound sequences of a song heard casually once are enough to recognize it later (Brand & Markowitsch, 2009).

Cognitive Development

Many psychologists say that human intellectual development passes through a series of stages from birth to adulthood, most notably the Swiss scientist Piaget.

Piaget (1896-1980) studied child psychology and education at the University of Zurich and explored in his research the question of the development and progression of children's intelligence. According to Piaget, human cognitive development goes through the following stages:

Stage one from birth to 2 years:

In the stage from birth to 2 years infants think using their senses and motor actions. For this, it is called sensorimotor stage. Children explore the world by touching, looking, listening or biting things. This way children develop simple concepts of things. This stage is identified by motor activities without use of symbols. The major basis of learning method in this stage is trial and error. Cognitive activities at this stage is expressed by goal directed behaviour, object permanence concept, mental representation, cause and effect relationship and coordinated space.

In early childhood there are three simple reflexes: sucking, following objects with the eyes, and grasping with the hand. However this reflexive action changes to voluntary goal directed action like intentional grasping around six weeks of life. At this stage, the child begins to become aware that things continue to exist even when they are hidden from view, and the child now has the ability to retain a mental image of an event even after direct experience. Also children are able now to know cause and effect relationship. E.g. a child may make different sounds to get the attention from caregivers.

During this stage, children develop concept that coordination occurs among different objects and between objects and the body. For example, they begin to learn that a rattle makes sounds when shaken. Children, in this stage, establish the concept that self are not an extension with surrounding, and they recognize the existence of a boundary between self and the surrounding.

Stage two from 2 to 7 years:

The development at this stage is characterized by Egocentrism, transductive reasoning, Anthropomorphism, Artificialism, animism, Symbolic Functioning, Centration, Irreversibility, Curiosity and Seriation. Piaget calls preschool-age thinking preoperational thinking.

- Logical operations are not yet possible, but the child has the ability to reason about things.
- Also, the ability to use and manipulate symbols (Lego-bricks = bed/car/...)
- Thinking leads to language; new language = new thinking.

They believe that inanimate objects have life and are capable of actions, and that environmental objects are controlled by people. During this level, children believe that others see, feel and think exactly the same as them, and they develop the ability to make use of symbols in communication. Children develop the ability to focus attention on only one aspect of a situation at a time, but they cannot reverse in mind what they do or know.

Child begins to develop curiosity and ask a lot of questions. But child still does not have the ability to put things into categories. In this stage, child develops the ability to think on two levels simultaneously- imaginative and realistic.

Imitation (Mimicing someone's behaviour), symbolic play (Using objects as symbols), mental imagery (Imagining many objects in minds), and verbal evacation events (Using language to describe events, people or objects) are important behaviors that developed in this stage.

Stage three from 7 to 11:

This stage is the Concrete Operational Stage:

Children at this level start using logical thinking. Cognitive development at this stage is characterized by Logical thinking, Decentration, Reversibility, Cause Classification, and Transitivity Egocentrism.

Decentration: Now child is able to focus his attention on many aspects of a situation simultaneously.

Reversibility: Now children can reverse thoughts in their minds. If they know the way from home to school, they can imagine the opposite way back from school to home.

Cause and Effect relationship: Children develop the concept that there is a cause for some event. They can understand the relationship between clouds and rain.

Classification: Being able to focus on the relations1hip between a general category and two specific categories simultaneously, develop ability to name or identify a group of objects based on their appearance, size, or other characteristic.

Transitivity: Children are able to do some conclusions by combining relations logically.

Elimination of Egocentrism: Now it is possible for the child to see things from someone else's point of view as well.

- Concepts of stage 2 disappear at the end of the preoperational period, individual speed.
- Almost all of the preoperational period is overcome by the time children start school.
- Child is capable of multiple operations.
- Cognitive deficiencies of the preoperational period slowly disappear under the influence of concrete experiences and give way to a realistic, logical view of the world.
- At this age, children begin to enjoy collecting.

The fourth stage is the formal operational stage (Age 12 and Beyond):

At this stage cognitive development is characterised by: Abstract thinking, Hypothetical thinking, Adolescent Ego-centrism, Imaginary Audience, Deductive reasoning, and Problem solving.

Abstract Thinking: Here, children develop the ability to predict the possible outcomes and plan for long-term.

Deductive Reasoning: The child are able to develop general rules and identifies specific outcomes. For example, if A > B and B > C, then A > C.

Problem Solving: Now, the child is able to solve a problem logically and in methodical way.

Hypothetical Thinking: The child can identify possible outcomes.

Adolescent Ego-Centrism: The children at this stage develop a high self-consciousness. They believe that others are interested in them. They belief that others are watching them, and that they are the center of attention.

Critical Thinking, Piaget's Concept and Neuropsychology

Piaget's concept can be related to the structural concept of cognition in neuropsychology. The neuropsychological approach provides a foundation for understanding Piaget's concepts of cognitive development and how brain processes and neural structures influence the patterns of thinking and learning described by Piaget, and vice versa. Piaget's theory focuses on the qualitative development of thought processes at specific stages, while neuropsychology studies the neural basis of these developmental stages.

Piaget's theory of cognitive development does not directly address "critical thinking" in the modern sense in education and psychology today. Rather, it focuses on the stages of development of thinking and growth, and how children develop more complex ways of thinking through the stages of development of their brains and interaction with their environment. Critical thinking skills, such as analysis, interpretation, reasoning, and evaluation, are not fully and effectively formed until later stages of development, particularly in formal procedural reasoning and logical reasoning. However, this developmental perspective, when reinforced by the concept of brain development, allows for better identification of methods and approaches to support the development of children's neurological and psychological foundations for more effective later assimilation of critical thinking skills.

From an early age, children demonstrate interest and curiosity about themselves and the things and people around them. To develop their cognitive abilities and, later, critical thinking skills, it's important to support their curiosity and give them space to explore themselves and their surroundings with all their senses. It's also noticeable that this curiosity for exploration and sensory experience develops in line with their developing mental abilities and stages of growth. These developments can be summarized as follows:

3rd month: The child follows small, colorful objects with their eyes for a short time and only for a short distance.

6th month: The baby grasps toys and objects with both hands, puts them in their mouth, and chews on them. However, they still observe them indistinctly and without any focus.

8th month: The child is wary of strangers.

9th month: The child is familiar with daily routines such as eating, changing diapers, bathing, or small games and knows how they work. They reach for favorite toys. The baby imitates small gestures and facial expressions, such as waving or "bake cake."

12th month: The child pulls a cloth away from hidden objects. They follow their mother's finger when she wants to show or explain something. The child points to an object, toy, or person. They are already learning short children's rhymes and what behavior is and is not desired.

15th month The child tries out the simplest ways of using objects, e.g. hitting them against each other, shaking them or lining them up. They already know that animals, humans, and plants are living beings that behave differently than objects.

18th month: The child engages in role-playing. They imitate everyday activities of adults. They can occupy themselves for 10 to 20 minutes by putting objects in and out, examining them, or looking at them closely.

2nd year: They can stack at least three building blocks or similar objects on top of each other. The child develops a concentrated ability to observe, touch, or put toys and objects in and out of containers (over 15 minutes). They play small role-playing games, e.g., with dolls, toys, cars, etc.

3rd year: The child draws and scribbles. Although they are not yet painting representationally, they do comment on who or what they have drawn. They develop concentrated and intensive "pretend play," e.g., with dolls, cars, building blocks.

Year 4: The child begins the phase of asking W-questions (Why?, How come?, Where?, When?, Where from?). They can distinguish and name identical objects of different sizes or colors, e.g., small and large pears, red colored pencils, or red building blocks. The child can draw and describe houses, trees, and people (cephalopods) even more easily.

Year 5: The child recognizes and names the primary colors (blue, green, red, yellow, black, white). They also play intensive role-playing games with other children on themes such as father, mother, and child, dressing up, transforming into animals, childlike "heroes," and role models. They can construct three-dimensional objects with or without a template and create easily recognizable pictures and scenes.

Year 6: Construction play becomes more sophisticated. Children enjoy a variety of materials and use toys that increasingly require technical understanding. Children develop complex collaborative role-playing activities with themes such as family, school, or shopping. They show a keen interest in numbers and quantities (e.g., arranging objects by size; comparing shape, size, and quantity when sorting; creating patterns and rows). Colors are recognized and named, and sorted by shade into groups of reds, blues, etc.

What Should We Do to Develop Critical Thinking in Children?

We have to offer appropriate and proper educational opportunities e.g.:

- A wide range of play materials,e.g.,table games for language and math development, combination and strategy games,
- Supporting children's curiosity and interests,
- Comprehensive sensory experiences so that children learn about and understand their environment through their senses,
- Opportunities for physical activity so that children broaden their horizons, e.g., walks, games in the outdoor area and hallway, exercise rooms, psychomotor group, swimming, horseback riding, forest days,
- Mixed-age and developmental groups - children learn from one another,
- Planning and decision-making together,
- Projects on a variety of subject topics,
- Enable experiences with the cultural environment, e.g., road traffic, shopping, post office, library, museum,
- Nature experiences,

The Family Environment

Especially the parents, can also support their children's cognitive development at home by:

- Supporting children's curiosity in exploring their environment
- Providing opportunities for experimentation
- Time and space for free, focused play without interruptions
- Developmentally appropriate play and activities that neither over- nor under-challenge your child

The Effective Role of Social and Educational Institutions for Children

It is also necessary that the goals of social and educational institutions for children, such as nurseries, kindergartens and schools, be:

- Discover and experience the world around you with fun
- Support, develop, and guide the child's natural curiosity for knowledge and learning
- Improve concentration and perseverance
- Develop the child's memory
- Improve the ability to understand logical connections
- Gain experience in scientific areas
- Plan and make decisions

Start Teaching Critical Thinking From Childhood

It is important and essential to begin teaching critical thinking from childhood. A child who receives this upbringing from the start within their family will later stand out from their peers who do not. This will enable him to make more balanced decisions, which will bring him comfort and enjoyment of the results of his decisions.

There are good reasons why critical thinking is important for children, the most important of which are listed below:

First is that critical thinking helps people understand the world and the environment around them. In order to survive and thrive in the society, it is essential to understand the world. What are the principles that govern life? What is our role, and what can we contribute? What is permitted? What is prohibited, and why is it prohibited? If children are empowered to understand this, they will also be able to act responsibly and independently! Life operates according to specific rules and norms. For example, lying to others is unacceptable. Of course, a child can be constantly reminded: "Don't lie!" and perhaps they will listen! But only when they truly understand why lying is harmful will they grow into honest and upright adults. Following rules isn't difficult, but when children understand why they must follow certain rules, they can internalize and support them. And that is the heart of the matter: the rules and principles of life must be questioned critically in order to understand them. This helps children navigate the world and integrate into society.

Second, children need to learn how to solve problems with critical thinking. All of humanity's most groundbreaking inventions and discoveries came about after someone recognized a situation or problem and found a solution. Thus, inventors used critical thinking skills to improve and advance the world. Without critical thinking skills, they wouldn't have noticed a problem. As an example, the Swiss Georges de Mestral observed and copied his invention from nature. He was walking his dog and noticed that the fruits of the burdock plant often stuck to his dog's fur. At home, he investigated why they were stuck there. To do this, he placed the burdock burrs under a microscope. He noticed that burdock burr have lots of small, flexible hooks at the end of their spines. These can easily catch on hairy surfaces. This gave him the idea of using his discovery for fasteners. In 1951, his Velcro fastener was completed.

A child doesn't have to make a groundbreaking discovery right away, but they will also benefit from the ability to solve problems in school and later prepare to solve even bigger problems! Critical thinking, for example, helps students cope with and improve their poor performance in class by asking themselves: Why did I fail the test? What mistakes did I make? What can I do to avoid repeating these mistakes on the next test? What material do I need to study more carefully?

Third, critical thinking helps building a solid, independent personality and protect against influence. It is especially important for children, in the digital age,-

to be equipped with critical thinking skills. Today, the internet and social media apps offer vast amount of information -much of it are false and misleading, so it must be carefully examined and studied. But this apply to all media outlets convey information- including newspapers, television, and books- and must be examined and critically thoughtful. The information we receive influences us. This happens unconsciously, but through critical thinking, we can recognize this influence. This has to be done by reviewing and evaluating information, comparing it with other sources, and ultimately deciding for ourselves: Does this work for me? Or: Does this not seem right? In this way, children simultaneously learn self-confidence and develop their own goals and ideas!

Fourth critical thinking teaches children to say "no" when appropriate. Knowing their own strengths and weaknesses, as well as their personal boundaries, is crucial! Other people's ideas or suggestions shouldn't be copied or adopted thoughtlessly. Rather, they should be carefully scrutinized and evaluated first. This way, children learn to say "no"! This reduces the likelihood of being tricked into doing something they don't really want to do. Critical thinking supports children's development of self-confidence and the ability to defend their opinions.

But what are the practical measures that enable us to develop the critical thinking skills in children? Before answering this question, it must be realized that a child's cognition develops as he grows and his age. Humans, and children in particular, must be protected from brain damage and developmental disorders that may affect their decision-making ability and personality development.

DEVELOPMENTAL BRAIN DISORDERS

During the period of human formation and the rapid growth of the brain, at this stage, as Swaab explains, brain cells are highly susceptible to various factors. The brain requires sufficient and adequate nutrition to develop properly, and the thyroid gland must function properly. At this stage, brain development is generally determined by our genetic background and, in detail, by the activity of our neurons. These, in turn, are influenced by the availability of necessary nutrients, as well as the regularity of chemical messages from other brain cells (neurotransmitters), growth regulators, and hormones. At this stage, the fetus's sex hormones regulate the sexual differentiation of the brain. There is a possibility that substances may enter the fetus's body through the placenta that could disrupt the delicate process of brain development. These substances may come from the environment or through the pregnant mother's consumption (for example, alcohol, nicotine, and other addictive substances and medications, as well as environmental pollutants and harmful radiation) (Swaab, 2014).

Our world is not ideal. We live daily in dangerous transformations that threaten the intellectual development of millions of children and people. We find the spread of environmental pollution as a result of government negligence, corporate greed, wars, and the use of weapons that pollute the air, water, and soil. Blockades also result in famines, especially among children, affecting their mental and neurological development. The threat of climate change also poses challenges to children's mental and neurological growth.

Heavy metals entering the mother's and child's bodies can also impede fetal brain development. Lead, added to gasoline burned by cars and other materials used in industry and daily life in today's technological civilization, causes more children to be born with mental disabilities. It was only in the 1950s that the dangers of mercury to the brain and nervous system became clear when cats in fishing villages around Minamata Bay in Japan began behaving strangely and dying, and fish began swimming in strange patterns. Fishermen would sell their best fish and save the worst for the family store. As a result of the high levels of organic mercury in the fish—mercury proven to have originated from a plastics factory -6% of children in the surrounding villages suffered severe prenatal brain damage. The mercury impeded the formation of brain cells and the growth of brain tissue, leading to mental retardation. Adults in these villages also suffered various forms of paralysis (Swaab, 2014).

Swaab wrote: "Many chemical substances can reach the fetus and threaten its developing brain. Heavy metals in the environment, nicotine, alcohol, cocaine, and other addictive substances, as well as medication taken during pregnancy, can disrupt the rapid development of the brain. Children exposed before birth to the drugs taken by their mothers not only display withdrawal symptoms after birth but can also be left with permanent brain damage." To further explore these effects, we recommend referencing (Swaab, 2014). Drugs are essentially chemicals that interfere with normal brain function. They can disrupt the transmission of signals between nerves and the brain and impair the brain's ability to process information.

Alcohol is a cytotoxic substance, which is why it is also used as an antiseptic. Pure ethyl alcohol, i.e., potable alcohol, is therefore only safe in small quantities. Severe alcohol poisoning leads to the death of brain cells and can be fatal. Even regular consumption of small amounts can cause significant brain damage. One of the most serious illnesses is Korsakoff syndrome, in which entire regions of the brain die. Those affected can no longer remember anything, are severely demented (mental decline), and disoriented. However, this is only the final stage. With regular consumption of quantities that are no longer low-risk, mental decline sets in gradually. A blackout after a night of heavy drinking, for example, should be considered a warning sign.

Ecstasy affects the concentration of serotonin, an important neurotransmitter in the brain. Recent research on this topic has provided increasing evidence that it can cause serious brain damage. This is very likely dose-dependent: the more consumed, the greater the damage. The damage primarily manifests itself as memory problems. According to a recent animal study, ecstasy also damages the blood-brain barrier. This is the brain's protective barrier that normally prevents harmful substances and pathogens from entering the brain.

Cannabis consumption, especially regular and long-term use, has negative effects on brain performance. Impairments in short-term memory and impairments in logical thinking and judgment have been observed. Current findings indicate that this does not cause permanent brain damage, as the brain recovers after discontinuation of use. However, the ability to learn new information appears to be permanently impaired. Neurotoxic effects (damage to nerve cells) are well documented with amphetamines.

The most toxic is methamphetamine, also known as crystal meth. Difficulty concentrating and attention deficits are the more benign consequences. More serious are cerebral hemorrhages and strokes with sudden paralysis. The consequences of long-term amphetamine use are also visible in behavior. Those affected often tend to repeat the same activities over and over again, for example, repeatedly opening a drawer and becoming fixated on a particular thought. Nicotine affects the brain by stimulating the release of dopamine and other neurotransmitters, resulting in a range of psychological and physical effects. These include stimulation, increased attention and memory, and possible appetite suppression.

Physical Influences of Devices on the Neural System

Physical influences can damage the nervous system, for example, traumatic brain injury (TBI). Noise, vibration, radiation, ultrasound, and electromagnetic fields can also cause damage. The consequences range from temporary functional impairments to permanent disabilities.

Excessive use of smartphones can negatively impact children's brain development, especially when these devices are used at an early age. This can lead to problems related to cognitive abilities, mental health, and social interaction. Television can have both positive and negative effects on the brain. While it stimulates the brain in general, excessive television viewing can lead to a deterioration in cognitive abilities, particularly verbal memory.

Noise (machine noise, traffic noise, etc.) can negatively impact brain function by releasing stress hormones that impair cognitive abilities and increase the risk of various diseases. Noise exposure can lead to stress, fatigue, increased irritability, and difficulty concentrating and paying attention.

Intense urban light, especially artificial light, has significant effects on the brain. It can disrupt circadian rhythms, leading to sleep disturbances, increased melatonin production, and potentially impacting metabolism, mood, and even the risk of certain diseases.

Prolonged exposure to vibrations can cause various brain damage, especially when combined with hand, arm, and whole-body vibrations. Vibrations can cause brain damage indirectly, but not directly through the vibration itself. The main risks lie in the transmission of vibrations through the body, which can lead to neurological problems, or indirectly through other damage caused by vibrations.

Electric current or strong magnetic fields can cause brain damage. Electric current can cause unconsciousness, seizures, and even permanent neurological damage. Strong magnetic fields can cause DNA damage and brain cell death.

Overpressure and underpressure affect divers and workers in specialized underground construction. Pressure differences can lead to a buildup of respiratory gases in the body, damaging bones, muscles, circulatory systems, nervous system, and respiratory organs.

Judgments and Decision-Making Errors Due to Cognitive Distortions

Cognitive distortions are errors in thinking that influence our perception of reality. These distortions arise from various mental processes in the brain and can have a significant impact on our decisions and interactions in everyday life.

As already mentioned, the human brain is a complex organ composed of different regions that perform different functions. Two key areas involved in information processing and decision-making are the prefrontal cortex and the limbic system.

Prefrontal cortex: Responsible for higher cognitive functions such as planning, decision-making, and critical thinking. It helps us make rational decisions and control our impulses. Limbic system: Controls emotional reactions and the processing of memories. In stressful or emotional situations, it can promote impulsive, nonrational decisions.

Recent studies show that the interplay between these brain regions is crucial. A study by (Kahneman & Tversky, 1979) demonstrates that emotional influences on decision-making often lead to irrational judgments. Neuroscientific research has also shown that the limbic system is overactivated during emotional decisions, leading to cognitive biases. To save energy, our brains tend to simplify their work. Without this simplification and habit formation, our brains become overloaded. Fortunately, these simplifications relieve us of 50% of the burden of making decisions in our daily lives. However, this carries other risks and is, as they say, a double-edged sword. The brain uses heuristics, mental shortcuts, or rules of thumb to make decisions and judgments quickly and efficiently, especially in complex situations or when time is limited.

Heuristics: Heuristics are mental shortcuts that help us make quick decisions. However, they can also lead to biases, such as the availability heuristic or the anchoring effect, because they are based on limited information and do not always reflect reality.

Self-efficacy: The belief that one has the ability to overcome challenges influences our behavior and perception. People with high self-efficacy tend to approach challenges optimistically and are more likely to stick to their goals, which can lead to biased perceptions if they believe they can avoid all risks.

Emotional intelligence: Emotional intelligence is the ability to recognize, understand, and control one's own and others' emotions. People with high emotional intelligence can better regulate their emotions and are less prone to cognitive biases because they are able to consciously incorporate their emotions into decision-making processes and act more objectively.

Below you will find a brief overview of the most common cognitive distortions, their mechanisms and concrete examples from our daily lives:

- Confirmation Bias

Confirmation bias describes our basic tendency to focus on, notice, and give greater credence to evidence that fits our existing beliefs. Contextual bias is a form of confirmation bias and describes the way additional contextual information influences information processing (Oeberst & Imhoff, 2023).

Mechanism of confirmation bias: The brain rewards us with dopamine when we find information that supports our views. This leads to an incentive to seek out information that is similar to our viewpoint, which increases the tendency to seek out such information, which may be false.

Example: Teacher A believes that students are lazy and cannot be trusted to use tools. He focuses exclusively on cases where students fail to complete their tasks and use tools incorrectly, rather than investigating all cases of proper tool use.

- Availability Heuristic

The availability heuristic is a mental shortcut in our brain that causes us to judge the frequency of events based on how easily we can recall examples of them. The easier something comes to mind, the more likely it seems to us to happen. I.e: it is the assessment of the probability of events based on how easily similar events come to mind.

Mechanism of availability heuristic: Emotional experiences are more easily remembered, causing us to perceive certain events as more likely.

Example: A classic example is that people perceive shark attacks as more fatal than falling aircraft parts, even though the latter are much more likely to cause death.

- Anchoring Effect

It occurs when an initial piece of information, or "anchor," influences our perception and evaluation of subsequent information or offers, even if these anchors are irrelevant or inaccurate. This happens because our brain tends to orient itself around this starting point and make further decisions from there. The brain tends to use these rules, and here lies the risk of creating biases and possibly confirming and repeating them in decision-making in similar situations. It can be described as the tendency to rely too heavily on the first piece of information received (the "anchor").

Mechanism of the anchoring effect: The anchor acts as a reference point that influences subsequent judgments.

Example: In a study by Tversky and Kahneman (1974), it was shown that participants who were first presented with a high number (e.g., 1,000) reported a higher number when estimating a product's price than participants who started with a lower number (e.g., 10).

- Optimism Bias

Overoptimism is a phenomenon in which decision makers overestimate the chance that a future event will turn out positively or underestimate the risk that a future event may turn out negatively. It is a tendency to overestimate positive events and underestimate negative ones.

Mechanism of the optimism bias: Positive emotions promote optimistic perspectives in the brain, while negative events often receive less attention.

Example: A study by Weinstein (1980) shows that the majority of people believe they are less likely to become victims of illness or accidents than others. This leads to careless behavior, such as driving or smoking.

- Cognitive dissonance

Cognitive dissonance is the unpleasant feeling that arises when a person holds contradictory beliefs or thoughts. To reduce emotional stress, the person often tries to change their beliefs or behavior. It means that contradictions between one's own thoughts, beliefs, and actions cause unpleasant feelings in the brain. This feeling leads the brain to develop strategies to reduce the dissonance, for example, by changing his beliefs or trying to justifying actions.

Mechanism of cognitive dissonance: When dissonances arise, a feeling of tension or discomfort arises. This discomfort motivates the individual to reduce the dissonance and restore a sense of balance.

Example: Someone smokes despite knowing that smoking is harmful to their health. To reduce the dissonance, they might try to quit smoking or downplay the risks of smoking.

How to Avoid Cognitive Distortions

Overcoming cognitive distortions (biases) means recognizing and correcting systematic errors in thinking that can lead to incorrect decisions and judgments. This can be achieved through conscious reflection, sharing with others, and collecting data.

To overcome cognitive biases, you need to be able to recognize and name them. Then, through self-reflection and a little practice, you can overcome most irrational thought patterns. When you find yourself in an unpleasant situation, remember that it's not the situation itself that's causing you discomfort, but your thoughts about it. While you can't always control external circumstances, you have the power to change your own perception of the situation. Observe your thoughts closely and look for patterns to identify the type of distorted thinking that's occurring. When you notice a negative thought, ask yourself if there is evidence to confirm or refute that perception. Are there other possible explanations for the situation or the feelings you're experiencing? Are you perhaps exaggerating the seriousness of the situation? How might someone else, such as a close friend, interpret the situation?

Below are some guidelines for reducing and avoiding cognitive biases:

- Mindfulness and self-reflection: Consciously pay attention to your own thoughts and judgments to identify errors in thinking.
- Changing perspectives: Seeking the opinions of others and considering other perspectives to identify “blind spots” in your own thinking.
- Cognitive behavioral therapy (CBT): In CBT, errors in thinking are identified and replaced with realistic and helpful thoughts.
- Ask questions: Question your own thoughts with questions like “What is the evidence for this?” or “Are there other possibilities?”
- Training: Targeted training can help you identify and overcome certain distortions in specific contexts.
- Sources of information: Inform yourself about various sources of information and make your own opinion-forming process transparent.
- Seek dialogue: Talk to others about negative thoughts and seek support.

- Change environmental conditions: Change the types of information you are exposed to to reduce distortions.
- Metacognition: Strengthen your ability to think about thinking to better identify errors in thinking.

Professional help: Seek professional help if needed, especially in cases of more severe distortions or mental illness.

When we think critically, we reflect on an object and want to think consciously and reflectively. Often, however, this thinking is untrained, so it can become one-sided, fragmented, or even distorted. One must actually acquire and cultivate this thinking. This is certainly strenuous, but worthwhile. Critical thinking means: One critically engages with knowledge about the world. At its core, critical thinking is to take responsibility for the quality of our own thinking. In this context following questions can be raised: What do I do when I think?, What makes a claim credible?, What is a judgment, and how can I make scientifically sound judgments?, How do I support my opinion with arguments?, How do I counter the arguments of others?, What are facts? What is knowledge?, How does a thought change when I write it down?

Critical thinking is not an innate trait. Mastering critical thinking skills helps a person make decisions and solve problems more effectively. Consequently, the results of their decisions are satisfactory, contributing to their comfort and stability.

In the literature, critical thinking is often viewed as a skill. This includes, for example, "conscious, self-regulatory judgment, which includes interpretation, analysis, evaluation, and inference" (Facione, 1990). What's especially important here is independent research (searching for information, analyzing, drawing conclusions) without bias - i.e., without, for example, favoring information that corresponds to one's own opinion (confirmation bias, I try to confirm what I already believe to be true instead of actively searching for possible refutations) or neglecting or devaluing opposing positions (myside bias, I am not objective but argue for my position).

There are many important factors that act to maintain and enhance mental and psychological health.The most important is a healthy lifestyle, which should be cultivated from childhood. This includes adequate sleep, a balanced diet, regular physical activity, mental stimulation, and social interaction. Negative thinking and stress should be avoided, and positive thoughts and feelings should be encouraged. Avoid drugs and alcohol. The environment also affects mental health, so we must strive to ensure a clean environment for the society.

REFERENCES

Aldrich, R. (2013). Neuroscience, education and evolution of the human brain. *History of Education, 42*(3), 396–410. DOI: 10.1080/0046760X.2012.749543

Baker, S. T. E., Lubman, D. I., Yücel, M., Allen, N. B., Whittle, S., Fulcher, B. D., Zalesky, A., & Fornito, A. (2015). Developmental Changes in Brain Network Hub Connectivity in Late Adolescence. *The Journal of Neuroscience : The Official Journal of the Society for Neuroscience, 35*(24), 9078–9087.

Bassett, D. S., & Gazzaniga, M. S. (2011). Understanding complexity in the human brain. *Trends in Cognitive Sciences, 15*(5), 200–209.

Birbaumer, N., & Schmidt, R. F. (2007). Lernen und Gedächtnis, in: Schmidt, R. F., Lang, F. (Hrsg.): Physiologie des Menschen, 30. Aufl., Springer Medizin Verlag, Heidelberg, 223– 238.

Blakemore, S.-J., & Frith, U. (2006). *Wie wir lernen. Was die Hirnforschung darüber weiß.* Deutsche Verlags-Anstalt.

Brodbeck, K.H. (1997). praxis perspektiven Band 2, Jahrbuch des Vereins für betriebswirtschaftlichen Wissenstransfer am Fachbereich Betriebswirtschaft der Fachhochschule Würzburg-Schweinfurt-Aschaffenburg, Verlag BWT Würzburg

Dumontheil, I. (2015). Development of the social brain during adolescence. *Psicologia Educativa, 21*(2), 117–124. DOI: 10.1016/j.pse.2015.08.001

Facione, P. A. (1990). *Critical thinking/ A statement of expert consensus for purposes of educational assessment and instruction.* The California Academic Press.

Gassen, H. G. (2008). *Das Gehirn.* Verlag Wissenschaftliche Buchgesellschaft.

Gasser, P. (2008). *Neuropsychologische Grundlagen des Lehrens und Lernens, hep Verlag.*

Gerrig, R. J. (2015). *Psychologie* (20th ed.). Pearson Studium, Hallbergmoos.

Goswami, U. (2008). Principles of Learning, Implications for Teaching: A Cognitive Neuroscience Perspective. *Journal of Philosophy of Education, 42*(3–4), 381–399. DOI: 10.1111/j.1467-9752.2008.00639.x

Greenfield, S. A. (2003). *Reiseführer Gehirn.* Spektrum Akademischer Verlag.

Herrmann, U. (2012). Lernen findet im Gehirn statt. Die Herausforderung der Pädagogik durch die Gehirnforschung. In Caspary, R. (Ed.), *Lernen und Gehirn* (7th ed., pp. 85–98). Nikol Verlag.

Herrmann, U. (Ed.), *Neurodidaktik. Grundlagen und Vorschläge für gehirngerechtes Lehren und Lernen* (2nd ed., pp. 69–85). Beltz Verlag.

Hoffmann, J., & Engelkamp, J. (2013). Lern- und Gedächtnispsychologie, Springer-Verlag, Berlin Heidelberg.

Hüther, G. (2012). Wie lernen Kinder? Voraussetzungen für gelingende Bildungsprozesse aus neurobiologischer Sicht. In Caspary, R. (Ed.), *Lernen und Gehirn. Der Weg zu einer neuen Pädagogik* (7th ed., pp. 70–84). Nikol Verlag.

Kahneman, D. (2011). *Thinking, Fast and Slow*. Farrar, Straus & Giroux.

Konrad, K., Firk, C., & Uhlhaas, P. J. (2013). Brain Development During Adolescence. Neuroscientific Insights Into This Developmental Period. *Deutsches Ärzteblatt International, 110*(25), 425–431.

Kraus, J. (2012). Was hat Bildung mit Gehirnforschung zu tun? Schule zwischen neurobiologischer Vision und bodenständiger Pädagogik. In Caspary, R. (Ed.), *Lernen und Gehirn. Der Weg zu einer neuen Pädagogik* (7th ed.). Nikol Verlag.

Lorenz, K. (1965). *Über tierisches und menschliches Verhalten. Aus dem Werdegang der Verhaltenslehre* (Vol. i). Piper.

Markowitsch, H. J. (2003). Psychogenic amnesia. *NeuroImage, 20*, 132–138. DOI: 10.1016/j.neuroimage.2003.09.010 PMID: 14597306

Oeberst, A., & Imhoff, R. (2023). Toward Parsimony in Bias Research: A Proposed Common Framework of Belief-Consistent Information Processing for a Set of Biases. In: Perspectives on Psychological Science. DOI: 10.1177/17456916221148147

Roth, G. (2003). *Fühlen, Denken, Handeln. Wie das Gehirn unser Verhalten steuert.* Suhrkamp Verlag.

Sălceanu, C. (2021). Big-Five Personality Traits and Cognitive Skills in Higher Education, the Pandemic Context, Vol. 12 No. 3: Postmodern Openings, DOI: https://doi.org/DOI: 10.18662/po/12.3

Schachl, H. (2012). *Was haben wir im Kopf? Die Grundlagen für gehirngerechtes Lehren und Lernen* (3rd ed.). Veritas-Verlag.

Spitzer, M. (2007). *Lernen. Gehirnforschung und die Schule des Lebens* (2nd ed.). Springer Verlag.

Stern, E. (2012). Wieviel Hirn braucht die Schule? Chancen und Grenzen einer neuropsychologischen Lehr-Lern-Forschung. In Caspary, R. (Ed.), *Lernen und Gehirn. Der Weg zu einer neuen Pädagogik* (7th ed., pp. 128–141). Nikol Verlag.

Swaab, D. F. (2014). *We are our brains: a neurobiography of the brain, from the womb to Alzheimer's.* Spiegel & Grau a Penguin Random House Company.

Tulving, E., & Markowitsch, H. J. (1998). Episodic and declarative memory: Role of the hippocampus. *Hippocampus*, *8*, 198–204.

Tversky, A., & Kahneman, D. (1974). Judgment under Uncertainty: Heuristics and Biases. *Science*, *185*(4157), 1124–1131. DOI: 10.1126/science.185.4157.1124 PMID: 17835457

Vester, F. (2012). *Denken, Lernen, Vergessen. Was geht in unserem Kopf vor, wie lernt das Gehirn und wann lässt es uns im Stich? 35.* Aufl, Deutscher Taschenbuch Verlag.

Weinstein, N. D. (1980). Unrealistic Optimism about Future Life Events. *Journal of Personality and Social Psychology*, *39*(5), 806–820. DOI: 10.1037/0022-3514.39.5.806

Wittmann, S., & Edelmann, W. (2012). *Lernpsychologie: Mit Online Materialien* (7th ed.). Beltz Verlag.

World Health Organization. (2015). Recognizing Adolescence._https://www.who.int/publications/i/item/WHO-FWC-MCA-14.05 [visited on 9 June 2025]

Chapter 9

The Influence of Obstructive Sleep Apnea on Longevity and Well-Being

Md. Nurul Huda
Armed Forces Medical Institute, Bangladesh

Mohammad Badruddoza Talukder
https://orcid.org/0009-0008-1662-9221
International University of Business Agriculture and Technology, Bangladesh

ABSTRACT

This study aims to discover the intricate connection between obstructive sleep apnea and lifespan, as well as the numerous ways in which it impacts overall health and wellness. The following is our goal: One of the most prevalent sleep disorders, obstructive sleep apnea (OSA), is characterized by frequent pauses in breathing that occur while the individual sleeps. With the help of secondary data based on literature reviews and previously published articles, we carried out an exhaustive investigation to shed light on the complex implications of OSA in several different environments. We highlight the potential benefits of prompt intervention in minimizing the harmful effects of OSA on health and quality of life by synthesizing the findings from previous studies and secondary data analysis. This study provides valuable insights into OSA's multidimensional influence on longevity and well-being. It also highlights the need for early detection, effective management, and holistic care methods in optimizing health outcomes for people who are affected by this prevalent sleep disease.

DOI: 10.4018/979-8-3373-1812-7.ch009

INTRODUCTION

Periodic disturbances in breathing characterize a common sleep disorder known as obstructive sleep apnea (OSA) while the individual is asleep. In most cases, these disruptions are brought on by the temporary collapse of the upper airway that occurs multiple times throughout the night (Sweetman et al., 2023). This illness can significantly impact a person's health and well-being, affecting their physical and mental functioning. Considering this, it is of the utmost importance to examine the impact of obstructive sleep apnea on the longevity of people and their overall well-being. Apneas, which are disruptions in breathing, are to blame for oxygen deficiency and disrupted sleep patterns. “Apneas” refers to obstructions restricting breathing (Svedmyr et al., 2023). These abnormalities set off a chain reaction of physiological responses, each of which has the potential to contribute to a variety of health issues. Changes in mood, cardiovascular difficulties, metabolic irregularities, and cognitive impairments are some health issues associated with this condition. To gain a better understanding of the effects of this illness, it is necessary first to acknowledge the potential impact that obstructive sleep apnea may have on the health of the cardiovascular system, the regulation of the metabolic system, cognitive function, mood and mental well-being, general quality of life, and even longevity (Samadi et al., 2024). To solve these issues, it is necessary to take a holistic approach, which encompasses everything from the early identification and diagnosis of the problem to the implementation of efficient management strategies.

This study's objective on obstructive sleep apnea's effects on longevity and well-being is to shed light on the intricate relationships between sleep, health, and the general enjoyment one derives from life (Ap & B, 2023). The dissection of these connections makes it possible for individuals and medical professionals to work towards promoting healthy sleep and minimizing the potential adverse effects of obstructive sleep apnea on a person's lifespan and quality of life. Sleep apnea, sometimes called OSA, is a complicated health issue with ramifications that go beyond the typical headaches associated with sleeping during the night (Lin et al., 2024). The consequences of OSA can emerge across various physiological systems, affecting both the short-term well-being and the long-term health outcomes of those who experience frequent interruptions in their breathing while experiencing the condition. Untreated obstructive sleep apnea has several consequences, one of the most well-known of which is its impact on the cardiovascular system. Because of the intermittent drops in oxygen levels that occur during these episodes and the burden that is placed on the cardiovascular system, apneas are related to an increased risk of hypertension, coronary artery disease, and stroke (S. Lee et al., 2024). This is because apneas put a strain on the cardiovascular system. This could, over time, culminate in an increased likelihood of unfavorable cardiac events, which could potentially impact an individual's lifetime. The repercussions for the metabolism, Insulin resistance, and an increased risk of developing type 2 diabetes are two metabolic abnormalities that have been connected to obstructive sleep apnea, which has been linked to metabolic abnormalities (Sowho et al., 2023). OSA can cause dysregulation in glucose metabolism due to disrupted sleep patterns and altered hormonal control that are characteristic of the condition. This knowledge highlights the importance of comprehending the relationship between sleep, metabolic health, and overall well-being. Figure 01 shows the possible causes of obstructive sleep apnea.

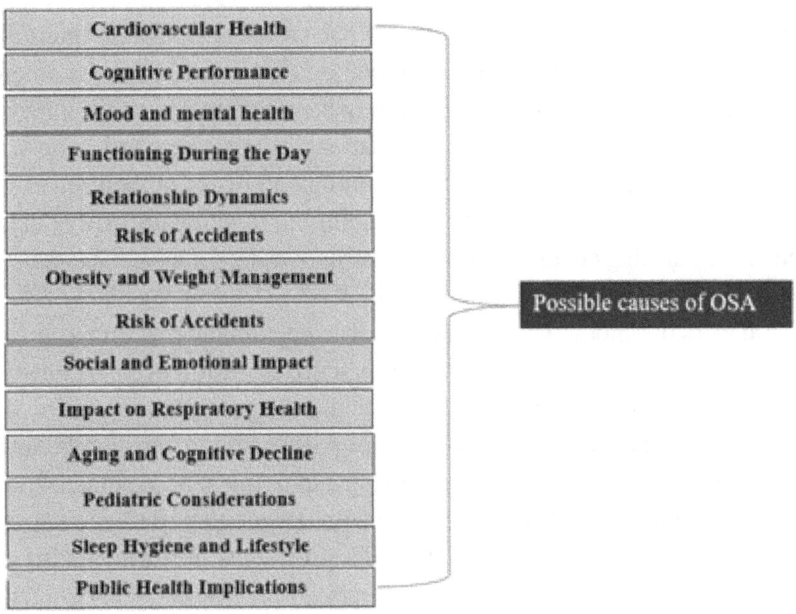

Source: Authors' compilation

Obstructive sleep apnea, also known as OSA, is a condition that can result in persistent sleep disruptions, which can cause daytime sleepiness and difficulties with cognitive function. Several cognitive problems are associated with people who have obstructive sleep apnea but have not received treatment for it (Berik Safçi, 2024). These problems include memory deficiencies, a shorter attention span, and a diminished decision-making ability. These aspects can potentially impact an individual's overall quality of life and capacity to participate in day-to-day situations effectively. Obstructive sleep apnea, often known as OSA, has been linked to an elevated risk of mood disorders like anxiety and depression, according to several studies. It is likely that mood fluctuations, which may affect mental well-being, can be caused by chronic weariness and anomalies in sleep patterns (Peker, 2023). When it comes to OSA, it is necessary to treat the psychological aspects of the condition to provide comprehensive care and enhance an individual's overall quality of life. In addition to the physiological effects, the symptoms of OSA, which include loud snoring and frequent awakenings, can have a significant impact on the quality of life of the individual who is affected by the condition as well as the health of their spouse who sleeps with them (Chalem, 2023). As a result of the strain that is placed on relationships, the tiredness experienced throughout the day, and the limitations in functioning, there is a general reduction in the quality of life. Even though obstructive sleep apnea substantially influences longevity and well-being, it is essential to recognize that effective preventative measures and management choices are available. Continuous positive airway pressure (CPAP) therapy is one of the appropriate interventions that has the potential to significantly improve outcomes and reduce the potential detrimental effects of OSA. It is essential to make a timely diagnosis, adjust one's lifestyle, and implement appropriate interventions. When a person has obstructive sleep apnea, the symptoms of the disorder continue to manifest themselves during the waking hours, which might hinder their ability to function normally during the day. One of the defining characteristics of obstructive sleep apnea that is not treated is excessive daytime sleepiness (Sowho et al., 2022). This can negatively affect performance at work or school, increase the risk of accidents, and make it more difficult to concentrate on tasks. A general loss in one's sense of well-being and contentment in day-to-day living may result from these challenges, contributing to the overall decline. As far as the dynamics of relationships are concerned, the disruptive nature of OSA symptoms, which include loud snoring and frequent awakenings, can place a strain on the connections that people have with one another. Bedmates may have trouble sleeping, which may lead to potential disagreements and influence the overall quality of their relationships. There is a probability that they will encounter sleep problems. In order to ensure the health and happiness of both the affected individual and their partner, it is necessary to address the impact that obstructive sleep apnea has on the dynamics of their relationship (Fridgeirsdottir et al., 2024). People who suffer from OSA are more likely to have daytime sleepiness and poor cognitive function, both of which can increase the likelihood of being involved in a car accident or participating in a variety of activities that they do while going about their daily lives. People who have obstructive sleep apnea that has not been treated may have a higher risk of being involved in accidents occurring at their place of employment or in collisions with motor vehicles (Bikov et al., 2024). Not only does this put them in danger, but it also puts the safety of others in immediate jeopardy. In both ways, there is a connection between obstructive sleep apnea and obesity. This connection is a two-way street. Both the control of weight and the prevention of obesity are intertwined. OSA can be made worse by being overweight, particularly around the neck. This can lead to the collapse of the airway during sleep, which can make the condition even more distressing. On the other hand, OSA, characterized by irregular metabolic processes, may contribute to weight gain (Argel, 2023). To effectively cure obstructive sleep apnea and improve overall health, it is vital to modify one's lifestyle to help manage one's weight. Influence on the health of one's social and emotional life, the challenges arising from obstructive sleep apnea extend beyond the physical realm, affecting the social and emotional well-being of an individual affected by it. When coping with a prolonged sleep disorder, it is possible to have sentiments of annoyance, helplessness, or loneliness. The individual can experience these sensations (Hendy et al., 2024). Improving awareness of OSA's social and emotional components is essential to providing comprehensive care and enhancing an individual's level of pleasure.

It is possible for obstructive sleep apnea to have immediate consequences, such as the obstruction of the airway, and to impact the respiratory system's health. People who suffer from obstructive sleep apnea may have a higher risk of contracting respiratory infections, which can make respiratory diseases that are already present much worse. It is essential to have a holistic approach to the health of the respiratory system since the occasional hypoxia that happens during apneas can create inflammation in the respiratory system (Çiftçi & Çiftçi, 2023). This further emphasizes the significance of taking a comprehensive approach to asthma management. In the context of aging and cognitive decline, there is a growing body of data that suggests that untreated OSA may lead to an accelerated rate of cognitive loss, which may have an influence on brain health in the long run. This is a concern because OSA is associated with more rapid cognitive decline. Because of this association, some problems need to be solved that are of the utmost importance about the likely role that obstructive sleep apnea plays in age-related neurodegenerative illnesses such as Alzheimer's disease, unpredictable Changes to the Sleep Architecture. Individuals who suffer from OSA cannot achieve and sustain sleep phases that are more restorative and deeper because the disorder creates disturbances to the standard architecture of sleep. The capacity of the body to repair and regenerate can be significantly damaged due to this disruption, which may have ramifications for the function of the immune system, the regulation of hormones, and the overall health of human cells (Duksal & Eren, 2023). Children can also be affected by obstructive sleep apnea, even though adults are more likely to be diagnosed with this condition. Considerations about children are necessary in this regard. When present in a child, OSA can impact the child's growth, cognitive development, and behavior. For children to attain and maintain healthy development and well-being throughout their lives, it is necessary to recognize and treat obstructive sleep apnea in children.

Individuals with obstructive sleep apnea that has not been treated may have higher utilization of healthcare services due to the management of associated comorbidities (Šmon et al., 2023). By understanding the more profound consequences of OSA on healthcare systems, it is possible to gain a better appreciation for the relevance of preventative measures, early diagnosis, and effective management to reduce the strain placed on healthcare resources. Not only does the management of obstructive sleep apnea involve the application of medical interventions, but it also requires an emphasis on general sleep hygiene and the evaluation of lifestyle factors. Several elements can work in conjunction with medical treatments and promote the health and well-being of an individual (Huang et al., 2024). Establishing a regular sleep schedule, creating an environment conducive to sleep, and adopting healthy sleep preferences are some essential elements with implications for the Health of the Public. There are more substantial implications for public health when one considers the incidence of obstructive sleep apnea as well as the potential influence that it may have on a variety of aspects of health. There is the possibility for improved health outcomes at the population level to be accomplished through implementing approaches for early identification and intervention, promoting education, and raising awareness.

The influence that obstructive sleep apnea has on a person's longevity and general well-being can have several effects on a person's physical, mental, and social well-being (Adekolu & Zinchuk, 2022). When these multifaceted effects are considered, it becomes clear how important it is to take a holistic and individualized approach to the diagnosis, treatment, and ongoing management of people with the illness. By addressing the many aspects of obstructive sleep apnea, medical professionals can work towards enhancing not only the quality of life but also the quality of life for individuals who are plagued with this frequent sleep disorder.

OBJECTIVES OF THE STUDY

To measure the relationship between health outcomes and OSA severity
To assess the effects of OSA therapy on health and lifespan
To investigate adjustable OSA elements and remedies for better health

LITERATURE REVIEW

A wide range of research has been conducted on the impact of OSA on longevity and well-being (Seda & Shrivastava, 2023). This study pertains to various fields, such as sleep medicine, cardiology, pulmonology, neurology, psychology, and public health. Figure 1 shows the burden of comorbidities in obstructive sleep apnea and the pathophysiologic mechanisms and effects. The following is a summary of the most important discoveries and trends that have been observed in the research literature:

Figure 2.

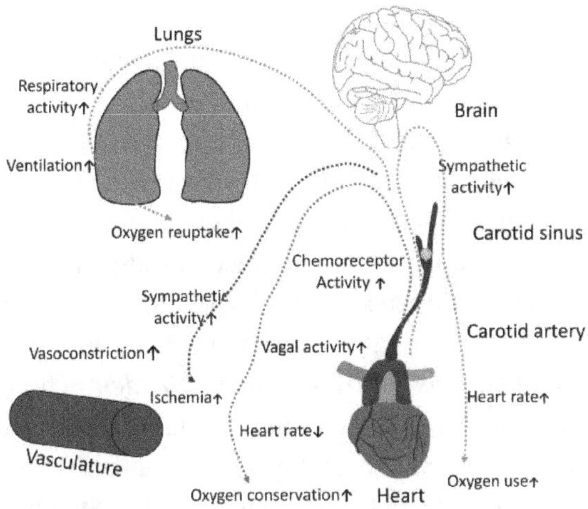

Source: *Authors compiled from Victoria Sircu et al., 2023*

***OSA and Cardiovascular Health*:** There is a strong correlation between obstructive sleep apnea and poor cardiovascular events, such as hypertension, coronary artery disease, stroke, and heart failure, according to a collection of research that has been conducted (Khan, 2023). The intermittent hypoxia, sympathetic activation, and oxidative stress that are associated with OSA lead to endothelial dysfunction, arterial stiffness, and atherosclerosis, which in turn increase the risk of cardiovascular events and mortality.

***Metabolic Consequences of OSA*:** Individuals who suffer from obstructive sleep apnea are more likely to develop metabolic disorders such as insulin resistance, dyslipidemia, and glucose intolerance (Heffernan et al., 2024). These metabolic disorders put people at a greater risk of developing type 2 diabetes mellitus and metabolic syndrome. Alterations in adipokine levels, cortisol production, and systemic inflammation are the mechanisms that underlie these relationships. These pathways illustrate the complex interaction between sleep-disordered breathing and the regulation of metabolic processes.

***Cognitive Impairment and Neurocognitive Disorders*:** OSA has been linked to cognitive dysfunction, namely lack of concentration, executive function, and memory (Kallel et al., 2023). Chronic sleep fragmentation and intermittent hypoxia, both of which are characteristics of OSA, have been involved in this dysfunction. Untreated OSA may hasten the deterioration of cognitive abilities and raise the risk of neurocognitive disorders such as Alzheimer's disease and vascular dementia, according to studies that have been conducted over an extended period.

***Psychological and Emotional Impact*:** There is a correlation between obstructive sleep apnea and an increased prevalence of mood disorders, such as anxiety and depression, as well as a decrease in quality of life and daily functioning (Votteler et al., 2023). Frequent sleep disruptions and excessive daytime sleepiness are factors that lead to emotional instability, decreased social engagement, and a general decline in well-being in those who are affected by this condition.

Impact of OSA Treatment on Health Outcomes: In addition to improving cardiovascular parameters, metabolic control, cognitive function, and mood stability, it has been demonstrated that effective management of OSA with continuous positive airway pressure (CPAP) therapy, dental appliances, or surgical therapies can enhance these areas. Nevertheless, adherence to treatment remains a substantial difficulty, highlighting the necessity of personalized treatments and comprehensive care models.

Public Health Implications and Healthcare Burden: The high incidence of OSA and its significant impact on morbidity, mortality, and healthcare utilization highlight the significance of public health programs that aim to increase awareness, promote early identification, and optimize management techniques (Oh et al., 2023). Comorbidities connected to OSA should be addressed, and multidisciplinary care pathways should be implemented to reduce the socioeconomic burden of this prevalent sleep disease.

The literature on OSA and its influence on longevity and well-being highlights the multifaceted nature of this sleep disorder. It emphasizes the critical role that early diagnosis, tailored interventions, and holistic care approaches play in optimizing health outcomes and improving the quality of life for affected individuals.

METHODOLOGY

Data Collection: We will draw from various sources to gather secondary data for our investigation. These sources will include research publications subjected to peer review, meta-analyses, systematic reviews, and pertinent databases such as PubMed, Scopus, and Web of Science (Miyahara et al., 2019). A complete understanding of the impact that OSA has on longevity and well-being will also be gathered through the utilization of data obtained from national health surveys, registries, and longitudinal cohort studies.

Inclusion and Exclusion Criteria: Specific criteria will be met by the studies included in the analysis. These criteria include relevance to the research issue, publishing in journals that have been subjected to peer review, availability of precise information on the diagnosis and severity of obstructive sleep apnea, and evaluation of health outcomes related to longer life spans and overall well-being (Subramaniam et al., 2023). Studies with insufficient sample sizes, incomplete data, or methodological restrictions will be eliminated to ensure the analysis is as reliable as possible.

Limitations: The variety of the studies that were included in the investigation, the variability in the diagnostic criteria and outcome measures for obstructive sleep apnea, and the retrospective nature of the analysis of secondary data are all potential limitations of the study (Ercolano et al., 2023). Sensitivity and subgroup analyses can address heterogeneity and investigate probable sources of bias.

FINDINGS

The results of the research indicate that there are strong connections between OSA and a variety of health outcomes that are associated with extended life and overall well-being(M.-K. Lee et al., 2024). As a result of doing an exhaustive investigation of secondary data, several important discoveries have been made:

Cardiovascular Health: The findings of this study demonstrate that there is a significant correlation between the severity of obstructive sleep apnea and poor cardiovascular events, such as hypertension, coronary artery disease, stroke, and chest pain. A greater incidence of cardiovascular events and death is observed in individuals who have untreated OSA in comparison to those who do not have OSA (Sehr et al., 2024). This highlights the significant role of sleep-disordered breathing in the cardiovascular system's health.

Metabolic Regulation: Various metabolic abnormalities, including insulin resistance, dyslipidemia, and glucose intolerance, are intimately associated with OSA. Through the use of longitudinal studies, it has been demonstrated that untreated OSA raises the likelihood of acquiring metabolic syndrome and type 2 diabetes mellitus (Wu & Cheng, 2023). This highlights the need to address sleep apnea in managing metabolic health.

Cognitive Function: As a result of OSA, individuals have chronic sleep fragmentation and intermittent hypoxia, both of which contribute to cognitive impairment, including deficiencies in attention, executive function, and memory. According to the study's findings, OSA that is not treated may hasten decreased mental function and raise the risk of neurocognitive disorders (Wojnowski et al., 2022). This highlights the importance of early detection and intervention to maintain cognitive function.

Psychological Well-being: There is a correlation between obstructive sleep apnea and an increased prevalence of mood disorders such as anxiety and depression, as well as a decrease in quality of life and diminished daytime functioning (Kaczmarski et al., 2023). A significant impact of sleep-disordered breathing on mental well-being is highlighted by the fact that individuals who suffer from obstructive sleep apnea and who have not received treatment report poorer levels of life satisfaction and social involvement.

Effectiveness of OSA Treatment: According to the findings, improved cardiovascular parameters, metabolic control, cognitive function, and mood stability can be achieved with the appropriate management of OSA through the use of continuous positive airway pressure (CPAP) therapy, lifestyle adjustments, or intervention through surgical procedures (Hoang-Anh et al., 2023). People with obstructive sleep apnea need to adhere to their therapy to maximize their health advantages and improve their general well-being.

Public Health Implications: The study highlights the significance of OSA to public health, its consequences for healthcare utilization, and the socioeconomic burden. Implementing multidisciplinary care pathways, promoting early identification, and raising awareness are all crucial components in reducing the negative consequences of OSA on the health and well-being of the population.

Impact on Quality of Life: The research sheds light on the significant influence that OSA has on a variety of elements of quality of life, such as physical functioning, social interactions, and emotional well-being. In comparison to people who do not have obstructive sleep apnea, those who have it and do not receive treatment for it report lower health-related quality of life ratings and more impairment in everyday activities (Hoang-Anh et al., 2023). Taking action to treat sleep-disordered breathing is essential for improving the overall quality of life and fostering optimal functioning in people impacted by this condition.

Role of Lifestyle Interventions: The findings highlight the significance of lifestyle modifications in managing obstructive sleep apnea and improving well-being. It is possible to boost the effectiveness of medical therapies by incorporating lifestyle changes such as losing weight, engaging in regular physical activity, and avoiding sedatives and alcohol (Alkhalifah et al., 2024). It is crucial to promote good lifestyle behaviors when optimizing sleep health and overall well-being in people with OSA.

Long-term Health Outcomes: Studies that follow patients over time shed light on the long-term effects of untreated obstructive sleep apnea on health outcomes and mortality risk. Individuals who suffer from severe obstructive sleep apnea have a greater risk of acquiring chronic health disorders and incurring premature mortality in comparison to individuals who do not have obstructive sleep aversion (Shi et al., 2023). Early intervention and ongoing care are necessary to reduce the adverse effects of sleep-disordered breathing on a person's health over the long run.

Health Disparities and Access to Care: The research points out significant differences in the diagnosis, treatment, and consequences of OSA among various demographic groups. These categories include racial and ethnic minorities, socioeconomically disadvantaged populations, and rural regions. Disparities in healthcare access and access obstacles to sleep medicine services lead to inequities in managing obstructive sleep apnea and health consequences (AliYeva, 2023). One of the most important things that can be done to ensure that all people who are impacted by obstructive sleep apnea have equal health outcomes is to address health disparities and improve access to care.

Interdisciplinary Collaboration: The findings make clear the significance of multidisciplinary teamwork in meeting the multifaceted requirements of people with obstructive sleep apnea. When providing comprehensive and patient-centered treatment, it is necessary to have coordinated care that includes sleep specialists, primary care doctors, cardiologists, pulmonologists, psychologists, and other professionals working in the healthcare environment (Kumar et al., 2024). Interdisciplinary teamwork makes conducting holistic assessments easier, developing individualized treatment plans, and providing continuous care for OSA patients.

Impact on Occupational Performance: This study aims to investigate the impact of obstructive sleep apnea on workers' performance and productivity in the workplace. Untreated OSA can cause individuals to struggle with focus, memory recall, and decision-making, resulting in lower job satisfaction, increased absenteeism, and worse job performance (Lombo et al., 2022). To establish workplace adjustments and interventions that will support affected people and boost productivity, it is vital to have a solid understanding of the impact of OSA on occupational functioning.

Social and Economic Burden: In light of these findings, the social and economic burden that obstructive sleep apnea places on individuals, families, and society should be better understood. The costs associated with untreated obstructive sleep apnea, including medical expenses, lost productivity, and decreased quality of life, constitute a considerable burden on the economy (Nguyen et al., 2024). The treatment of sleep-disordered breathing is the most critical factor in lowering healthcare expenses, increasing workforce productivity, and improving society's overall well-being.

Role of Sleep Environment: This study investigates how the environment in which one sleeps affects obstructive sleep apnea and overall health and wellness. Ambient noise, temperature, lighting, and the quality of the mattress are all factors that can have an impact on the quality of sleep and make symptoms of obstructive sleep apnea worse (Johnson, 2023). When medical therapies are combined with the optimization of the sleeping environment through the reduction of noise, the regulation of temperature, and the provision of comfortable bedding, it may be possible to achieve excellent sleep hygiene and general well-being.

Educational Interventions: These findings underline the significance of educational interventions in encouraging preventative measures and increasing knowledge about obstructive sleep apnea through disseminating information (Bonacina et al., 2024). Increased understanding of OSA risk factors, symptoms, and accessible treatments can be achieved by implementing public health campaigns, community outreach programs, and educational materials directed at individuals, healthcare professionals, and politicians. It is necessary to increase public awareness and comprehension of sleep-disordered breathing to facilitate early detection, timely management, and improved health outcomes.

Family Dynamics and Support: This study aims to investigate the effects of obstructive sleep apnea on the dynamics of families and support networks. There is a possibility that bed companions of people who have obstructive sleep apnea will face sleep problems, relational difficulties, and caregiver stress. There is potential for improved communication, decreased stress levels among carers, and strengthened social support networks if impacted families are provided with educational opportunities, counseling, and support services (Camañes-Gonzalvo et al., 2024). When it comes to addressing the holistic needs of people who have obstructive sleep apnea and their loved ones, family-centered treatment approaches are necessary.

Health Literacy and Self-management: To effectively manage obstructive sleep apnea and promote overall well-being, the findings highlight the significance of health literacy and the ability to self-manage medical conditions. To optimize treatment outcomes and improve the overall quality of life, providing people with obstructive sleep apnea with the skills necessary to participate in their care actively, adhere to treatment regimens, and adopt healthy lifestyle behaviors (Pun et al., 2023). Self-management can be made more accessible, and individuals can be empowered to take charge of their health and well-being by implementing services such as peer support programs, self-care treatments, and health education.

DISCUSSION

Considering the findings, the debate sheds light on the myriad ways in which OSA affects the health and well-being of individuals, as well as the more significant societal variables at play. The findings of this study highlight the strong correlations between untreated obstructive sleep apnea and unfavorable health consequences, such as cardiovascular disease, metabolic abnormalities, cognitive impairment, and mental health difficulties. In addition, the research sheds light on the socioeconomic burden of obstructive sleep apnea, including medical care expenditures, the loss of productivity, and decreased quality of life. It is necessary to take a comprehensive and interdisciplinary strategy to address the intricate relationship between obstructive sleep apnea and the various aspects of well-being (Theorell-Haglöw et al., 2023). This approach should involve healthcare providers, legislators, employers, and the general community. To mitigate the negative consequences of sleep-disordered breathing on people and society, it is vital to implement strategies that include increasing knowledge of OSA, improving access to diagnostic and treatment services, and promoting healthy lifestyle behaviors. In addition, the research emphasizes the significance of individualized care plans, individualized therapies, and continuing support for people with obstructive sleep apnea and their families (Roeder et al., 2024). Stakeholders can contribute towards minimizing the burden of OSA and improving overall health outcomes and well-being for all individuals by addressing the holistic needs of afflicted individuals and implementing preventive interventions at the individual, community, and population levels.

As an additional point of interest, the debate digs into the implications of the study's findings for clinical practice and public health policy. Because of the considerable correlations that have been found between obstructive sleep apnea and a variety of health outcomes, it is essential for clinical settings to implement early detection and intervention strategies. The screening of people at risk for OSA, the performance of complete examinations, and the implementation of suitable management techniques are all essential roles that healthcare providers play (ZU „Pulmo S" Teslić & Glišić, 2023). Furthermore, the study underscores the necessity of interdisciplinary collaboration among healthcare providers to treat the complicated needs of people with OSA. This collaboration should include sleep specialists, cardiologists, pulmonologists, psychologists, and other specialists with the appropriate expertise.

The research highlights the significance of implementing preventative interventions at the population level and increasing knowledge about OSA from the point of view of public health professionals. Individuals can be empowered to seek timely care by increasing their understanding of OSA's risk factors, symptoms, and treatments by implementing public health campaigns, educational efforts, and community outreach programs (Gu et al., 2023). Reducing inequities in the management of OSA and improving health equality depend on the efforts to enhance access to diagnostic services and treatment alternatives, particularly for underserved groups.

Furthermore, the study highlights the necessity of policies and initiatives to create supportive environments for individuals with OSA, both in clinical settings and the wider community. This includes campaigning for accommodations in the workplace, promoting healthy sleep practices in educational settings, and establishing policies to eliminate environmental variables that exacerbate symptoms of OSA, such as air pollution and noise pollution.

The study's findings shed light on the intricate relationship between OSA, health outcomes, and societal issues. This fact highlights the significance of adopting holistic strategies to tackle the myriad challenges of sleep-disordered breathing (S. Lee et al., 2024). Stakeholders can contribute towards improving outcomes for individuals with OSA and increasing general health and well-being for all parts of society by integrating clinical care, public health initiatives, and policy interventions.

PRACTICAL IMPLICATIONS

The study's findings have varied consequences for many stakeholders, including healthcare professionals, policymakers, employers, and individuals with OSA (Sharafkhaneh et al., 2023). These implications are far-reaching and have ramifications for those affected by OSA.

Healthcare Providers

Enhancement of Screening: Healthcare practitioners can establish more systematic screening methods to identify people who are at risk for OSA, particularly those who have concomitant disorders such as hypertension, obesity, or diabetes.

Misdiagnosis and the Role of Critical Thinking in Achieving Accurate Diagnosis and Effective Intervention

Misdiagnosis can lead to serious consequences, especially when it comes to conditions like OSA. This is where critical thinking becomes vital. It helps clinicians take a deeper, more thoughtful approach to evaluating symptoms, considering patient histories, and interpreting diagnostic tests. Clinicians can pinpoint OSA more accurately by carefully analyzing all the available information (Hai et al., 2024). When an accurate diagnosis is prioritized, it ensures that OSA is addressed correctly, avoiding the complications that can arise when the condition goes undiagnosed or untreated.

Critical thinking also guides clinicians in choosing the proper treatment approach. With a good understanding of the various options available, they can make informed decisions about the best course of action for each patient. This may include referring patients to sleep specialists like sleep physicians or surgeons when necessary. Treatment could involve methods like continuous positive airway pressure (CPAP) therapy, which helps manage OSA, or using oral appliances to keep the airway open during sleep. Surgery may be the best option to tackle the root cause of airway obstruction in some cases. By considering each patient's unique situation, clinicians can tailor their interventions to ensure the most effective treatment, ultimately improving their quality of life and overall health.

Patient Education: A significant part of the responsibility for teaching patients about the dangers of untreated OSA and the significance of medication adherence, lifestyle adjustments, and frequent follow-up care falls on the shoulders of healthcare practitioners.

Policymakers

Health Policy Initiatives: Policies that are designed to increase access to services for the diagnosis and treatment of OSA can be supported by policymakers (Sequeira et al., 2019). These initiatives can include coverage for sleep studies and CPAP equipment through public and commercial health insurance policies.

Workplace Regulations: Those in positions of authority can lobby for workplace rules that encourage healthy sleeping patterns, provide accommodations for people who suffer from obstructive sleep apnea, and lessen the risks associated with sleep loss and exhaustion.

Employers

Workplace Accommodations: Employers can implement various workplace accommodations to accommodate employees who have OSA (Qin et al., 2024). These accommodations include flexible work hours, designated nap rooms, and ergonomic improvements to improve sleep quality and productivity.

Employee Education: Employees can get education and resources from their employers regarding maintaining good sleep hygiene, recognizing the symptoms of OSA, and promptly obtaining medical examination and treatment.

Individuals with OSA

Treatment Adherence: Patients diagnosed with OSA should prioritize adhering to their treatment regimens to obtain the best possible health outcomes and quality of life (Jaromirska et al., 2023). Keeping up with the ongoing use of CPAP therapy or any other prescription therapies is included in this description.

Lifestyle Modifications: Complementing medical therapies and improving symptoms of OSA can be accomplished by adopting good lifestyle behaviors such as managing one's weight, engaging in regular exercise, and avoiding alcohol and sedatives before bed.

Support Networks: To provide emotional support, encouragement, and resources for coping with the challenges of living with OSA, it is possible to build a support network consisting of family members, friends, and healthcare practitioners.

The study's practical implications highlight the significance of a multidisciplinary approach to addressing OSA (Chiang et al., 2024). This approach should involve healthcare providers, policymakers, employers, and individuals to improve diagnosis, treatment, and support for those affected by this common sleep disorder. By implementing these practical solutions, stakeholders can collaborate to reduce the adverse effects of OSA on health, well-being, and productivity for individuals and society.

Suggestions

The following are some recommendations for further research and interventions that can be implemented in the real world based on the findings of the study:

Interventional Trials: It is essential to conduct randomized controlled trials to assess the efficacy of novel interventions in managing OSA and improving well-being. These interventions may include behavioral therapy, alternative treatments, or digital health solutions (Nadeem et al., 2023). The development of comparative effectiveness research could assist in determining the most effective and economical methods for managing obstructive sleep apnea in various populations.

Health Education Programs: Providers of healthcare, people who suffer from OSA, and members of the general public should all be included in health education programs designed to raise knowledge about the significance of sleep health, OSA risk factors, and the various available treatment options. Individuals could be empowered to recognize symptoms, seek immediate diagnosis and treatment, and adopt healthy lifestyle behaviors to improve the quality of their sleep through education campaigns.

Telemedicine Services: Telemedicine services should be implemented for remote diagnosis, monitoring, and management of OSA, particularly in locations that are underserved or for people who have restricted access to sleep medicine specialists. To improve patient outcomes and access to OSA services, telehealth platforms could enable virtual consultations, sleep apnea testing at home, and remote follow-up care.

Workplace Wellness Programs: Workplace wellness programs that prioritize the health of employees' sleep and help those who suffer from obstructive sleep apnea should be developed in collaboration with employers (Yang et al., 2024). Workshops on sleep education, ergonomic improvements, flexible work schedules, and employee assistance programs are all examples of workplace interventions that can treat sleep-related concerns and increase general well-being.

Community Outreach Initiatives: To increase awareness about OSA and to give resources for prevention, screening, and treatment, you should participate in community outreach programs. Through the formation of partnerships with local healthcare organizations, community centers, schools, and faith-based organizations, outreach efforts might be facilitated, and varied audiences could be reached with messages that are specifically targeted to talk about the importance of sleep health.

Policy Advocacy: It is essential to advocate for legislation and regulations that will increase access to OSA care, promote healthy sleep, and address environmental factors that contribute to sleep disruptions (Zaffanello et al., 2024). The funding of healthcare services for sleep services, the provision of accommodations in the workplace for those who suffer from sleep disorders, and the implementation of zoning restrictions to reduce noise pollution in residential areas should be among the policy priorities.

Remote Monitoring Technologies: For real-time monitoring of OSA symptoms, treatment adherence, and health outcomes, it is recommended to investigate the utilization of remote monitoring technologies, such as wearable devices and smartphone applications. These technologies may enable people with obstructive sleep apnea to receive proactive intervention, personalized feedback, and remote support, improving engagement and outcomes.

Culturally Tailored Interventions: To address the cultural beliefs, linguistic preferences, and social norms associated with sleep health and obstructive sleep apnea, it is necessary to develop interventions and instructional materials that are culturally adapted for varied groups (Isaac et al., 2024). Approaches that are sensitive to different cultures have the potential to improve the relevance and effectiveness of interventions, as well as to boost involvement among underserved communities.

Family-Based Interventions: Family-based interventions should be designed or developed to involve and educate family members about OSA, its impact on health and well-being, and techniques for helping affected people. By facilitating treatment adherence, providing emotional support, and creating an atmosphere that is supportive of lifestyle changes, family participation has the potential to improve outcomes for people who suffer from OSA.

Peer Support Networks: Create online forums or peer support networks for people with obstructive sleep apnea so they can connect, discuss their experiences, and offer support to one another. Individuals negotiating the obstacles of living with obstructive sleep apnea may benefit from peer support networks because they can provide practical advice, emotional encouragement, and a sense of community, fostering resilience and empowerment.

Sleep Health Education in Schools: Education regarding sleep health should be incorporated into the schools' curriculum to encourage good sleeping patterns and create knowledge about sleep's significance for general health and effective academic performance. Educators and students should be empowered to prioritize sleep health by implementing school-based programs that include interactive workshops, instructional resources, and instructions for proper sleep hygiene.

Health System Integration: It is important to include sleep medicine services in primary care settings to enhance access to obstructive sleep apnea screening, diagnosis, and management for people with comorbid disorders or restricted access to specialist care treatments (Prikladnicki et al., 2024). Streamlining the delivery of care and improving outcomes for people with OSA could be accomplished by implementing collaborative care models involving primary care clinicians, sleep specialists, and allied health professionals.

Research on Vulnerable Populations: Researchers should focus their attention on disadvantaged populations that are disproportionately impacted by OSA, such as racial and ethnic minorities, people with poor incomes, and people who are suffering from homelessness. Investigating socioeconomic determinants of health, barriers to care, and culturally relevant interventions could provide valuable insights that could inspire focused measures to reduce inequities and enhance outcomes in these patient populations.

Public Awareness Campaigns: Initiate public awareness campaigns with the goals of reducing the stigma associated with OSA, enhancing comprehension of the impact it has on health and well-being, and encouraging early detection and treatment-seeking behaviors (Baycheva et al., 2024). Increasing awareness of OSA as a public health concern and encouraging proactive participation in sleep health could be accomplished through mass media campaigns, social media outreach, and community activities.

Stakeholders can contribute to advancing research, improving clinical practice, and enhancing support for individuals impacted by obstructive sleep apnea if they implement these ideas (Zhang et al., 2024). Engaging in collaborative efforts across many sectors is vital to solving the complex problems that OSA poses and promoting optimal sleep health for everyone.

CONCLUSION AND FUTURE RESEARCH DIRECTION

In conclusion, the research offers persuasive evidence of how OSA can affect a person's longevity and overall well-being. The study elucidates strong connections between untreated obstructive sleep apnea and adverse health outcomes across various domains, including cardiovascular health, metabolic regulation, cognitive function, mental well-being, and quality of life. A comprehensive examination of secondary data accomplishes this. In addition to this, the research highlights the socioeconomic cost that OSA places on individuals, families, and society as a whole, highlighting the necessity of proactive therapies to address this prevalent sleep disease.

When optimizing health outcomes and improving the quality of life for people with OSA, the findings underline the significance of early detection, personalized therapies, and holistic care methods. Stakeholders can work towards minimizing the impact of OSA on health, well-being, and productivity for affected individuals and society by integrating clinical care, public health initiatives, and policy interventions.

Future Research Directions

Future research on OSA should concentrate on enhancing our understanding of this complicated sleep disorder and discovering novel techniques to diagnose better, treat, and manage the condition. It is necessary to conduct longitudinal studies to evaluate the long-term effects of OSA treatment on health outcomes, mortality risk, and quality of life. These studies will provide insights into the advantages sustained over time due to intervention treatment. The effectiveness of innovative interventions, such as behavioral therapies, digital health solutions, and community-based interventions, in managing obesity-related OSA and enhancing well-being should be investigated through interventional trials. Health equity research is vital to address disparities in the diagnosis, treatment, and consequences of OSA across various groups. This study can inform targeted initiatives for lowering inequalities and promoting health equity.

Furthermore, research on telemedicine, wearable devices, and smartphone applications can increase remote monitoring and self-management of OSA, enhancing access to care and supporting healthy behaviors. It is essential to advocate for policies to improve access to care for OSA, promote healthy sleep, and create surroundings that help people with OSA. The advancement of information regarding OSA and, ultimately, the improvement of outcomes for those affected by this prevalent sleep disorder can be accomplished by pursuing these prospective research paths.

REFERENCES

Adekolu, O., & Zinchuk, A. (2022). Sleep Deficiency in Obstructive Sleep Apnea. *Clinics in Chest Medicine*, *43*(2), 353–371. DOI: 10.1016/j.ccm.2022.02.013 PMID: 35659030

Alİyeva, A.AlİYeva. (2023). Obstructive Sleep Apnea and Circadian Rhythms. *Kulak Burun Boğaz ve Baş Boyun Cerrahisi Dergisi*, *31*(3), 179–188. DOI: 10.24179/kbbbbc.2023-98095

Alkhalifah, K., Alsalhi, S., Alrashed, A., Almagushi, S., Alharbi, M., Almutairi, A., Alghanim, S., Alkharraz, A., Alnasser, A., & Alradhi, M. (2024). Worldwide Prevalence of obstructive sleep apnea among pediatrics: A Systematic Review and Meta-Analysis. *International Journal of Medicine in Developing Countries*, *455–459*, 455–459. DOI: 10.24911/IJMDC.51-1701581085

Ap, K., & B, K. (2023). Pharyngeal Fascia and its Relationship with Obstructive Sleep Apnea. *Acta Scientific Neurology*, 26–31. DOI: 10.31080/ASNE.2023.06.0679

Argel, M. (2023). Sleep Obstructive Apnea Syndrome. In Esquinas, A. M., De Vito, A., & Barbetakis, N. (Eds.), *Upper Airway Disorders and Noninvasive Mechanical Ventilation* (pp. 269–276). Springer International Publishing., DOI: 10.1007/978-3-031-32487-1_29

Baycheva, S., Georgieva, G., Stoykov, M., Milkov, M., & Enchev, M. (2024). Impact of obstructive sleep apnea on patients'' quality of life. *Romanian Journal of Rhinology*, *14*(53), 24–28. DOI: 10.2478/rjr-2024-0005

Berik Safçi, S. (2024). The prevalence and polysomnographic characteristics of treatment-emergent central sleep apnea with obstructive sleep apnea. *Sleep and Breathing*, *28*(3), 1245–1250. DOI: 10.1007/s11325-024-02999-1 PMID: 38308750

Bikov, A., Bailly, S., Testelmans, D., Fanfulla, F., Pataka, A., Bouloukaki, I., Hein, H., Dogas, Z., Basoglu, O. K., Staats, R., Parati, G., Lombardi, C., Grote, L., & Mihaicuta, S.ESADA study group. (2024). The relationship between periodic limb movement during sleep and dyslipidaemia in patients with obstructive sleep apnea. *Journal of Sleep Research*, *33*(2), e14012. DOI: 10.1111/jsr.14012 PMID: 37596874

Bonacina, C. F., Soster, L. M. S. F. A., Bueno, C., Diniz, J. S., Bozzini, M. F., Di Francesco, R. C., Olegário, I. C., & De Oliveira Lira, A. (2024). Sleep bruxism and associated physiological events in children with obstructive sleep apnea: A polysomnographic study. *Journal of Clinical Sleep Medicine : JCSM : Official Publication of the American Academy of Sleep Medicine*, *20*(4), 565–573. DOI: 10.5664/jcsm.10950 PMID: 38059335

Camañes-Gonzalvo, S., Montiel-Company, J. M., Paredes-Gallardo, V., Puertas-Cuesta, F. J., Marco-Pitarch, R., García-Selva, M., Bellot-Arcís, C., & Casaña-Ruiz, M. D. (2024). Relationship of ankyloglossia and obstructive sleep apnea: Systematic review and meta-analysis. *Sleep and Breathing*, *28*(3), 1067–1078. DOI: 10.1007/s11325-024-03021-4 PMID: 38478208

Chalem, P. (2023). Obstructive Sleep Apnea and Systemic Autoimmune Diseases. In Baptista, P. M., Lugo Saldaña, R., & Amado, S. (Eds.), *Obstructive Sleep Apnea* (pp. 143–156). Springer International Publishing., DOI: 10.1007/978-3-031-35225-6_8

Chiang, J.-K., Lin, Y.-C., Kao, H.-H., & Kao, Y.-H. (2024). Surge of Sympathetic Activity during Hyperventilation at the End of Apnea for Patients with Obstructive Sleep Apnea. *Medicina*, *60*(3), 366. DOI: 10.3390/medicina60030366 PMID: 38541092

Çiftçi, B., & Çiftçi, T. U. (2023). Obstructive Sleep Apnea Syndrome: A Pulmonology Perspective. In Cingi, C., Yorgancıoğlu, A., Bayar Muluk, N., & Cruz, A. A. (Eds.), *Airway diseases* (pp. 1–17). Springer International Publishing., DOI: 10.1007/978-3-031-22483-6_129-1

Duksal, F., & Eren, F. (2023). Evaluation of thyroid functions and obesity in obstructive sleep apnea syndrome. *Revista da Associação Médica Brasileira*, *69*(9), e20230376. DOI: 10.1590/1806-9282.20230376 PMID: 37729367

Ercolano, E., Bencivenga, L., Palaia, M. E., Carbone, G., Scognamiglio, F., Rengo, G., & Femminella, G. D. (2023). Intricate relationship between obstructive sleep apnea and dementia in older adults. *GeroScience*, *46*(1), 99–111. DOI: 10.1007/s11357-023-00958-4 PMID: 37814196

Freire, C., Sennes, L. U., & Polotsky, V. Y. (2022). Opioids and obstructive sleep apnea. *Journal of Clinical Sleep Medicine : JCSM : Official Publication of the American Academy of Sleep Medicine*, *18*(2), 647–652. DOI: 10.5664/jcsm.9730 PMID: 34672945

Fridgeirsdottir, K. Y., Ólafsdóttir, K. A., Islind, A. S., Leppänen, T., Arnardottir, E. S., & Saavedra, J. M. (2024). The role of physical activity on obstructive sleep apnea severity and hypoxic load, and the mismatch between subjective and objective physical activity assessments. *Journal of Sleep Research*, *14195*(6), e14195. DOI: 10.1111/jsr.14195 PMID: 38480993

Gu, Y., Gagnon, J., & Kaminska, M. (2023). Sleep electroencephalography biomarkers of cognition in obstructive sleep apnea. *Journal of Sleep Research*, *32*(5), e13831. DOI: 10.1111/jsr.13831 PMID: 36941194

Hai, Y., Kou, W., Gu, Z., Zhang, C., Zou, Q., Wang, F., Yao, H., & Wei, P. (2024). Obstructive sleep apnea affects the psychological and behavioural development of children–a case–control study. *Journal of Sleep Research, 33*(1), e13924. DOI: 10.1111/jsr.13924 PMID: 37194421

Heffernan, A., Lalande, A., Chadha, R., MacNeill, A., & Chadha, N. K. (2024). Carbon savings potential of virtual care in obstructive sleep apnea and otitis media with effusion. *Laryngoscope Investigative Otolaryngology, 9*(2), e1221. DOI: 10.1002/lio2.1221 PMID: 38623079

Hendy, R. M., Elawady, M. A., Nasr, H. E., & Sarhan, R. S. R. (2024). Correlation of obstructive sleep apnea severity and lipid profile level. *The Egyptian Journal of Bronchology, 18*(1), 7. DOI: 10.1186/s43168-024-00260-7

Hoang-Anh, T., Duong-Minh, Q., Nguyen-Thi-Y, N., & Duong-Quy, S. (2023). Study of the obstructive sleep apnea syndrome in cerebral infarction patients. *Frontiers in Neurology, 14*, 1132014. DOI: 10.3389/fneur.2023.1132014 PMID: 37416312

Huang, B., Huang, Y., Zhai, M., Zhou, Q., Ji, S., Liu, H., Zhuang, X., Zhang, Y., & Zhang, J. (2024). Association of Sex With Cardiovascular Outcomes in Heart Failure Patients With Obstructive or Central Sleep Apnea. *Journal of the American Heart Association, 13*(5), e031186. DOI: 10.1161/JAHA.123.031186 PMID: 38410942

Isaac, M., ElBeshlawy, D. M., Elsobki, A., Ahmed, D. F., & Kenawy, S. M. (2024). Correlation between cone-beam computed tomographic findings and the apnea-hypopnea index in obstructive sleep apnea patients: A cross-sectional study. *Imaging Science in Dentistry, 54*(2), e17. DOI: 10.5624/isd.20230249 PMID: 38948186

Jaromirska, J., Kaczmarski, P., Strzelecki, D., Sochal, M., Białasiewicz, P., & Gabryelska, A. (2023). Shedding light on neurofilament involvement in cognitive decline in obstructive sleep apnea and its possible role as a biomarker. *Frontiers in Psychiatry, 14*, 1289367. DOI: 10.3389/fpsyt.2023.1289367 PMID: 38098628

Johnson, K. G. (2023). Obstructive Sleep Apnea. *Continuum (Minneapolis, Minn.), 29*(4), 1071–1091. DOI: 10.1212/CON.0000000000001264 PMID: 37590823

Kaczmarski, P., Sochal, M., Strzelecki, D., Białasiewicz, P., & Gabryelska, A. (2023). Influence of glutamatergic and GABAergic neurotransmission on obstructive sleep apnea. *Frontiers in Neuroscience, 17*, 1213971. DOI: 10.3389/fnins.2023.1213971 PMID: 37521710

Kallel, S., Kchaou, K., Kharrat, I., Chaabouni, M. A., Ayedi, S., & Charfeddine, I. (2023). Association between mean platelet volume and cardiovascular disease in obstructive sleep apnea syndrome. *SAGE Open Medicine*, *11*, 20503121231181634. DOI: 10.1177/20503121231181634 PMID: 37388904

Khan, A. F. (2023). Obstructive Sleep Apnea In An Indian Population: A Cross Sectional Study. *International Journal of Medical Students*, *S108*, S108. DOI: 10.5195/ijms.2023.2367

Kumar, R., Kaushik, R., Ish, P., Gupta, N., Hirekar, D. J., & Talukdar, T. (2024). Precision Medicine in Obstructive Sleep Apnea. *Indian Journal of Sleep Medicine*, *19*(1), 11–12. DOI: 10.5005/jp-journals-10069-0127

Lee, M.-K., Choi, J. H., & Lee, J. Y. (2024). Validity of Modified STOP-Bang Questionnaire as a Screening Tool for Obstructive Sleep Apnea. *The Annals of Otology, Rhinology, and Laryngology*, *00034894241234156*(6), 554–559. DOI: 10.1177/00034894241234156 PMID: 38384241

Lee, S., Noh, S., & Lee, W. H. (2024). Association of obstructive sleep apnea and diurnal variation of cystatin C. *BMC Nephrology*, *25*(1), 40. DOI: 10.1186/s12882-024-03472-7 PMID: 38287274

Lin, W., Wu, M., Wang, Y., Lin, C., & Wei, J. C. (2024). The prevalence of obstructive sleep apnea syndrome after COVID-19 infection. *Journal of Medical Virology*, *96*(1), e29392. DOI: 10.1002/jmv.29392 PMID: 38235910

Miyahara, L. K., Stefanini, R., Suguri, V. M., Wawginiak, G. H., Balsalobre, R. D. A., & Haddad, F. L. M. (2019). Evaluation of sleep quality and risk of obstructive sleep apnea in patients referred for aesthetic rhinoplasty. *Sleep Science*, *12*(03), 126–131. DOI: 10.5935/1984-0063.20190077 PMID: 31890086

Nadeem, W., Qayum, A., Jahangiri, R. H., Hasnain, S., & Jahangiri, F. R. (2023). *Exploring the Efficacy of Hypoglossal Nerve Monitoring and Stimulation in Treating Obstructive Sleep Apnea*. DOI: 10.5281/ZENODO.10214346

Nguyen, T. T. H., Pham, V. H., Ngo, Q. C., Pham, M. H., Vũ, V. G., & Phan, T. P. (2024). Clinical characteristics of obstructive sleep apnea in patients with heart failure. *T p Chí Ph u Thu t Tim M ch và L ng Ng c Vi t Nam*, *45*, 74–81. DOI: 10.47972/vjcts.v45i.1103

Oh, Y., Kim, J., Lyoo, C. H., & Kim, H. (2023). Obstructive Sleep Apnea and Striatal Dopamine Availability in Parkinson's Disease. *Movement Disorders*, *38*(6), 1068–1076. DOI: 10.1002/mds.29402 PMID: 37046390

Peker, Y. (2023). Obstructive Sleep Apnea and Cardiovascular Disease: Where Do We Stand? *The Anatolian Journal of Cardiology*. DOI: 10.14744/AnatolJCardiol.2023.3307 PMID: 37284828

Prikladnicki, A., Gomes, E., Sousa, L. C. C. R., Gonçalves, S. C., & Martinez, D. (2024). Cheeks appearance as a novel predictor of obstructive sleep apnea: The CASA score study. *Journal of Clinical Sleep Medicine*, jcsm.11022. DOI: 10.5664/jcsm.11022

Pun, M., Guadagni, V., Longman, R. S., Hanly, P. J., Hill, M. D., Anderson, T. J., Hogan, D. B., Rawling, J. M., & Poulin, M. (2023). Sex differences in the association of sleep spindle density and cognitive performance among community-dwelling middle-aged and older adults with obstructive sleep apnea. *Journal of Sleep Research, 14095*. DOI: 10.1111/jsr.14095 PMID: 37963455

Qin, H., Fietze, I., Mazzotti, D. R., Steenbergen, N., Kraemer, J. F., Glos, M., Wessel, N., Song, L., Penzel, T., & Zhang, X. (2024). Obstructive sleep apnea heterogeneity and autonomic function: A role for heart rate variability in therapy selection and efficacy monitoring. *Journal of Sleep Research, 33*(1), e14020. DOI: 10.1111/jsr.14020 PMID: 37709966

Roeder, M., Sievi, N. A., Frei, N., Schwarz, E. I., Steinack, C., Gaisl, T., & Kohler, M. (2024). The effect of longitudinal sleep monitoring on clinician agreement in obstructive sleep apnea diagnosis: The ELSA study. *Journal of Sleep Research, 33*(2), e13943. DOI: 10.1111/jsr.13943 PMID: 37197997

Samadi, S., Mehrain, A., Kheirollahi, A., Baradaran, M., & Arab Bafrani, M. (2024). Efficacy of Acupuncture in the Treatment of Obstructive Sleep Apnea: A Review. *Archives of Neuroscience, 11*(2). DOI: 10.5812/ans-144231

Seda, G., & Shrivastava, S. (2023). Effects of Obstructive Sleep Apnea and Insomnia on Cognitive Function. *Medical Research Archives, 11*(2). DOI: 10.18103/mra.v11i2.3578

Sehr, T., Akgün, K., Benkert, P., Kuhle, J., Ziemssen, T., & Brandt, M. D. (2024). Effects of obstructive sleep apnea treatment on neurodegenerative biomarker neurofilament light chain and cognitive performance. *Journal of Sleep Research, 14164*(5), e14164. DOI: 10.1111/jsr.14164 PMID: 38351662

Sequeira, V. C. C., Bandeira, P. M., & Azevedo, J. C. M. (2019). Heart rate variability in adults with obstructive sleep apnea: A systematic review. *Sleep Science, 12*(03), 214–221. DOI: 10.5935/1984-0063.20190082 PMID: 31890098

Sharafkhaneh, A., Agrawal, R., Nambi, V., BaHammam, A., & Razjouyan, J. (2023). Obesity paradox or hypoxia preconditioning: How obstructive sleep apnea modifies the Obesity-MI relationship. *Sleep Medicine, 110*, 132–136. DOI: 10.1016/j.sleep.2023.07.035 PMID: 37574613

Shi, N., Pang, F., Chen, J., Lin, M., & Liang, J. (2023). Abnormal interaction between cortical regions of obstructive sleep apnea hypopnea syndrome children. *Cerebral Cortex (New York, N.Y.), 33*(19), 10332–10340. DOI: 10.1093/cercor/bhad285 PMID: 37566916

Sircu, V., Colesnic, S.-I., Covantsev, S., Corlateanu, O., Sukhotko, A., Popovici, C., & Corlateanu, A. (2023). The Burden of Comorbidities in Obstructive Sleep Apnea and the Pathophysiologic Mechanisms and Effects of CPAP. *Clocks & Sleep, 5*(2), 333–349. DOI: 10.3390/clockssleep5020025 PMID: 37366660

Šmon, J., Kočar, E., Pintar, T., Dolenc-Grošelj, L., & Rozman, D. (2023). Is obstructive sleep apnea a circadian rhythm disorder? *Journal of Sleep Research, 32*(4), e13875. DOI: 10.1111/jsr.13875 PMID: 36922163

Sowho, M. O., Koehl, R., Shade, R., Judge, E., Woo, H., Wu, T. D., Brigham, E. P., Hansel, N. N., Tversky, J., Sterni, L. M., & McCormack, M. C. (2023). Obstructive sleep apnea screening in children with asthma. *Pediatric Pulmonology, 58*(6), 1683–1690. DOI: 10.1002/ppul.26375 PMID: 36852547

Sowho, M. O., Koehl, R., Shade, R., Judge, E., Woo, H. J., Wu, T. D., Brigham, E. P., Hansel, N. N., Tversky, J., Sterni, L., & McCormack, M. (2022). *Obstructive sleep apnea screening in children with asthma.* DOI: 10.22541/au.167035324.41591416/v1

Steffen, A., Schöbel, C., Vogler, J., Bruchhage, K.-L., & Tilz, R. R. (2023). Concurrent hypoglossal and phrenic nerve stimulation in patients with obstructive and treatment emergent central sleep apnea. *Sleep and Breathing*. DOI: 10.1007/s11325-023-02939-5 PMID: 37926800

Subramaniam, M., Rajaram Mohan, K., Fenn, S. M., & Pethagounder Thangavelu, R. (2023). Obstructive Sleep Apnea: A Case Report. *Cureus*. DOI: 10.7759/cureus.38644 PMID: 37284371

Svedmyr, S., Hedner, J., Bonsignore, M. R., Lombardi, C., Parati, G., Ludka, O., Zou, D., & Grote, L.European Sleep Apnea Database (ESADA) study group. (2023). Hypertension treatment in patients with sleep apnea from the European Sleep Apnea Database (ESADA) cohort – towards precision medicine. *Journal of Sleep Research, 32*(4), e13811. DOI: 10.1111/jsr.13811 PMID: 36539972

Sweetman, A., Osman, A., Lack, L., Crawford, M., & Wallace, D. (2023). Comorbid insomnia and sleep apnea (COMISA): Recent research and future directions. *Current Opinion in Pulmonary Medicine, 29*(6), 567–573. DOI: 10.1097/MCP.0000000000001007 PMID: 37642477

Theorell-Haglöw, J., Zhou, X., Wittert, G., Adams, R., Appleton, S., Reynolds, A., Ljunggren, M., & Marshall, N. (2023). Does obstructive sleep apnea increase the risk of cancer and cancer mortality in combined community-based cohorts? *Journal of Sleep Research, 14089*. DOI: 10.1111/jsr.14089 PMID: 37990480

Votteler, S., Knaack, L., Janicki, J., Fink, G. R., & Burghaus, L. (2023). Sex differences in polysomnographic findings in patients with obstructive sleep apnea. *Sleep Medicine, 101*, 429–436. DOI: 10.1016/j.sleep.2022.11.025 PMID: 36516599

Wojnowski, K., Mayo, M., Blanco, J. C. G., Abreu, A. R., & Chediak, A. D. (2022). Comorbid Narcolepsy and Obstructive Sleep Apnea: A Review. *Current Pulmonology Reports, 11*(4), 160–165. DOI: 10.1007/s13665-022-00297-3

Wu, Y., & Cheng, X. (2023). *Causal relationship between obstructive sleep apnea and asthma: A Mendelian randomization study*. DOI: 10.21203/rs.3.rs-3226417/v1

Yang, Q., Huang, X., Lin, Y., Chen, K., Lu, Q., Lin, W., Wang, X., Teng, Y., Jiang, P., Patil, S., & Zheng, Y. (2024). Exploring the Multifaceted Landscape of Pediatric Obstructive Sleep Apnea: Insights into Prevalence, Severity, and Coexisting Conditions. *Nature and Science of Sleep, 16*, 359–368. DOI: 10.2147/NSS.S452221 PMID: 38617037

Yu, P. K., Radcliffe, J., Gerry Taylor, H., Amin, R. S., Baldassari, C. M., Boswick, T., Chervin, R. D., Elden, L. M., Furth, S. L., Garetz, S. L., George, A., Ishman, S. L., Kirkham, E. M., Liu, C., Mitchell, R. B., Kamal Naqvi, S., Rosen, C. L., Ross, K. R., Shah, J. R., & Redline, S. (2022). Neurobehavioral morbidity of pediatric mild sleep-disordered breathing and obstructive sleep apnea. *Sleep (Basel), 45*(5), zsac035. DOI: 10.1093/sleep/zsac035 PMID: 35554583

Zaffanello, M., Ersu, R. H., Nosetti, L., Beretta, G., Agosti, M., & Piacentini, G. (2024). Cardiac Implications of Adenotonsillar Hypertrophy and Obstructive Sleep Apnea in Pediatric Patients: A Comprehensive Systematic Review. *Children (Basel, Switzerland), 11*(2), 208. DOI: 10.3390/children11020208 PMID: 38397319

Zhang, E., Yao, Y., Zhou, N., Chen, Y., Zhang, H., Guo, J., & Teng, F. (2024). A fine-grained convolutional recurrent model for obstructive sleep apnea detection. *International Journal of Machine Learning and Cybernetics, 15*(7), 3043–3056. DOI: 10.1007/s13042-023-02080-5

Chapter 10
The Link Between Choosing a Field of Study: Critically and Wisely and Overall Well-Being and Satisfaction

Raad Kadhum
https://orcid.org/0009-0003-3097-4121
Independent Researcher, Bahrain

ABSTRACT

The chapter aims to provide students and stakeholders with understanding of the problem of choosing a university major and to help them make an informed decision, taking into account the various influencing factors. It explains the nature and importance of the relationship between this choice and critical thinking. It presents a concept for developing critical thinking based on models and research on the development of thought and cognition in children and individuals. Specifically, and based on Tutt's concept of study choice and Jean Piaget's view of children's mental and intellectual development, a conceptual proposal is developed to prepare individuals to make sound decisions and select an appropriate study program. The chapter addresses the relationship and interaction between the Big Five personality factors and the careers an individual needs, as well as their impact on personal satisfaction and well-being. Proper preparation for individuals impacts not only the decision-making stage but also the course of study and the chances of future success.

DOI: 10.4018/979-8-3373-1812-7.ch010

INTRODUCTION

For many who complete their schooling, the most important question they face is, What's next? Work or university? The transition from school to university is a crucial change that shapes young people's futures and lives. Choosing a major is vital for many students, resulting in significant consequences.

The individual is ultimately the one who determines and elects his/her own future. To meet his or her needs and interests, he or she must make sound choices, taking into account numerous influencing factors. However, individuals and the factors influencing their decisions are subject to change, whether these changes and influences are external or internal.

Although most students have a clear desire to choose a subject that suits their interests, inclinations, and abilities and that prepares them for a career that also suits them, they are often unable to identify these courses and feel overwhelmed by this task (Heublein & Sommer, 2002). The fact that the choice of subject is not always successful is shown, for example, in the statistics on changes of subject and dropouts. Almost 40% of students have to revise their first choice of subject and either switch to a different subject or drop out of their studies altogether (Friebertshäuser, 2008).

Numerous surveys of schoolchildren, prospective students, and new students indicate that a major factor in the uncertainty and overwhelm caused by choosing a course of study is that students do not feel adequately prepared for their studies (Hachmeister, 2007; Mutz & Daniel, 2008; Heine et al., 2005).

The extent to which information influences the decision-making process is demonstrated by a survey where students who had already decided on a set of subjects felt significantly more informed than students who did not yet know what they wanted to study (Hachmeister, 2007). This illustrates how important it is to be informed about the study options for decision-making because only those who know the options available to them and what conditions or consequences they entail are able to evaluate the options that best fit their ideas. This is in addition to the ability to identify sources of information, determine what is useful, and discard what is unnecessary.

Providing and accessing information is important, but it is not sufficient. Mastering the skill of analyzing information not only influences the decision-making process but also impacts the course of study and its chances of success. This information relates to the nature and circumstances of the study, as well as subsequent job and employment opportunities. Part of this information also relates to the importance of understanding an individual's personality type, which helps them choose their academic and professional specializations later on. Not every personality type is suitable for every profession or study. A high degree of congruence between professional identity and professional self-concept leads to professional success, well-being, satisfaction, and job stability.

It is noted that a large percentage of students drop out of study due to their poor choices. These findings underscore the need for better preparation for this crucial stage of choosing an academic major. Many students are ill-prepared for this stage. Incorrect decisions regarding their study selection and subsequent career choices will lead to discomfort in their work and therefore their lives.

The results of the studies and research confirm the need for a better approach to preparing students from an early age for this critical stage in choosing an appropriate academic major. The skills of searching for accurate and useful information, analyzing it, and utilizing it to make sound and appropriate decisions are essential parts of critical thinking skills. Empowering students with these skills from an early age will be the foundation for their success in discovering their potential and interacting successfully with their environment.

The development of these skills occurs in tandem with the development of the human cognitive stages, which influence the formation of personality, as highlighted below. This chapter will discuss their importance. Deficits in sound decision-making skills can be a result of deviation and failure to consider these developmental stages.

In this chapter, we will discuss all the factors and elements mentioned above that influence the quality of choice of study course, and consequently the career and job an individual will pursue later. We emphasize the importance of preparing students from an early age to make sound decisions by equipping them with critical thinking skills. But what is critical thinking? Let's first look at the topic in more detail.

WHAT IS CRITICAL THINKING?

The general, fundamental goal of thinking is to "understand the essence and core of things." We all face multiple choices on a daily basis, so we need the best information, methods, and analytical tools to make sound decisions. The best of these analytical methods and tools is critical thinking. It can be said that critical thinking is a type of thinking that improves the quality of thinking by skillfully tracking, measuring, and comparing underlying inherent thought structures according to intellectual standards, according to Elder and Paul (Elder & Paul, 2006) "Critical thinking is the disciplined art of ensuring that you use the best thinking you are capable of in any given set of circumstances."

Critical thinking skills are used to address and overcome the challenges of life, work, and learning. It is a skill that can be learned and developed. Critical thinking is not just "thinking," but rather a tool that can be used, developed, and applied to solve problems. Skills can be understood as self-regulating behaviors that enable self-organized action under ambiguous conditions. This concept has become a near-universal reference term for educational performance, contributing to a comprehensive educational improvement process.

People strive and desire to practice critical thinking and try to think about things consciously and reflectively. However, their thinking is often untrained, so it can become one-sided, fragmented, or even distorted. Therefore, it is necessary for students to acquire and cultivate this thinking constantly and diligently. At its core, critical thinking means taking responsibility for the quality of our thinking. Mastering critical thinking skills helps a person make decisions and solve problems more effectively. This will lead to more satisfying and effective results, which will contribute to their well-being, comfort, and satisfaction. After this presentation, which gives us some background on the concept of critical thinking, let us return to addressing our main topic.

COMMON CONCEPTS FOR STUDY AND CAREER CHOICE

The decision to accept or reject any study program is not made at a specific point in time; rather, it is a process influenced by multiple factors, during which the basic decision regarding any subject or university is made. These factors include changes and development of the brain during growth and maturation, as well as the accumulation of experiences, knowledge, and interaction with the surrounding environment. This means that the decision-making process regarding career choice and future studies is a complex process, not a one-dimensional one.

Concepts based on the theory of congruence and development are based on the basic assumption that each individual has unique personality traits and that each professional field and academic discipline has different and specific requirements. Given this background, the process of choosing a career path and academic discipline is interpreted as a type of individual adaptation effort (Bußhoff, 1984; Forßbohm, 2010; Beyer, 1992). The assumption here is that people choose their career or educational paths in accordance with their talents, interests, and personal inclinations. In this regard, Holland (Holland, 1985) seeks to understand vocational interest as a form of personality expression and self-control (see Weinrauch & Srebalus, 1994) and conceives vocational choice as a process of matching personality type with professional work environments.

Holland postulates six ideal types in his personality model. He distinguishes between the realistic (technical-practical orientation), the investigative (intellectual-research orientation), the artistic (artistic-linguistic orientation), the social (helpful teaching orientation), the enterprising (predominant entrepreneurial orientation), and the conventional (organized, rule-based orientation). He also describes the professional environments with ideal types: The realistic, the investigative, the artistic, the social, the enterprising, and the conventional. According to his assumptions, people with a predominantly investigative intellectual orientation would be particularly interested in studying at university, and a more practice-oriented interest would lead to a suitable career choice.

Others look deeper into the influences, arguing that drives and incentives acquired in childhood (Kratz, 1969), needs (Vroom, 1964), and conflicts between internal drives and social norms (Freud, 1930) in particular have been identified as effective aspects of career decision-making.

The perspective and concept in developmental psychology have changed. It no longer views the emergence of personality traits as a specific, short-term phenomenon, but rather as a process of growth over time. The focus is on the question of which stage of individual development occurs at which age.

According to Ginzberg's stage model (Ginzberg, 1988), career choice is an irreversible, cumulative developmental process, which he divided into three developmental stages, beginning in childhood between approximately seven and eleven years of age and becoming more specific and precise with age. Based on an increasingly clearer connection with reality, career choice is irreversibly completed around the age of seventeen (Ginzberg, 1988). The developmental process is largely completed by career choice (Ginzberg et el., 1951).

Super (Super, 1953; Super 1980) also followed a step-by-step approach (lifespan and life-space approach to career development). In his framework model (the career rainbow), the phases of growth were described: exploration, consolidation, maintenance, and decline, which are aligned with a career and linked to standardized life story patterns.

A person's life roles change according to the stage of development. The choice of career is assigned to the phase of exploration and is made in comparison with professional self-concepts. Similar to Holland (1985), Super also assumes that the individual follows individual aspirations to create congruence between self-concept and professional requirements. Unlike Ginzberg (1988), Super, however, does not consider career decisions to end with the first career choice. Rather, professional personality development is described as a process that extends over the entire span of working life.

Professional Identity & Professional Self-Concept, Overall Well-Being and Satisfaction

We note that there is a constant effort to align professional identity with professional self-concept. Professional identity is defined here as an objective view of oneself- a stable image of one's goals, interests, and talents (Pfuhl, 2010). Professional self-concept also includes a level of self-reflection and indicates the personal significance of interests, values, and decisions (Super, 1980). A high congruence between professional identity and professional self-concept leads to professional success, well-being, satisfaction, and job stability. Therefore, professional success depends primarily on the individual's willingness and ability to manage the assigned task effectively in terms of related development tasks (Pfuhl, 2010).

Tutt's Selection Process

Based on the Rubicon model of action motivation, Lars Tutt (1997) developed his study of the selection process. The Rubicon model is a central model of motivation. It is developed by the German psychologists Heinz Heckhausen and Peter Gollwitzer (1987). The primary focus of it is on the four central questions listed below:

How are goals selected?
How is the achievement of goals planned?
How is action taken to achieve the goal?
How is the action evaluated afterward?

In short, this model tries to show why a person acts the way he does and what leads or motivates him to do certain actions.

Lars Tutt interpreted study selection as a process that is divided into various decision-making stages. He emphasizes the importance of gathering information at each stage separately, inspired by this model. The marketing sector's insights are used by him to view the future student as a client of the university institution (Tutt, 1997). He views the study decision as a multistage process of decision-making.

Figure 1. Stages of study selection

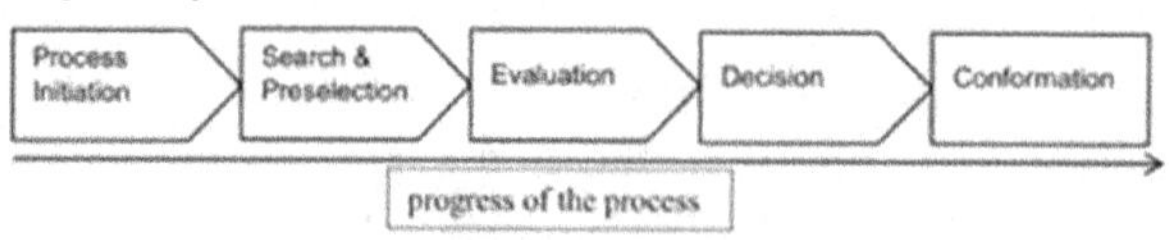

According to Tutt (1997); prepared by the author

As shown in Figure 1, Tutt distinguishes five essential stages. The first stage is the initiation of the process. In many cultures, particularly industrialized cultures, it was typically the parents of the future student who made the majority of the decisions regarding their child's career path up to this point. The first years of a person's life are crucial to the development of his or her personality. External influences after birth, however, will have a significant impact. The local culture in which the child is raised has a significant impact on the intensity of these influences. For instance, the size and extent of a family can vary from culture to culture. After that, the future student is faced with the decision of how he or she wants to lead the rest of his or her life (here we encounter the influence of the cultural factor of society once again. In some societies, potential future jobs are determined by gender). Tutt makes it clear that the high school graduate does not need to undertake extensive information-gathering measures on his or her own at first, as he or she will initially receive initial information from family, school, friends, and the media (Tutt, 1997).

In the next stage of orientation, the student will need specific information and advice from a specialized party. For this purpose, in some countries, career advisors from employment agencies are consulted. Today, however, the internet and various guidance, options, and offers play an important role, especially during this introductory stage. Furthermore, most universities send detailed information themselves, either to promote the program in an attractive manner or to provide only basic information. That assumes that a student is generally interested in studying a particular major. In this case, the research and pre-selection phase begins. This stage also involves gathering a variety of information. Therefore, from the perspective of universities, technical colleges, and vocational academies, it is important to arouse the student's interest in studying at the university in principle and to explain the advantages of its location. “The universities play a very important role in this evaluation phase” (Tutt, 1997). It can be assumed that the student has received all the information about the desired major and only needs to decide on the university location. As a rule, a prospective student does not apply to just one university to preserve the opportunity to start studying at another in case of rejection.

After this decision-making phase comes the confirmation phase: the student has chosen the major and the university but also has doubts, especially if the place of study or the majors he/she rejected are considered particularly attractive. Now it is the responsibility of universities to enter the reinforcement phase: the prospective student must be encouraged to make their choice even after the university has been chosen. It is now much easier for universities to provide interested parties with information, as it can be specifically addressed (Tutt, 1997).

START DEVELOPING INDIVIDUAL ABILITIES AND SKILLS FROM EARLY CHILDHOOD

Undoubtedly, making sound decisions and choices depends on an individual's ability to think clearly and possess appropriate skills and abilities. This requires obtaining the cognitive abilities necessary to understand the structure of problems, deal with them efficiently, construct a position, and solve existing problems. The concepts of thinking and cognitive abilities will be discussed in more detail later. However, as previously mentioned, the family and social environment play a vital role in shaping a child's personality and developing their skills and abilities. Critical thinking is one of the most important of these skills. Those who possess it will be distinguished by their ability to make successful decisions and achieve results that align with their aspirations and desires, leading to well-being and satisfaction.

Based on what will be explained below, one can imagine that the process of preparing an individual to make a sound decision and choose an appropriate study program runs roughly parallel to the processes envisioned by Tutt, beginning before the child is born.

Tutt called the first stage "the initiation stage" (in this stage, the foundations for building critical thinking have to be formed). According to Tut, the study selection stage represents the true conscious beginning of this process (and is the first stage of using critical thinking). Then the second stage (the evaluation) requires higher critical thinking skills and the ability to use them correctly. The final stages, the decision-making, and the confirmation stages, require a much higher level of critical thinking skills and the ability to apply them effectively.

Today, based on the experiences and research of many specialists, one knows that individuals' personalities and mental and intellectual abilities begin to crystallize from the moment of birth, and even before that, in the mother's womb. This justifies emphasizing the importance of the family, parents, and primary educational institutions in building critical thinking skills in children in their early years. The beginning of the growth and development of the elements and factors that influence the formation of a child's personality and mental abilities can be traced back to the period before birth, as agreed upon by experts.

In his book "We are our brains: a neurobiography of the brain, from the womb to Alzheimer's" Swaab confirms the interaction between the mother's brain and her child's brain (Swaab, 2014). In several chapters of his book, he details the reciprocal relationship between mother and child, which significantly influences the formation of a child's personality and mind later on. Swaab also refers to the influence of the father. In this regard, he says, "As children grow up, their fathers may inspire them and affect the course of their lives. This can take many different forms." (Swaab, 2014).

Swaab emphasizes the importance of a child growing up under parental care to develop his mental abilities and intelligence. "Studies have shown that orphans adopted before the age of two go on to develop normal IQs (averaging 100), while children who are not adopted until between the ages of two and six attain average IQs of 80." (Swaab, 2014). Swaab refers also to the influence of the environment on human development from childhood, specifically referring to language and communication skills (Swaab, 2014).

Generally, human memory is formed in the first years of life and develops thereafter. However, this does not mean that the period before that has no influence. Human brain development can be affected in the womb, during childhood, and beyond due to a lack of necessary and adequate nutrition, stress, or environmental pollution (e.g., heavy metals); (Swaab, 2014) (chapter 2).

Swaab concept expands the scope of the first-stage influence beyond what Tutt addressed in his model. This encourages us to deepen our understanding of it and its impact and perhaps link it to subsequent decisive factors in the university choice process.

Several studies suggest a relationship between an individual's personality and critical thinking skills (Acevedo & Hess, 2022), so we will discuss the concept of personality in more detail, depending on what the chapter allows.

INDIVIDUAL PERSONALITY, COGNITIVE ABILITIES, DECISION MAKING

"Understand yourself!" is an ancient wisdom. It is important, but not easy. To achieve this, we must possess the necessary skills. It has also been said: "Self-knowledge is the first step towards improvement!" However, life experiences tell us and teach us that such self-knowledge is usually only available in a specific place and time, and may occur in a completely different context. Even in this case, we can ask ourselves: "What took me so long?" We need to start immediately to understand ourselves. It is widely accepted that possessing critical thinking skills give us a good chance of understanding our-self. Therefore, in this section, we will discuss the most important component of the self: personality.

Human personality and the way it influences and is influenced by the environment and the individual are important factors in decision-making. This factor is not easy to understand and assess, as it is subject to change, development, and influence by various factors.

Some Important Concepts in Personality

In experimental, empirical personality psychology, there has been a debate for decades about the best terminology to describe personality and which "basic types" it can be divided into. Individuals react and behave differently when faced with similar life situations. Among the many factors that contribute to individual behavioral variation, such as physiological and psychological characteristics, personality significantly influences individuals' self-determination. Personality is a pattern of an individual's behavioral, temperamental, emotional, and mental traits. People with different personalities have distinctive behavioral characteristics.

To facilitate and simplify the understanding of the diversity in cognitive and behavioral abilities and emotional responses of individuals, an OCEAN (Openness, Conscientiousness, Extraversion, Agreeableness, Neuroticism) personality model was developed and adopted by many behavioral psychologists to investigate the different decision preferences of heterogeneous individuals. For example, according to an assessment (McCrae & Costa, 1987), there is a convergence between different personality models toward identifying five basic factors, the Big Five, that determine personality. A visual illustration of these factors is shown in Figure 2.

Figure 2. The basic big five factors

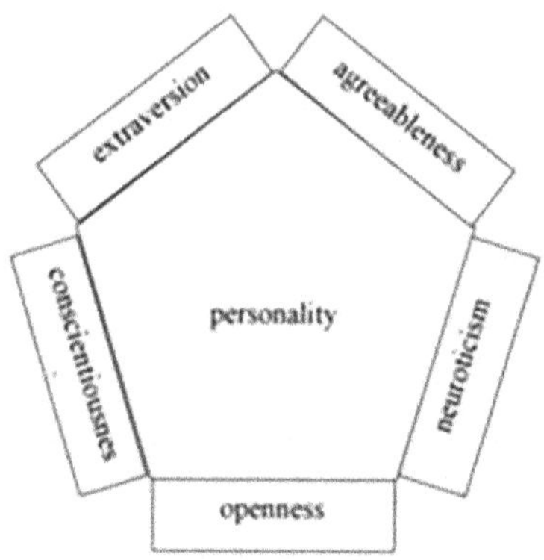

One finds many authors who believe in the necessity of studying and understanding the biological foundations of personality theory, and this is interesting. Amelang and Bartussek point out that for a number of personality traits, "individuals differ in their biological determined reactions, and that these differences influence social behavior." (Amelang & Bartussek, 1997). A complete understanding of personality differences cannot be achieved without recourse to biopsychological concepts. They also emphasize the continuing importance of research into the biological causes of personality. Personality psychology, which aims not only to describe but also to explain differences between individuals, must begin by relying on the biological basis of behavior.

Are Human Behavior and Personality Largely Determined by Genetic Factors, or Does the Environment Play a Major Role?

Since ancient times, the debate has raged over whether human personality is innate or shaped by environmental conditions. It is pointless to attempt to trace the history of this "nature versus environment" debate in detail. In biology and the behavioral sciences, opinions on this topic are sometimes extremely opposed. While American behaviorism assumes that all cognitive, emotional, and behavioral characteristics of animals and humans are completely determined by the environment, the Austrian Lorenz and his supporters, as well as representatives of sociobiology and behavioral ecology, believe that human behavior is largely genetically determined.

Amid this debate, Freud occupies an important intermediate position. He believed that individual thinking, feeling, and behavior are largely determined, but at the same time, he postulated various reasons for this determination. Freud argued that some determinants of individual behavior are genetic or phylogenetic in nature and therefore innate, while others arise from imprinting processes in early childhood, and still others from formative pubertal experiences. According to Freud, there is a gradual process of determining personality, beginning with genes, continuing through the early postnatal period, and continuing through early adolescence (Freud, 1930).

Furthermore, from a modern biological perspective, we must also assume that several factors shape an individual's personality. Some factors are undoubtedly genetic, an individual inherits them from their parents. These factors, including genetic factors, influence individuals subsequent decision-making.

However, the concrete significance of this factor in our question remains unclear. Following the sequencing of the human genome, it is surprising that humans possess so few genes. To date, no geneticist or developmental biologist knows precisely what a gene or set of genes means for brain function, particularly with regard to an individual's complex cognitive and emotional characteristics.

In the past, it has been shown that even the simplest anatomical and physiological characteristics of the human brain, which can be considered largely independent of the environment, depend to a large extent on the extremely complex interplay of numerous genes and a large number of so-called epigenetic processes. These are highly complex interactions between different types of neural tissue during brain development. Very little is known about the genetic-epigenetic determination of the brain at a more complex level.

Another important factor is environmental influences that, in one way or another, whether specific or random, affect the fetal brain. These include influences absorbed by the fetus through its body and functioning sensory organs; substances (such as oxygen, nutrients, and possibly nicotine, alcohol, and other drugs) that pass through the mother's bloodstream; and mechanical injuries in the event of accidents or acts of violence against the pregnant woman. This also includes the physiological and mechanical effects of the birth process, which are obviously very intense. It is believed that traumatic events immediately preceding, during, and after childbirth—such as exposure to violence, obstructed labor, severe illness, drug abuse, or excessive maternal alcohol and nicotine use during pregnancy—are strongly associated with later self-harm behavior, including an increased risk of suicide. (Anand & Scalzo, 2000).

The third, and perhaps most important, factor is the newborn's experiences in the first hours, days, and weeks after birth, particularly the "first experiences" of the mother's warmth, smell, sight, voice, skin-to-skin contact, and food. All evidence indicates that severe disruptions during these first experiences have significant negative consequences for the child's psychological development and subsequent personality formation.

The qualitative importance of these three factors in personality development is undeniable, but it is difficult to estimate quantitatively and, at least in humans, to test them directly experimentally for ethical reasons. For this reason, psychology has pursued a method of comparing the cognitive and emotional characteristics of identical twins who were separated shortly after birth and raised in different families or environments. It is known and assumed that identical twins carry the same genes, and the basic idea is that their similarities and differences can be used to estimate the degree of genetic or environmental determination of certain characteristics, such as intelligence, talents, and personality traits. This is done using a correlation analysis as a statistical measure of the relationship between two or more variables. A correlation coefficient of 0 means that the variables examined have nothing to do with each other, a value of i means complete agreement and a value of -i means an "anti-correlation" (i.e., two variables behave in exactly the opposite way) (Roth, 2001).

A correlation coefficient of about 0.3 indicates a weak association and a correlation coefficient of about 0.8 indicates a strong association. These data can then be compared with the results of research on non-identical twins (who are genetically related), on "normal" siblings, and on adopted children who are not genetically related to their parents. In particular, the latter can reveal to what extent the influence of the parental upbringing is (Roth, 2001).

The number of identical twins who grew up apart is, of course, very small. (Amelang & Bartussek, 1997) mention a number of 117 pairs on which trustworthy studies of the type mentioned were carried out between 1937 and 1990, and they faced all sorts of methodological and evaluative problems. What is even more surprising is the high level of agreement found, for example, in IQ scores between identical twins raised separately. The result was a correlation coefficient of between 0.67 and 0.78. This means that intelligence, as measured by common intelligence tests, is not exactly the same between identical twins raised separately, but there is a clear correlation between them.

Studies show that IQ generally increases with age (see Figure 3), and then an individual's intelligence begins to "stabilize" (Amelange & Bartosek, 1997). Here, the correlation coefficient between intelligence at age four and fourteen is about 0.65, which is already surprisingly high. The correlation between intelligence at age fourteen and twenty-nine is about 0.85, despite the long time interval, which is also very high (and, of course, we find that correlation coefficients are higher the shorter the time interval between tests). According to the results of some researchers, intelligence at age six is related to intelligence at age forty by a coefficient of 0.6. This is an astonishingly high value and means that, based on knowledge of a child's intelligence at age six, their intelligence at age forty can be predicted with a good approximation.

Figure 3. Changes in intelligence during childhood adolescence

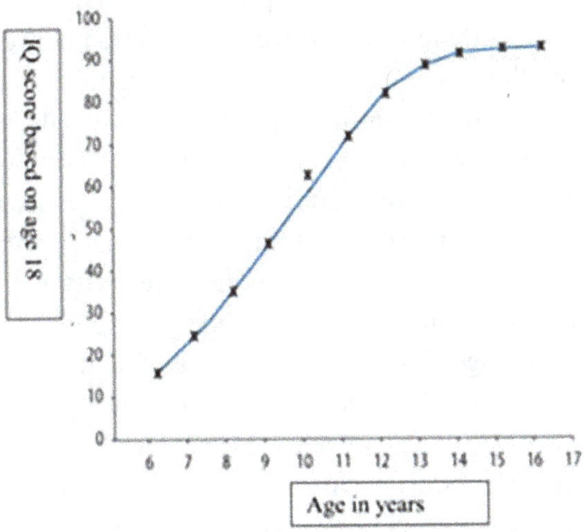

Asendorpf (2007)

This does not necessarily mean that intelligence is largely innate and simply matures with age, as is the case with many purely physical characteristics and functions. While intelligence is presumed to be largely genetically determined, in addition to early, unguided imprinting, intelligence also develops and stabilizes through the cumulative acquisition of knowledge and skills in increasingly stable environments with age. Exercise, training, and experience contribute to the development and growth of an individual's intelligence.

In general, many personality psychologists believe that intelligence is related to the environment, accounting for approximately 20 IQ points (Amelange & Bartosek, 1997). According to specialists, education represents only 20% of total intelligence from an IQ statistical perspective. Intelligence, of course, is only one personality trait, albeit a very important one.

For the Big Five, corresponding studies on identical twins who grew up apart have shown correlation coefficients that are lower than for the intelligence quotient but still lie around 0.5, i.e., show a medium-strong correlation. Based on these research results, we must therefore assume that a significant part of our personality traits also develops depending on our environment (Roth, 2001). The environment here also includes upbringing, experiences, education, and the type of culture to which a person is exposed.

Another way to estimate the influence of the environment on intelligence and the Big Five is to examine the correlation between genetically unrelated adopted children and their adoptive parents compared to the correlation between parents and their biological children who were given up for adoption and therefore not raised by them. In the first case, there is a very weak correlation between 0.09 and 0.15 with regard to the intelligence quotient, and in the second case, a medium-strong correlation of 0.4 (Amelang & Bartussek, 1997). This would mean that raising children by (genetically unrelated) adoptive parents has a very weak effect on IQ, while the genetic basis prevails over different upbringings, at least in part.

What about creativity as a personality trait alongside intelligence? Here, too, the question arises as to whether, and to what extent, creativity is innate. Long-term studies show a picture similar to that of intelligence, namely that creative potential stabilizes markedly with age. This suggests that the foundations of creativity are partly innate and partly established very early on. However, parental behavior, such as a non-authoritarian home or an independent parent-child relationship, appears to be particularly beneficial for the development of creativity (Roth, 2001).

So, if we compare the results of these studies together, we find that the different environments in which identical twins, who were separated very early, were raised do not have the effect that behaviorism assumed, as was often attributed to them in educational theories in the 1970s and 1980s. If intelligence and personality were strongly and closely related to the environment, there would be a much stronger correlation between adoptive parents and their adopted children and a much smaller correlation between biological parents and their biological children who were raised separately, as well as between identical twins who were raised separately, than studies have found.

However, these studies show a strong "genetic" factor in intelligence and personality and a relatively small environmental influence. Is this really true? The answer is not necessarily. Concordance among identical twins takes into account genetic identity and its influence on the brain, intelligence, and personality (but we know nothing about its actual makeup), as well as virtually all the identical influences on twins during pregnancy, birth, and early postnatal development. Identical twins not only have identical genomes, but they are also exposed to very similar environmental influences in what may be the most important period of their lives: the period immediately before, during, and immediately after birth. The extent of these influences before, during, and after birth can be estimated by comparing identical twins with fraternal twins who were exposed to these influences in more or less the same way but have genomes that correspond to those of siblings born at different times. As expected, the correlation coefficient of the IQs of fraternal twins lies between that of identical twins and "normal" siblings (Roth, 2001).

A report published in the German Frankfurter Allgemeine Zeitung on September 26, 2000, emphasized the importance of the "first three years." A long-term study of more than 1,000 New Zealand children and young people between the ages of three and twenty-one highlighted the importance of the "first three years." The study, conducted by London-based psychologist Avshalom Caspi, concluded that "personality remains stable from childhood to adulthood. This means that basic personality traits (such as the Big Five traits mentioned above) do not change, or do not change significantly. Children who were categorized as "maladapted" and "antisocial" early in life were more likely to experience serious social difficulties or to engage in crime later, while those who were well-adjusted early on also became "amiable" and "well-adjusted" later.

There has been much debate about the importance of the first years of life in personality development. Some psychologists and educators have dismissed the great importance usually attributed to this early stage of life, considering it a fantasy and assuming that people change throughout their lives. However, many experts assume that the first three to five years constitute an important formative stage for a person's subsequent life. These are called "sensitive periods" or "imprinting periods," that is, periods of development when the individual is particularly receptive ("sensitive") to certain environmental stimuli as a result of genetically controlled processes, which then "imprint" themselves on the central nervous system like a seal on sealing wax. Such imprinting periods are known in the animal kingdom, especially in the field of vocal communication and the sexual behavior of birds (Lorenz, 1965).

It can also be assumed that such genetic imprinting processes occur in humans, as in the development of language. It is also assumed that mothers and newborns copy and imprint on each other. However, we do not know much about the extent and strength of these processes in humans, and there are difficulties in studying them experimentally, which is why they are controversial. Most experts who assume that such genetic imprinting processes occur simultaneously in the fetus, infant, and young child point out that, as in animals, there may be critical periods of varying length for different characteristics and abilities.

People are not typically influenced by randomly changing social factors, but they typically grow up in homes that provide a relatively stable environment for children and adolescents. In most countries, they also attend formal educational institutions. The subsequent environment is often determined and influenced by factors already prevailing in the parents' home, as well as factors prevailing in the educational system. However, in some regions of the world, the climate surrounding an individual is affected by economic instability, unemployment, and political unrest such as wars and displacement.

LINKING TUTT'S MODEL WITH SKILLS DEVELOPMENT AND HUMAN COGNITION

The Practical Importance of This Link

Individuals must focus on achieving their goals, commit to them, and take action. This also means distinguishing between important and unimportant steps and aligning their goals accordingly. This is where critical thinking comes in. It helps us achieve our goals with determination and resolve, and helps us understand and differentiate between personal and situational factors. Furthermore, critical thinking helps us overcome the challenges of the circumstances around us. However, this requires a certain level of development and sufficient cognitive abilities. Critical thinking skills are not an inherited mental ability; they cannot be inherited, but must be learned.

Certainly, cognitive abilities are the foundation and cornerstone of knowledge acquisition, learning, and problem-solving, and the extent to which they are developed largely determines people's success as students. (Alloway & Allowa, 2010; de Abreu, Gathercole, & Martin, 2011; Hornung, Schiltz, Brunner, & Martin, 2014).

If Tutt's model of the study selection process is viewed from the perspective of the process of human cognition development over time and age, as previously mentioned, and if the two processes are linked, one can conclude that the importance of critical thinking skills and the ability to use them increases as the process proposed by Tutt progresses. Accordingly, we can conclude that the need to master and use critical thinking skills increases as these stages progress, and thus as the decision crystallizes and matures. Figure 4 illustrates this. The practical importance of this conclusion lies in its application in raising and educating children and preparing them for future choices.

Figure 4. The importance and development of critical thinking skills increases with the process progresses

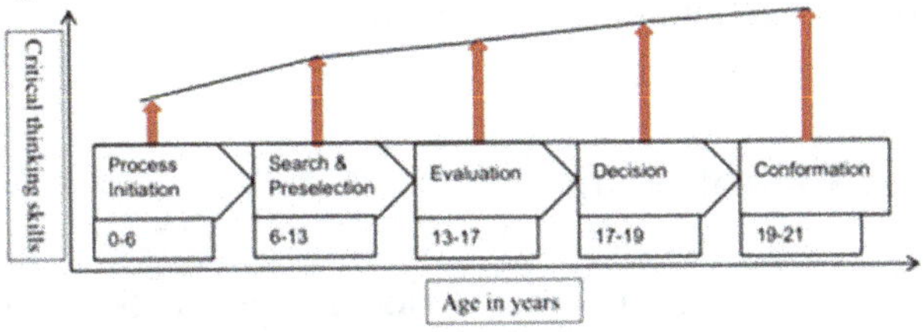

In Figure 4, we see that the influence of external factors (such as parents and the environment) is dominant in the first stage. At this stage, personality is not clearly developed and does not play a major role; rather, it undergoes a period of growth and development. However, it is a crucial stage for subsequent development, as mentioned before. If we relate this growth to the development of IQ, as shown in Figure 3, we find that this process develops as personality and cognitive abilities become increasingly crystallized.

In the early stages of the decision-making process given by Tutt, families, and later also educational institutions, can contribute to providing children with the opportunity to learn and develop their critical thinking skills. This education and training will effectively empower children, enhance their abilities and skills, and enable them to make sound decisions about their future studies. This enables them to fulfill their wishes and achieve self-satisfaction. For this reason, it's very beneficial to begin teaching critical thinking at an early age. A child raised with this type of upbringing will later outperform their peers who don't receive it. This will enable them to make more balanced decisions, which will bring them comfort and enjoyment.

To support the suggestion that Tutt's model of study selection is related to the development of human cognition and reasoning over time and age, and the importance of critical thinking, as illustrated in Figure 4 above, research examining the stages of mental development in children through adulthood could be useful. One of the most important of these studies is the work of Jean Piaget, who explored the development and progression of children's thinking and cognitive abilities.

The Work of Jean Piaget

Piaget's research helps us develop appropriate practical measures and procedures to serve this purpose. Adult teaching methods and approaches should not be imposed on different age groups. One must take into account the stages of children's cognitive development. Children's abilities and educational needs pass through stages. Therefore, we must recognize that each age group requires appropriate measures commensurate with its level of cognitive development. To achieve this goal, we can draw on the expertise gained from researchers to provide educational programs and methods that teach critical thinking in a way that is appropriate to the child's age, needs, and abilities at the specific stage.

Terms Used by Piaget Mean

Decentration: Children are now able to focus their attention on several aspects of a situation at the same time.

Reversibility: At this stage, children of this age can reverse their thoughts. If they know and learn the route from home to school, they can now imagine the opposite route back home.

Cause-and-effect relationship: At this age, children can now develop the concept of a cause for an event. They can understand the relationship between the appearance of clouds in the sky and rain.

Classification: Now, children can relate and distinguish the relationship between a general category and two specific categories at the same time and can name or identify a group of objects based on their appearance, size, or other characteristics.

Transitivity: At this stage, the child is able to reach some conclusions by linking relationships logically.

Elimination of Egocentrism: At this age, it is possible for a child to see things from someone else's point of view as well.

Abstract Thinking: Now children have developed abilities to predict possible outcomes and plan for the future.

Deductive Reasoning: The child is able to define general rules, develop relations, and identify specific outcomes. For example, if $A > B$ and $B > C$, then $A > C$.

Problem Solving: At this stage, children have the ability to solve problems logically and in a methodical way.

Hypothetical Thinking: children are able to identify and determine possible outcomes.

Adolescent Ego-Centrism: The children at this stage develop a high self-consciousness. They believe that others are interested in them and that others are watching them, and they are at the center of attention.

Stages According to Piaget

According to Piaget, human cognitive development goes through the following stages (Reimann, 2021):

-Piaget tells us that in the period extending from birth to the age of two, infants think using their senses and motor actions. That's why it's called the sensorimotor stage. In this stage, babies explore the world by listening to sounds, looking at, biting, or touching things. In this way, children interact and evolve simple thoughts of things. Trial and error is the main basis for learning at this stage. In early infancy, three simple reflexes are present: sucking, eye tracking, and grasping. These reflexes then transform into voluntary goal-directed actions, such as intentional grasping, at about six weeks of age. At this stage, infants begin to realize that objects still exist even when they are out of sight. Children are able to retain a mental image of an event even after direct experience. They also become able to perceive cause-and-effect relationships. For example, an infant may make different sounds to attract caregivers' attention. They begin to learn that a rattle makes sounds when shaken. The children, in this stage, establish the concept that the self is not an extension of the environment, and they recognize the existence of a boundary between self and the surroundings.

-Then comes the next stage (from two to seven years), which Piaget called the pre-operational stage. The development at this stage is manifested by ego-centrism, transductive reasoning, anthropomorphism, artificialism, animism, symbolic functioning, centration, irreversibility, curiosity, and seriation. In this age, logical operations are not yet possible, but the child has the ability to reason about things and also has the ability to use and manipulate symbols (Lego bricks = bed/car/...). The children's language abilities develop, and thinking leads to language; new language = new thinking. Children now believe that inanimate objects have life and are capable of acting and that environmental objects are controlled by people. At this age, children believe that others see, feel, and think just like them, and they develop the ability to use symbols to communicate. Children develop the ability to focus attention on only one aspect of a situation at a time, but they cannot reverse in their minds what they do or know. They begin to develop curiosity and start to ask a lot of questions. But the child still does not have the ability to put things into categories. In this stage, a child develops the ability to think on two levels simultaneously—imaginative and realistic. Imitation (imitating someone's behavior), symbolic play (using objects as symbols), mental imagery (imagining many objects in mind), and verbal evacuation events (using language to describe events, people, or things) are obvious behaviors that develop at this stage.

- The third stage, according to Piaget, is the Concrete Operational Stage: 7 to 11 years. Children at this level start using logical thinking. Cognitive development at this stage is characterized by logical thinking, decentration, reversibility, cause classification, and transitivity egocentrism.

- He called the fourth stage the formal operational stage (from 12 years and above): In this stage, cognitive development is able to carry out abstract thinking, hypothetical thinking, the adolescent ego, the imaginary audience, deductive thinking, and problem-solving.

The concepts of the second stage disappear at the end of the pre-operational period, but at a speed that varies from one individual to another. The pre-operational stage almost completely ends with children entering school. Thus, the cognitive deficits disappear gradually in this stage under the influence of concrete experiences, giving way to a realistic and logical perception of the world. Children begin to enjoy collecting objects at this stage; they also become able to perform multiple operations at this age.

Piaget's perspective cannot be fully generalized. It is noted that some children were more developed at certain stages than Piaget described (Bauer, Larkina, & Deocampo, 2011). Moreover, transitions between stages do not occur suddenly but rather continuously and consistently. It is found that not all adolescents approach the formal operational stage (Martin *et al.*, 2010). In addition, it has been observed that cultural differences and the nature of communication play an important role in the development of children's abilities. In any case, it is essential to encourage families and educational institutions to use discovery-based learning and inductive teaching methods from an early age, which help children understand concepts and principles and acquire critical thinking skills. These competencies will help future students make mature and informed decisions later in their lives and careers. It is worth noting here that the methods and approaches to applying critical thinking vary depending on personality traits. Furthermore, thinking skills and inclinations intertwine when thinking skills are combined with personal talents for acting critically (Facioni, 1990).

THE INTERRELATIONSHIP BETWEEN PERSONALITY, ACADEMIC SPECIALIZATION, AND PROFESSION

Previously in this chapter, the necessity and importance of critical thinking in decision-making have been emphasized. Personality, critical thinking, cognitive perception, and intelligence are also studied, and the theories and concepts associated with the development of these phenomena are reviewed. However, our journey will continue to explore and provide answers to questions that have been targeted: Is there a relationship or influence between personality traits and the type of academic and professional major an individual subsequently chooses? More specifically, does this choice impact their well-being and satisfaction? If the answer is yes, then individuals with appropriate decision-making skills will be able to achieve satisfaction and well-being after making intelligent and critical choices in their field of study.

Not only academic achievement, family history, and interests are important, but personality traits also influence student's behavior, well-being, performance, and creativity at work. Numerous studies have examined the relationship between personality and student's major choices based on the Big Five factors. These studies have been conducted in various countries, from Spain to Canada and the United States, and have found similar results.

Various researchers have studied the relationship between personality traits and the choice and suitability of a field of study. In her research, Claudia Sălceanu (Sălceanu 2021) identified links between cognitive skills and personality traits. She found that analytical thinking is closely related to conscientiousness, awareness, and emotional stability, and that text comprehension is related to emotional stability.

Results of a meta-analysis in 2002 showed that occupations that favor and require creative and scientific research are associated with high levels of personality openness (Larson et al., 2002). A personality with a high level of extraversion and agreeableness is more likely to be associated with jobs that require frequent human contact, e.g., sales or childcare (Larson et al., 2002).

It may be appropriate here to point out that certain personality traits also influence motivations and other factors in choosing a field of study. For example, emotionally unstable individuals tend to be more influenced by their parents in their choices, as demonstrated by Datu's work on the relationship between neuroticism and career choice (Datu 2012).

Datu's research focused on limited occupational categories. His studies demonstrated the significant influence of different levels of the Big Five factors on study choice and subsequent career path. One can find a lot of research on this topic, especially in the field of medicine; for example, Young Kwon and Youn Park investigated the links between the Big Five factors and the chosen specialty of Korean physicians (Young Kwon and Youn Park 2016). They concluded that there was a positive relationship between agreeableness and clinical career path. Open-minded and conscientious physicians were primarily guided by their personal interests in their career decisions, rather than material incentives.

Research on the choice of medical specialization among young doctors from Mexico produced similar results: The results show that above-average extroverted, conscientious, and emotionally stable physicians tend to choose a career in the surgical field. A career in a clinical context, on the other hand, was more favored by doctors with a high level of agreeableness (Barbosa-Camacho et al., 2020). Anna Vedel presented a study for Denmark. Some of the findings—and what this means specifically for choice of study and career orientation, as well as for developing personal strengths—are presented in (Vedel & Poropat, 2017).

ASSOCIATIONS BETWEEN PERSONALITY TRAITS, ACADEMIC SPECIALIZATION, AREAS OF WORK, WELL-BEING, AND SATISFACTION

Below, the relationship between behavior and personality traits (the Big Five) and their importance in some academic and professional disciplines based on the results of relevant studies are presented:

Extroversion

People with high extroversion scores are more likely to choose technical careers (AlKhelil, 2016). They may also excel in marketing. Business-related majors generally attract extroverted students more than non-business majors.

What does this mean for well-being and overall satisfaction when choosing a course?

Of course, every discipline benefits from diversity and a good mix. However, it's natural to feel alienated, strange, and uncomfortable when everyone around you is different. This feeling of alienation undermines well-being and reduces self-confidence. This is particularly true during the personal development phase when it's difficult to deal with differences calmly and in a relaxed manner. Sales and marketing departments are typically busier and more hectic (more extroverted), while finance and IT departments are quieter (more introverted). Students should consider this when choosing their major.

Neuroticism/Instability

Some people claim that students who choose to study psychology often do it because they have a problem. This isn't as absurd as it looks: Students of education, psychology, and the humanities are generally much less emotionally stable than science students. This means they are more anxious, less resilient, and less risk-averse. Most observations have determined that economy and law students are more emotionally stable and therefore less neurotic. This extends to include medical students as well.

What does this mean for overall well-being and satisfaction by choosing a study program? These people should also acquire the necessary business knowledge in most fields and use their qualities to improve the world and make it a little better. A study found that neuroticism is negatively related to job satisfaction, showing that people who score high on neuroticism are generally less satisfied with their jobs (Knutas, 2021). Humanities students are often asked, “What would you do with this?” Given their high sensitivity, they are likely to react sensitively to this question. The outward response is disconcerting. The only way to overcome this is to remain calm and, better yet, to be rational from the outset rather than overthinking. Sensitivity can be a strength, especially when combined with introversion, which produces deeper thinking. We reiterate the need for students to practice developing their strengths early on to build self-confidence, such as by discussing their perspectives and building their self-esteem by exploring current and in-demand topics. They should also acquire and gather the necessary business knowledge in most fields and use their qualities to improve the world and make it a little better.

Openness to New Experiences

Those with a high degree of openness tend to choose research roles (Alkhelil, 2016). This applies to students in the humanities and natural sciences. This also applies to medical students, who tend to be more open-minded, indicating that they are more curious and thirsty for knowledge, and therefore more creative. They are constantly searching for the "other" and often have a strong interest in arts and philosophy. It is worth noting here that mathematicians, physicists, and biologists often tend to be interested in matters outside their specialties and fields of study. This can lead to mismatches, as many students in the natural sciences tend to follow alternative career paths.

What does this mean for overall well-being and satisfaction by choosing a study program? Certainly, less open fields would greatly benefit from students classified on openness. But it's also good to have conflicting tendencies between conservation and change—those concerned shouldn't cancel everything just because something new is more interesting (which is what open-minded scientists tend to do). Graduate students, in particular, who have increasingly struggled to find work, should consider interdisciplinary approaches and consider business-related disciplines like philosophy and computer science as alternatives.

Certainly, fields with low openness would greatly benefit from people with high levels of openness. It is also good that there are opposing tendencies between those who favor the status quo and those who favor change—those interested shouldn't throw everything out just because something new and more interesting comes along (which is what researchers with high levels of openness often do). Graduate students, in particular, who are increasingly finding it difficult to find work, should consider interdisciplinary approaches and studying business-related disciplines, such as graphic design, teaching, and computer science, as alternatives.

Agreeableness

Those who score high on agreeableness are best suited for jobs involving managerial and executive roles (Alkhelil, 2016). Several studies have shown that lawyers and economists have low levels of agreeableness, but psychology and humanities students are significantly more agreeable. Medical students and natural scientists also have a high level of agreeableness.

What does this mean for overall well-being and satisfaction by choosing a study program? Of course, anyone with a high level of friendliness and likability is friendly and likable, but there's another side that can lead to discomfort at work. People with this high level of friendliness may have difficulty making decisions or be easily taken advantage of, especially in a highly competitive work environment. They may tend to avoid conflict when confrontation is necessary. They may not be able to demonstrate the necessary assertiveness at work. But this shouldn't be discouraging. Students need to understand themselves well, build self-confidence, and be clear with their colleagues before venturing into areas that cause them stress.

Conscientiousness

Individuals who rate themselves highly in conscientiousness tend to prefer managerial and executive roles (Alkhelil, 2016). These individuals, who strive for organization, precision, and perfection, are best suited to the fields of management and organization. Although the level of conscientiousness is not precisely defined, it is usually average. Conscientiousness has a significant impact on job satisfaction. Studies indicate that the best jobs for this trait are those that require meticulous attention to detail. These individuals also strive to meet deadlines and adhere to agreed-upon schedules. Conscientious individuals can become leaders, supervisors, or independent managers, and their ability to be precise and thorough gives them an added advantage. Students with a high score in conscientiousness should consider careers such as entrepreneurship, freelancing, accounting, surgery, and IT management.

What does this mean for overall well-being and satisfaction by choosing a study program? This personality type requires and supports good organization and effective communication between employees and management. They can communicate information efficiently and understand the needs of others. They have a strong attention to detail and a strong work ethic and are motivated to use thoughtful and focused learning strategies. They are comfortable performing routine tasks, rarely deviate from the norm, and have difficulty adapting to constant and sudden changes. Their tendency to be highly organized also means they are stiff and find it difficult to adapt to change. They are often overly serious, so an office full of conscientious individuals may have a rigid and inflexible corporate culture. It is important to remember that conscientiousness, like the other Big Five personality traits, is a spectrum with varying intensities. In extreme cases, conscientious individuals may sometimes suffer from obsessive-compulsive disorder or perfectionism.

THE IMPORTANCE OF CRITICAL THINKING IN STUDY SELECTION AND SUCCESS

A student armed with critical thinking skills will realize the importance of understanding their personality and its characteristics. If they are unable to do so on their own, they will realize the importance of conducting a personal analysis before choosing an academic major to better understand themselves and their personality. Personality type significantly impacts success and comfort during study and future work. There are other factors to consider when determining a career path or academic major. The most prominent of these factors are the individual's skills, personal interests, social restrictions, family requirements, and economic conditions.

Students who grow up in an environment that supports the development of their personalities and thinking skills will be able to identify and provide appropriate answers to the following questions before making a decision and choosing their studies:

What are my interests, strengths, and abilities?
What does my future job mean to me?
How do I envision my future?
Who can I ask? Where can I get information?

They can also direct questions to the university, such as: What degree is achievable? What are the admission requirements? When are the application deadlines? What opportunities for in-depth study and specialization are available? What prior knowledge should or must the student have? Are preparatory courses offered? Does the chosen degree program match my expectations? What career options are open to me after graduation? What job market prospects does the degree offer?

People who possess critical thinking skills will certainly excel in making sound decisions and will enjoy satisfaction and success in their future studies and careers.

REFERENCES

Acevedo, E. C., & Hess, C. (2022) "The link between critical thinking and personality: individual differences in a concern for truth," Modern Psychological Studies: Vol. 27: No. 1, Article 9. Available at: https://scholar.utc.edu/mps/vol27/iss1/9

Alkhelil, A. H. (2016). The Relationship between Personality Traits and Career Choice: A Case Study of Secondary School Students. *International Journal of Academic Research in Progressive Education and Development*, *5*(2), 122–135. DOI: 10.6007/IJARPED/v5-i2/2132

Alloway, T. P., & Alloway, R. G. (2010). Investigating the Predictive Roles of Working Memory and IQ in Academic Attainment. *Journal of Experimental Child Psychology*, *106*(1), 20–29. DOI: 10.1016/j.jecp.2009.11.003 PMID: 20018296

Amelang, M., & Bartussek, D. (1997): Differentielle Psychologie und Persönlichkeitsforschung. Kohlhammer, Stuttgart, Berlin, Köln, 4.edition

Anand, K. J. S., & Scalzo, F. M. (2000). Can adverse neonatal experiences alter brain development and subsequent behavior? *Biology of the Neonate*, *77*(2), 69–82. DOI: 10.1159/000014197 PMID: 10657682

Asendorpf, J. B. (2007). *Psychologie der Persönlichkeit* (4th ed.). Springer Medizin Verlag Heidelberg. DOI: 10.1007/978-3-540-71685-3

Barbosa-Camacho, F. J., Miranda-Ackerman, R. C., Vázquez-Reyna, I., Jimenez-Ley, V. B., Barrera-López, F. J., Contreras-Cordero, V. S., Sánchez-López, V. A., Castillo-Valverde, T. J., Lamas-Abbadie, C. C., González-Adán, B. A., Cortes-Flores, A. O., Morgan-Villela, G., Cervantes-Cardona, G. A., Cervantes-Guevara, G., Fuentes-Orozco, C., & González-Ojeda, A. (2020). Association between HEXACO personality traits and medical specialty preferences in Mexican medical students: A cross-sectional survey. *BMC Psychology*, *8*(1), 23. DOI: 10.1186/s40359-020-0390-0 PMID: 32171327

Bauer, P. J., Larkina, M., & Deocampo, J. (2011). Early Memory Development. In Goswami, U. (Ed.), *The Wiley-Blackwell Handbook of Childhood Cognitive Development* (2nd ed.). Wiley-Blackwell.

Beyer, H. (1992). Die Berufswahl als Gegenstand sozialwissenschaftlicher Theoriebildung. Überlegungen zum theoretischen Rahmen sozialwissenschaftlicher Analysen der Berufswahl und zur Möglichkeit einer „verstehenden" Erkenntnisperspektive in der Theoriebildung sozialwissenschaftlicher Berufswahlforschung. Augsburg Universitätsschrift: Wirtschafts- und sozialwissenschaftliche Fakultät.

Bußhoff, L. (1984). *Berufswahl*. Kohlhammer.

Crites, J. (1969). *Vocational Psychology. The Study of Vocational Behavior and Development*. McGraw-Hill.

Datu, J. A. (2012, July). Personality Traits and Paternal Parenting Style as Predictive Factors of Career Choice. *Academic Research International, 3*(1), •••.

Elder, L., & Paul, R. (2006). *Critical Thinking: Tools for Taking Charge of Your Learning and Your Life. 2*. Pearson/Prentice Hall.

Engle de Abreu, P. M. J., Gathercole, S. E., & Martin, R. (2011). Disentangling the Relationship between Working Memory and Language: The Roles of Short-Term Storage and Cognitive Control. *Learning and Individual Differences, 21*(5), 569–574. DOI: 10.1016/j.lindif.2011.06.002

Facione, P. A. (1990). *Critical thinking: A statement of expert consensus for purposes of educational assessment and instruction*. The California Academic Press.

Forßbohm, D. (2010). *Berufswahl als Entscheidung. Eine Auseinandersetzung mit ausgewählten Konzepten zur Berufswahl unter geschlechtsspezifischer Perspektive*. Verlag Dr. Kovac.

Freud, S. (1930). *Das Unbehagen in der Kultur*. Internationaler Psychoanalytischer Verlag.

Friebertshäuser, B. (2008). Statuspassage von der Schule ins Studium. In Helsper, W., & Böhme, J. (Eds.), *Handbuch der Schulforschung* (pp. 611–627). VS Verlag für Sozialwissenschaften. DOI: 10.1007/978-3-531-91095-6_24

Ginzberg, E. (1988). Toward a Theory of Occupational Choice. (first appeared in 1952). *The Career Development Quarterly, 36*(4), 358–363. DOI: 10.1002/j.2161-0045.1988.tb00510.x

Ginzberg, E., Ginsburg Sol, W., Axelrad, S., & Herma, J. L. (1951). *Occupational Choice /An Approach to a General Theory*. Columbia University Press.

Hachmeister, C. D. (2008). Optimierung der Studienentscheidung durch verbesserte Studieninformation. In Schuler, H., & Hell, B. (Eds.), *Studierendenauswahl und Studienentscheidung* (pp. 57–66). Hogrefe.

Heckhausen, H., & Gollwitzer, P. M. (1987). Thought contents and cognitive functioning in motivational versus volitional states of mind. *Motivation and Emotion, 11*(2), 101–120. DOI: 10.1007/BF00992338

Heckhausen, H., & Heckhausen, J. (2018). *Motivation und Handeln* (5th ed.). Springer Verlag. DOI: 10.1007/978-3-662-53927-9

Heine, C., Spangenberg, H., Schreiber, J., & Sommer, D. (2005). Studienanfänger 2003/2004 und 2004/2005. Bildungswege, Motive der Studienentscheidung und Gründe der Hochschulwahl. HIS-Kurzinformation A, 15.

Heublein, U., & Sommer, D. (2002). *Studienanfänger 2000/2001. Hochschul-Informations System: Hannover Holland, J. L. (1985): Making Vocational Choices. A Theory of Vocational Personalities and Work Environments. Englewood-Cliffs.* Prentice-Hall.

Hornung, C., Schiltz, C., Brunner, M., & Martin, R. (2014). Predicting first-grade mathematics achievement: The contributions of domain-general cognitive abilities, nonverbal number sense, and early number competence. *Frontiers in Psychology, 5*, 272. DOI: 10.3389/fpsyg.2014.00272 PMID: 24772098

Knutas, F. (2021). Personality, Fields of Research, and Job Satisfaction Evidence from a Swedish University, (URN: urn:nbn:se:ltu:diva-85432) [thesis Basic level, degree of Bachelor, Luleå University of Technology, Department of Health, Learning and Technology]. https://www.diva-portal.org/smash/get/diva2:1566717/FULLTEXT01.pdf

Kwon, Y., & Park, Y. (2016). Specialty choice preference of medical students according to personality traits by Five-Factor Model. *Korean Journal of Medical Education, 28*(1), 95–102. DOI: 10.3946/kjme.2016.14 PMID: 26838573

Larson, L. M., Rottinghaus, P. J., & Borgen, F. H. (2002). Meta-analyses of Big Six Interests and Big Five Personality Factors. *Journal of Vocational Behavior, 61*(2), 217–239. DOI: 10.1006/jvbe.2001.1854

Lorenz, K. (1965). *Über tierisches und menschliches Verhalten. Aus dem Werdegang der Verhaltenslehre* (Vol. i). Piper.

Martin, G. N., Carlson, N. R., & Buskist, W. (2010). *Psychology*. Pearson.

McCrae, R. R., & Costa, P. T. (1987). Validation of the five-factor model of personality across instruments and observers. *Journal of Personality and Social Psychology, 1987*(52), 81–90. DOI: 10.1037/0022-3514.52.1.81 PMID: 3820081

Mutz, R., & Daniel, H.-D. (2008). Warum studiert man Psychologie? *Psychologische Rundschau, 59*(1), 47–51. DOI: 10.1026/0033-3042.59.1.47

Pfuhl, N. (2010). *Untersuchungen zur Bestimmung von typischen Merkmalen des Image von Studien fächern*. Waxmann.

Reimann, E. (2021). *Jean Piagets Theorie der kognitiven Entwicklung/ Die Grundlagen*. GRIN Verlag.

Roth G. (2001), Fühlen, Denken, Handeln:Wie das Gehirn unser Verhalten steuert. Suhrkarap Verlag Frankfurt am Main

SĂLCEANU C. (2021). Big-Five Personality Traits and Cognitive Skills in Higher Education, the Pandemic Context, 2021. *Postmodern Openings*, *12*(3). Advance online publication. DOI: 10.18662/po/12.3

Super, D. E. (1953). A Theory of Vocational Development. *The American Psychologist*, *1953*(8), 185–190. DOI: 10.1037/h0056046

Super, D. E. (1980). A Life-Span. Life-Space Approach to Career Development. *Journal of Vocational Behavior*, *1980*(13), 282–290. DOI: 10.1016/0001-8791(80)90056-1

Swaab, D. F. (2014). *We are our brains: a neurobiography of the brain, from the womb to Alzheimer's*. Spiegel & Grau a Penguin Random House Company.

Tutt, L. (1997): Der Studienentscheidungsprozess: Informationsquellen, Informationswünsche und Auswahlkriterien bei der Hochschulwahl. Diskussionsbeiträge des Fachbereichs Wirtschaftswissenschaften der Gerhard-Mercator- Universität Duisburg, Band 243. Duisburg

Vedel, A., & Poropat, A. E. (2017). Personality and Academic Performance. In Zeigler-Hill, V., & Shackelford, T. (Eds.), *Encyclopedia of Personality and Individual Differences*. Springer., DOI: 10.1007/978-3-319-28099-8_989-1

Vroom, V. (1964). *Work and Motivation*. Wiley.

Weinrauch, S. G., & Srebalus, D. J. (1994). Die Berufswahltheorie von Holland. In: Brown, D./Brooks, L. (Hrsg.): Karriere-Entwicklung. Stuttgart: Klett-Cotta, p. 43-74.

Chapter 11
Critical Thinking in Psychological Diagnosis and Treatment

S. Hemalatha
https://orcid.org/0009-0005-0397-8738
Panimalar Engineering College, India

Ajay S. Krithick
Panimalar Engineering College, India

ABSTRACT

Abstract Misdiagnosis in psychological practice remains a critical challenge, often leading to inappropriate treatment, patient distress, and ethical concerns. Many diagnostic errors stem from cognitive biases, time constraints, and reliance on traditional frameworks rather than a comprehensive analytical approach. Critical thinking enhances diagnostic accuracy by encouraging clinicians to systematically evaluate symptoms, challenge assumptions, and consider alternative explanations. By mitigating biases such as confirmation and anchoring bias, clinicians improve diagnostic reliability. Case studies highlight how critical thinking prevents misdiagnoses, such as distinguishing hypothyroidism from depression or recognizing cultural influences on symptoms. Research supports structured diagnostic frameworks and second opinions in reducing errors. Integrating critical thinking into diagnostic processes fosters ethical responsibility and enhances patient outcomes, making it essential for advancing mental health care.

DOI: 10.4018/979-8-3373-1812-7.ch011

1. INTRODUCTION: APPLYING CRITICAL THINKING TO REDUCE DIAGNOSTIC ERRORS

Accurate psychological diagnosis is the cornerstone of effective mental health treatment. However, misdiagnosis remains a pervasive issue, often leading to ineffective interventions, prolonged patient distress, and unnecessary healthcare costs. Research indicates that diagnostic errors in mental health care are frequently influenced by cognitive biases, clinician overconfidence, and an overreliance on subjective impressions rather than objective assessments. Given the complexity of psychological disorders—many of which share overlapping symptoms—practitioners must adopt a critical thinking approach to minimize errors and enhance the reliability of their diagnostic conclusions.

Critical thinking plays a vital role in improving diagnostic accuracy by encouraging clinicians to systematically analyze information, question initial assumptions, and consider multiple perspectives before reaching a conclusion. It enables practitioners to recognize and counteract cognitive biases such as confirmation bias (favoring information that supports an initial impression) and anchoring bias (sticking too rigidly to an early diagnostic hypothesis). By integrating evidence-based decision-making, structured reasoning, and reflective judgment, mental health professionals can refine their diagnostic skills and make more accurate assessments.

A real-world example highlights the dangers of diagnostic errors and the value of critical thinking. A 35-year-old woman presented with persistent fatigue, lack of motivation, and concentration difficulties. Based on these symptoms, she was diagnosed with Major Depressive Disorder (MDD) and prescribed antidepressant medication. However, when her condition did not improve over several months, a different clinician applied a more critical approach, questioning the initial diagnosis and ordering additional medical tests. The results revealed that the patient was suffering from hypothyroidism, a condition that can mimic symptoms of depression but requires a completely different treatment approach. This case underscores the importance of moving beyond surface-level symptoms and adopting a differential diagnostic approach to rule out medical conditions, comorbid disorders, and alternative explanations.

In this chapter, we will explore how critical thinking can enhance diagnostic accuracy, prevent common cognitive biases, and ensure ethical, culturally competent mental health assessments. By integrating structured reasoning techniques, evidence-based practices, and interdisciplinary collaboration, clinicians can strengthen their diagnostic decision-making and ultimately improve patient outcomes.

2. BACKGROUND AND LITERATURE REVIEW

Critical thinking plays a fundamental role in improving the accuracy and reliability of psychological diagnosis. Research indicates that diagnostic errors in mental health assessment are common, often resulting from cognitive biases and heuristic shortcuts. A review of key theories, empirical studies, and case examples provides insight into the necessity of critical thinking in psychological diagnosis and treatment planning. This section explores the prevalence of diagnostic errors, the impact of cognitive biases on clinical decision-making, and the role of evidence-based practices in mitigating these issues.

Prevalence of Diagnostic Errors in Mental Health

Psychological diagnosis is inherently complex due to overlapping symptoms across different disorders, patient variability, and the influence of subjective interpretation. Studies have shown that diagnostic discrepancies are common. For example, Smith et al. (2022) found that over 30% of initial psychiatric diagnoses changed after a second evaluation by another clinician, highlighting the fallibility of initial assessments. Similarly, a meta-analysis by Jones & Patel (2020) reported that clinicians frequently misdiagnose conditions such as Bipolar Disorder and Borderline Personality Disorder due to symptom overlap, leading to inappropriate treatment strategies. These findings underscore the need for a structured critical thinking framework to enhance diagnostic accuracy and reduce the risk of misdiagnosis.

Cognitive Biases and Their Impact on Diagnosis

Cognitive biases are systematic patterns of deviation from rationality that can unconsciously influence clinical judgment. Several biases have been identified as particularly problematic in mental health diagnosis:

1. Confirmation Bias – The tendency to favor information that confirms preexisting beliefs while ignoring contradictory evidence. A clinician who initially suspects Major Depressive Disorder may selectively focus on symptoms of sadness and fatigue while overlooking signs of an underlying medical condition such as hypothyroidism.
2. Anchoring Bias – The reliance on the first piece of information encountered (initial diagnosis) and failure to adjust judgments based on new evidence. For instance, if a patient has been previously diagnosed with anxiety, future clinicians may interpret new symptoms as anxiety-related rather than exploring alternative diagnoses like PTSD or OCD.

3. Availability Heuristic – The tendency to judge the probability of an event based on how easily similar cases come to mind. If a clinician recently treated multiple patients with ADHD, they may be more likely to diagnose a new patient with ADHD, even when symptoms align more closely with an autism spectrum disorder.
4. Overconfidence Bias – The belief that one's diagnostic accuracy is higher than it actually is, leading to reduced openness to alternative explanations. Studies have shown that experienced clinicians can sometimes be less likely to revise their diagnoses even when presented with conflicting evidence (Kahneman, 2011).

These biases can lead to inaccurate diagnoses and inappropriate treatment plans. Recognizing and mitigating them through structured critical thinking strategies can improve clinical judgment and patient outcomes.

Evidence-Based Approaches to Reducing Diagnostic Errors

The application of critical thinking in mental health diagnosis is closely tied to evidence-based practices. Research has shown that structured assessment tools, standardized diagnostic criteria, and collaborative decision-making can significantly improve diagnostic accuracy.

1. Structured Clinical Interviews – Tools such as the Structured Clinical Interview for DSM-5 (SCID-5) or Mini-International Neuropsychiatric Interview (MINI) provide a systematic approach to diagnosis, reducing reliance on subjective judgment. Studies have demonstrated that structured interviews lead to greater inter-rater reliability compared to unstructured assessments (First et al., 2016).
2. Differential Diagnosis Frameworks – The use of differential diagnosis strategies encourages clinicians to systematically rule out alternative explanations before confirming a diagnosis. The DSM-5 provides decision trees and diagnostic criteria checklists that support this approach.
3. Interdisciplinary Collaboration – Consulting with psychiatrists, neurologists, and medical professionals can help rule out organic causes of psychological symptoms. Research has found that interdisciplinary case reviews result in more accurate diagnoses and better patient outcomes (Lee & Thomas, 2018).
4. Reflective Practice and Decision-Support Tools – Encouraging clinicians to engage in reflective practice, where they critically evaluate their own thought processes, can improve diagnostic accuracy. Additionally, AI-driven decision-support tools are emerging as valuable resources for reducing diagnostic bias. Machine learning models have been shown to assist in identifying patterns in

mental health conditions, supporting more objective decision-making (Wang et al., 2021).

Case Studies Highlighting the Role of Critical Thinking in Diagnosis

Several case studies illustrate the consequences of diagnostic errors and the benefits of applying critical thinking strategies.

Case Study 1: Misdiagnosis of Schizophrenia

A 25-year-old male was diagnosed with schizophrenia after reporting auditory hallucinations. The initial clinician, influenced by availability bias, assumed a psychotic disorder based on recent similar cases. However, a second evaluation incorporating a broader critical thinking approach revealed that the hallucinations were related to severe obsessive-compulsive disorder (OCD), not schizophrenia. The revised diagnosis led to more appropriate treatment with cognitive-behavioral therapy (CBT) and selective serotonin reuptake inhibitors (SSRIs) rather than antipsychotic medication.

Case Study 2: Overlooking Medical Conditions in Psychological Assessment

A 40-year-old woman presented with extreme fatigue, brain fog, and depressive symptoms. She was initially diagnosed with Major Depressive Disorder and prescribed antidepressants. However, after applying a differential diagnosis approach and consulting with a medical specialist, the clinician discovered she had undiagnosed Hashimoto's thyroiditis, an autoimmune condition that causes depression-like symptoms. By addressing the underlying medical condition, the patient's symptoms significantly improved without psychiatric medication.

These cases demonstrate how critical thinking can challenge initial assumptions, incorporate alternative explanations, and lead to more accurate and effective treatment plans.

The literature on diagnostic errors and cognitive biases highlights the need for critical thinking in psychological assessment. Research shows that misdiagnosis is prevalent, often due to unconscious biases that affect clinical judgment. By integrating structured assessment tools, interdisciplinary collaboration, and evidence-based frameworks, mental health professionals can improve diagnostic accuracy and enhance patient outcomes. Future research should explore how emerging technologies, such as AI-driven diagnostic models and digital mental health tools, can further support critical thinking in mental health practice.

3. PRACTICAL APPLICATION: HOW TO USE CRITICAL THINKING IN DIAGNOSIS AND TREATMENT

Applying critical thinking in psychological diagnosis requires a structured approach that minimizes bias and enhances clinical accuracy. Many diagnostic errors stem from cognitive shortcuts, overreliance on intuition, and failure to consider alternative explanations. By systematically applying critical thinking strategies, mental health professionals can improve their decision-making, reduce misdiagnosis, and enhance treatment effectiveness. This section outlines practical steps for clinicians, tools to support diagnostic reasoning, and real-world case examples that illustrate the impact of critical thinking in mental health practice.

One of the most fundamental steps in critical thinking is questioning initial assumptions. Often, clinicians make premature conclusions based on surface-level symptoms without exploring deeper underlying causes. For instance, a patient presenting with anxiety might be quickly diagnosed with Generalized Anxiety Disorder (GAD) without considering medical conditions such as thyroid dysfunction, substance withdrawal, or trauma-related stress. A critical thinking approach encourages clinicians to ask: Could there be another explanation for these symptoms? Am I making assumptions based on past experiences rather than the patient's unique context? Have I considered both psychological and physiological factors? In one real-world case, a clinician diagnosed a patient with panic disorder due to frequent episodes of palpitations and breathlessness. However, after conducting a thorough assessment, it was discovered that the patient had an undiagnosed heart arrhythmia. By questioning initial assumptions, the clinician avoided a potentially serious medical misdiagnosis.

Another key strategy in critical thinking is seeking multiple perspectives. A single clinician's viewpoint can sometimes be limited by personal biases or past experiences. Consulting with colleagues, supervisors, or interdisciplinary teams can provide alternative viewpoints and prevent diagnostic blind spots. Peer case reviews, interdisciplinary collaboration with medical professionals, and including family perspectives in child and adolescent assessments can lead to more accurate diagnoses. For example, a child was initially diagnosed with Attention-Deficit/Hyperactivity Disorder (ADHD) due to hyperactivity and impulsive behavior. However, after a multidisciplinary review, a pediatric neurologist identified an underlying seizure disorder that had been misinterpreted as inattention. This case highlights the importance of integrating different perspectives into the diagnostic process.

Applying evidence-based guidelines is another essential component of critical thinking in mental health diagnosis. Instead of relying solely on intuition or clinical experience, practitioners must integrate scientific evidence to support their conclusions. Cross-checking symptoms with standardized diagnostic criteria from the DSM-5 or ICD-11, using empirically validated screening tools, and staying updated with the latest research can enhance diagnostic accuracy. For example, a clinician suspected bipolar disorder in a patient experiencing mood fluctuations. Instead of relying solely on patient self-reports, they administered the Mood Disorder Questionnaire (MDQ) and found that the symptoms aligned more closely with Borderline Personality Disorder (BPD) rather than Bipolar Disorder. By incorporating evidence-based assessment tools, the clinician avoided an incorrect mood disorder diagnosis and was able to recommend appropriate treatment.

In recent years, advancements in artificial intelligence (AI) and digital health tools have provided clinicians with powerful resources to enhance diagnostic accuracy. AI-driven diagnostic systems can analyze vast amounts of data and recognize patterns that may be overlooked by human clinicians. Many AI-powered decision-support tools can cross-check symptoms, leverage machine learning models to assess risk factors for disorders, and use natural language processing (NLP) systems to analyze patient history. For example, researchers have developed AI-based diagnostic models that can predict the likelihood of depression and anxiety based on voice tone, facial expressions, and linguistic patterns. In one clinical case, a psychiatrist used AI-assisted analysis to detect depressive speech patterns in a patient who was initially reluctant to disclose emotional distress. This early detection allowed for timely intervention and a more accurate treatment plan.

A real-world case study illustrates the impact of critical thinking in preventing misdiagnosis. A 42-year-old woman presented with persistent fatigue, weight gain, and low mood. A psychiatrist diagnosed her with Major Depressive Disorder (MDD) and prescribed antidepressants. However, after six months, her symptoms worsened rather than improved. A second clinician applied a critical thinking framework, questioning the initial diagnosis, consulting with an endocrinologist, and applying evidence-based guidelines. Additional testing revealed that the patient had undiagnosed hypothyroidism, a medical condition that mimics depression but requires hormonal treatment rather than psychiatric medication. This case highlights the importance of adopting a differential diagnostic approach, ruling out medical conditions, and avoiding premature conclusions.

To help clinicians integrate critical thinking into their practice, structured checklists can serve as valuable tools. A diagnostic accuracy checklist can include questions such as: Have I considered all possible diagnoses? Did I check for medical conditions that could mimic mental health symptoms? Have I reviewed past medical and psychiatric history thoroughly? Am I relying on scientific evidence rather than intuition? Similarly, an ethical considerations checklist can prompt clinicians to reflect on their biases, cultural influences, and commitment to patient-centered care.

In conclusion, integrating critical thinking into psychological diagnosis is essential for reducing errors, improving patient outcomes, and ensuring ethical treatment. By questioning assumptions, seeking multiple perspectives, applying evidence-based guidelines, and leveraging AI tools, clinicians can make more accurate and unbiased diagnostic decisions. A structured, analytical approach enhances clinical judgment, fosters better patient trust, and ultimately leads to more effective mental health interventions.

4. ETHICAL CONSIDERATIONS IN PSYCHOLOGICAL DIAGNOSIS

Ethical concerns are central to psychological diagnosis, as clinicians hold the responsibility of ensuring accuracy, fairness, and cultural sensitivity in their assessments. Misdiagnosis and overdiagnosis can have severe consequences, including inappropriate treatment, stigma, and patient distress. This section explores how critical thinking can safeguard against ethical dilemmas in mental health diagnosis, the role of cultural competence in reducing biases, and best practices for maintaining ethical integrity in clinical settings.

Addressing Biases in Psychological Diagnosis

Cognitive biases, both implicit and explicit, can lead to diagnostic errors that disproportionately affect certain populations. Research has shown that minority groups are more likely to be misdiagnosed with severe mental illnesses compared to non-minority groups. For instance, Jones & Lee (2021) found that African American men are diagnosed with schizophrenia at disproportionately higher rates than white patients, even when they present with mood disorder symptoms. This misclassification is often linked to cultural misunderstandings, clinician biases, and an overreliance on symptom presentation rather than a holistic patient history.

Common Biases in Mental Health Diagnosis

1. Implicit Bias – Unconscious stereotypes or preconceptions about a patient's background influencing diagnostic decisions.
2. Confirmation Bias – The tendency to focus on evidence that supports an initial diagnosis while ignoring contradictory information.

3. Overpathologizing – Misinterpreting culturally normative behaviors as symptoms of mental illness (e.g., labeling spiritual beliefs or emotional expressiveness as signs of psychosis).

Applying critical thinking in diagnostic assessments helps clinicians recognize and challenge these biases. Strategies such as structured interviews, cultural competence training, and consultation with diverse professional teams can improve diagnostic accuracy and reduce disparities in mental health care.

Safeguarding Against Misdiagnosis and Overdiagnosis

Misdiagnosis occurs when a clinician assigns an incorrect diagnosis, while overdiagnosis refers to labeling normal variations in behavior as pathological. Both errors can lead to inappropriate treatment, unnecessary medication use, and long-term psychological harm.

A critical example of overdiagnosis is the increasing rates of Attention-Deficit/Hyperactivity Disorder (ADHD) diagnoses in children. Research (Evans et al., 2020) suggests that some children diagnosed with ADHD may actually be experiencing normal developmental variations or environmental stressors rather than a clinical disorder. Overreliance on quick assessments and subjective interpretations contributes to this problem. By incorporating evidence-based criteria, conducting multi-informant assessments, and using objective rating scales, clinicians can mitigate the risk of overdiagnosis.

Conversely, underdiagnosis can also occur, particularly in populations where mental health symptoms manifest differently. Women and ethnic minorities, for example, are less likely to be diagnosed with Autism Spectrum Disorder (ASD) because their symptoms do not always align with traditional diagnostic frameworks. A critical thinking approach encourages clinicians to explore alternative symptom presentations, seek multiple data sources, and remain open to reconsidering initial assessments.

The Role of Cultural Competence in Ethical Diagnosis

Cultural competence—the ability to understand, respect, and integrate diverse cultural perspectives into clinical practice—is essential for ethical mental health diagnosis. Culture influences how symptoms are expressed, how individuals perceive mental illness, and how they seek help. A lack of cultural awareness can lead to misinterpretations of distress, further perpetuating diagnostic inaccuracies.

For example, in many Asian cultures, individuals experiencing depression may report somatic symptoms (such as headaches or fatigue) rather than emotional distress. A clinician unfamiliar with these cultural variations may overlook depression and instead diagnose an anxiety or physical disorder. By applying culturally informed diagnostic tools, engaging in open-ended discussions about the patient's background, and avoiding ethnocentric assumptions, clinicians can make more accurate and ethical assessments.

Best Practices for Ethical Diagnosis in Mental Health

To promote ethical decision-making in psychological diagnosis, clinicians should adhere to the following best practices:

1. Adopt a Critical Thinking Framework
    - Continuously question assumptions and avoid premature conclusions.
    - Cross-check diagnoses with multiple sources of information, including standardized assessments.
    - Engage in reflective practice to evaluate potential biases in clinical reasoning.
2. Ensure Cultural Sensitivity
    - Use culturally validated diagnostic tools and screening measures.
    - Seek supervision or consultation when working with populations outside one's expertise.
    - Recognize variations in symptom expression across different cultural backgrounds.
3. Utilize Evidence-Based Diagnostic Tools
    - Incorporate structured interviews (e.g., SCID-5, MINI) to minimize subjective interpretation.
    - Stay informed on the latest research and clinical guidelines to support diagnostic accuracy.
    - Use multiple assessment methods (clinical observation, patient self-report, and collateral reports).
4. Reduce Overdiagnosis and Misdiagnosis Risks
    - Consider environmental and contextual factors before diagnosing a disorder.
    - Rule out medical conditions that may mimic psychological symptoms (e.g., thyroid disorders, neurological conditions).
    - Avoid pathologizing normative developmental behaviors, especially in children and adolescents.
5. Promote Interdisciplinary Collaboration
    - Work alongside medical professionals, educators, and community leaders to gain a holistic understanding of a patient's condition.

- Encourage second opinions or team-based case reviews for complex diagnostic cases.

6. Maintain Ethical Transparency and Patient Involvement
   - Clearly explain the diagnostic process and criteria to patients and their families.
   - Engage patients in shared decision-making regarding treatment options.
   - Ensure informed consent and respect patient autonomy in mental health care.

Ethical considerations in psychological diagnosis demand vigilance against biases, cultural awareness, and a commitment to evidence-based practice. Cognitive biases can contribute to misdiagnosis and overdiagnosis, leading to significant ethical dilemmas in patient care. By integrating critical thinking, cultural competence, and structured diagnostic approaches, clinicians can minimize diagnostic errors and uphold the ethical principles of fairness, accuracy, and patient-centered care. Future efforts should focus on expanding training programs that emphasize critical thinking and ethical decision-making, ensuring that mental health professionals are well-equipped to navigate the complexities of psychological assessment.

5. CONCLUSION AND FUTURE DIRECTIONS

The integration of critical thinking into psychological diagnosis is essential for improving diagnostic accuracy, minimizing biases, and ensuring ethical mental health care. Throughout this chapter, we have explored the impact of cognitive biases, the importance of cultural competence, and the role of structured, evidence-based approaches in reducing diagnostic errors. By adopting a critical thinking mindset, mental health professionals can enhance patient outcomes, avoid premature conclusions, and foster a more ethical and reliable diagnostic process.

Strengthening Critical Thinking in Psychology Training

One of the most effective ways to advance critical thinking in psychological diagnosis is through education and training programs that emphasize analytical reasoning, reflective practice, and evidence-based decision-making. Current mental health curricula should include:

1. Case-Based Learning – Using real and hypothetical case studies to analyze diagnostic errors and alternative perspectives.

2. Bias Awareness Training – Teaching clinicians to recognize and counteract implicit biases in diagnostic decision-making.
3. Interdisciplinary Collaboration – Encouraging case discussions among psychiatrists, psychologists, and medical professionals to incorporate diverse viewpoints.
4. Ethical Decision-Making Frameworks – Providing structured guidelines to navigate complex diagnostic dilemmas.

By embedding critical thinking exercises in psychology programs, future mental health professionals will be better equipped to handle diagnostic challenges and ensure that patient care remains evidence-driven and ethically sound.

Future Research Directions on Critical Thinking in Diagnosis

Despite growing recognition of the importance of critical thinking in psychology, further research is needed to explore innovative approaches to improving diagnostic reasoning. Key areas for future investigation include:

- The Role of Artificial Intelligence (AI) in Clinical Decision-Making

AI-driven diagnostic tools are increasingly being integrated into mental health assessments. Future research should examine how AI can support (rather than replace) clinician judgment and whether it enhances diagnostic accuracy while reducing bias.

- The Long-Term Impact of Critical Thinking Training

While many psychology programs incorporate elements of critical thinking, studies should evaluate the effectiveness of structured critical thinking interventions in reducing misdiagnosis and improving patient outcomes.

- Cross-Cultural Variations in Diagnostic Bias

More research is needed to understand how cultural factors influence cognitive biases in diagnosis and how training programs can better prepare clinicians to navigate diverse mental health presentations.

- Neuroscientific Perspectives on Diagnostic Reasoning

Advances in neuroscience may help us better understand how mental health professionals process diagnostic information and identify cognitive patterns that contribute to errors.

Call to Action for Mental Health Professionals

As the field of mental health continues to evolve, critical thinking must remain at the core of diagnostic and treatment processes. Clinicians must actively engage in self-reflection, continuously seek updated research, and apply structured reasoning methods to prevent diagnostic errors. Institutions should prioritize ongoing education and professional development to ensure that practitioners are well-equipped with the skills necessary to think critically in complex diagnostic scenarios.

Ultimately, the future of psychological diagnosis depends on the ability of mental health professionals to apply critical thinking rigorously, adapt to new scientific advancements, and uphold the highest ethical standards. By doing so, we can foster a more accurate, compassionate, and culturally competent approach to mental health care—one that truly serves the needs of diverse populations and enhances patient well-being.

REFERENCES

Aas, M., & Høyer, G. (2021). Cognitive biases and their influence on clinical decision-making in psychiatry. *Journal of Psychiatric Research, 137*, 14–22. DOI: 10.1016/j.jpsychires.2021.02.021

American Psychological Association. (2017). *Diagnostic and statistical manual of mental disorders* (5th ed.). American Psychiatric Publishing.

Baer, M. (2019). Cognitive biases in diagnosis: Understanding their impact on clinical practice. *Journal of Psychology and Behavioral Sciences, 44*(2), 115–127. DOI: 10.1080/1744233X.2019.1642045

Barkley, R. A., & Murphy, K. R. (2018). *Attention-deficit hyperactivity disorder: A handbook for diagnosis and treatment* (3rd ed.). Guilford Press.

Becker, D., & Mehl, M. R. (2017). The role of heuristics in clinical decision-making: Biases and challenges in psychological diagnosis. *Clinical Psychology Review, 52*, 25–34. DOI: 10.1016/j.cpr.2017.01.004

Bisson, J. I., & Shepherd, J. (2018). Improving diagnostic accuracy: Critical thinking in the assessment of post-traumatic stress disorder. *Journal of Traumatic Stress, 31*(3), 457–466. DOI: 10.1002/jts.22335

Chavez, R. L., & Torres, S. (2020). The role of cultural competence in reducing diagnostic errors in minority populations. *Cultural Diversity & Ethnic Minority Psychology, 26*(3), 405–417. DOI: 10.1037/cdp0000351

Cook, J. M., & Heppner, P. P. (2020). Developing critical thinking skills in psychological practice: Implications for clinical training and practice. *Psychological Services, 17*(4), 468–475. DOI: 10.1037/ser0000350

Evans, C., Williams, R., & Green, M. (2020). Overdiagnosis of ADHD in children: Factors contributing to an increasing diagnosis rate. *Journal of Child Psychology and Psychiatry, and Allied Disciplines, 61*(5), 543–555. DOI: 10.1111/jcpp.13238

Garcia, J. L., & Figueira, M. A. (2019). Diagnostic errors in mental health: A critical review of challenges and solutions. *International Journal of Psychiatry, 56*(2), 109–116. DOI: 10.1080/00207594.2018.1495479

Green, A. R., & Carillo, J. E. (2018). Cultural competence and diagnostic decision-making: A systematic review of current practices. *Psychiatry Research, 270*, 635–641. DOI: 10.1016/j.psychres.2018.10.036

Harris, P., & Thomas, D. (2021). Overcoming biases in psychological assessments: A critical thinking approach. *Psychological Assessment*, *33*(1), 80–93. DOI: 10.1037/pas0001061

Huang, Y., & Zheng, Y. (2020). Cognitive biases in psychiatric diagnosis: Implications for clinical practice and training. *The Psychiatric Clinics of North America*, *43*(4), 663–674. DOI: 10.1016/j.psc.2020.07.003

Jones, A. R., & Lee, H. (2021). Implicit bias in psychiatric diagnoses: The case of schizophrenia among minority populations. *Cultural Psychiatry Review*, *38*(2), 227–239. DOI: 10.1016/j.cpr.2021.04.009

Kahneman, D. (2011). *Thinking, fast and slow*. Farrar, Straus and Giroux.

Kiger, D., & Stoner, J. (2017). The influence of cognitive biases on diagnostic decision-making in psychological practice. *Journal of Clinical Psychology*, *73*(2), 157–169. DOI: 10.1002/jclp.22373

Mayer, R. E., & Alexander, P. A. (2019). *Handbook of research on learning and instruction* (2nd ed.). Routledge.

Miller, W. R., & Rollnick, S. (2019). *Motivational interviewing: Helping people change* (3rd ed.). Guilford Press.

Rosenbaum, L. (2019). The role of reflective practice in improving diagnostic reasoning. *Journal of Medical Ethics*, *45*(2), 91–98. DOI: 10.1136/medethics-2018-105107

Smith, J., Brown, T., & White, S. (2022). The impact of second opinions in clinical psychology: A study on diagnostic changes. *Journal of Clinical Psychology*, *78*(3), 467–476. DOI: 10.1002/jclp.23055

Sommers-Flanagan, J., & Sommers-Flanagan, R. (2018). *Clinical interviewing* (6th ed.). Wiley.

Tversky, A., & Kahneman, D. (1974). Judgment under uncertainty: Heuristics and biases. *Science*, *185*(4157), 1124–1131. DOI: 10.1126/science.185.4157.1124 PMID: 17835457

Williams, C. T., & Anderson, S. L. (2020). Clinical decision-making in psychological diagnosis: Enhancing diagnostic accuracy with cognitive models and critical thinking. *Psychological Services*, *17*(1), 20–28. DOI: 10.1037/ser0000345

Compilation of References

Aas, M., & Høyer, G. (2021). Cognitive biases and their influence on clinical decision-making in psychiatry. *Journal of Psychiatric Research, 137*, 14–22. DOI: 10.1016/j.jpsychires.2021.02.021

Ab Hamid, M. R., Sami, W., & Sidek, M. M. (2017, September). Discriminant validity assessment: Use of Fornell & Larcker criterion versus HTMT criterion. [IOP Publishing.]. *Journal of Physics: Conference Series, 890*(1), 012163. DOI: 10.1088/1742-6596/890/1/012163

Abrami, P. C., Bernard, R. M., Borokhovski, E., Waddington, D. I., Wade, C. A., & Persson, T. (2015). Strategies for teaching students to think critically: A meta-analysis. *Review of Educational Research, 85*(2), 275–314. DOI: 10.3102/0034654314551063

Acevedo, E. C., & Hess, C. (2022) "The link between critical thinking and personality: individual differences in a concern for truth," Modern Psychological Studies: Vol. 27: No. 1, Article 9. Available at: https://scholar.utc.edu/mps/vol27/iss1/9

Adekolu, O., & Zinchuk, A. (2022). Sleep Deficiency in Obstructive Sleep Apnea. *Clinics in Chest Medicine, 43*(2), 353–371. DOI: 10.1016/j.ccm.2022.02.013 PMID: 35659030

Aggarwal, N. K., Nicasio, A. V., DeSilva, R., Boiler, M., & Lewis-Fernández, R. (2013). Barriers to implementing the DSM-5 cultural formulation interview: A qualitative study. *Culture, Medicine and Psychiatry, 37*(3), 505–533. DOI: 10.1007/s11013-013-9325-z PMID: 23836098

Aldrich, R. (2013). Neuroscience, education and evolution of the human brain. *History of Education, 42*(3), 396–410. DOI: 10.1080/0046760X.2012.749543

Ali̇yeva, A.Ali̇Yeva. (2023). Obstructive Sleep Apnea and Circadian Rhythms. *Kulak Burun Boğaz ve Baş Boyun Cerrahisi Dergisi, 31*(3), 179–188. DOI: 10.24179/kbbbbc.2023-98095

Alkhalifah, K., Alsalhi, S., Alrashed, A., Almagushi, S., Alharbi, M., Almutairi, A., Alghanim, S., Alkharraz, A., Alnasser, A., & Alradhi, M. (2024). Worldwide Prevalence of obstructive sleep apnea among pediatrics: A Systematic Review and Meta-Analysis. *International Journal of Medicine in Developing Countries, 455–459*, 455–459. DOI: 10.24911/IJMDC.51-1701581085

Alkhelil, A. H. (2016). The Relationship between Personality Traits and Career Choice: A Case Study of Secondary School Students. *International Journal of Academic Research in Progressive Education and Development*, *5*(2), 122–135. DOI: 10.6007/IJARPED/v5-i2/2132

Alloway, T. P., & Alloway, R. G. (2010). Investigating the Predictive Roles of Working Memory and IQ in Academic Attainment. *Journal of Experimental Child Psychology*, *106*(1), 20–29. DOI: 10.1016/j.jecp.2009.11.003 PMID: 20018296

Amelang, M., & Bartussek, D. (1997): Differentielle Psychologie und Persönlichkeitsforschung. Kohlhammer, Stuttgart, Berlin, Köln, 4.edition

American College of Obstetricians and Gynecologists (ACOG). (2017). *The importance of mental health in adolescents: Guidelines for assessment and intervention*. ACOG Clinical Updates.

American College of Obstetricians and Gynecologists. (2017). Mental health disorders in adolescents. Retrieved from https://www.acog.org/clinical/clinical-guidance/committee-opinion/articles/2017/07/mental-health-disorders-in-adolescents

American Educational Research Association, American Psychological Association, & National Council on Measurement in Education. (2014). *Standards for educational and psychological testing*. American Educational Research Association.

American Psychiatric Association. (2013). *Diagnostic and statistical manual of mental disorders* (5th ed.). Author.

American Psychiatric Association. (2013). *Diagnostic and statistical manual of mental disorders (DSM-5 (R))* (5th ed.). American Psychiatric Association Publishing.

American Psychiatric Association. (2022). Diagnostic and statistical manual of mental disorders (5th ed., text rev.). American Psychiatric Publishing., DSM-5-TR.

Anand, K. J. S., & Scalzo, F. M. (2000). Can adverse neonatal experiences alter brain development and subsequent behavior? *Biology of the Neonate*, *77*(2), 69–82. DOI: 10.1159/000014197 PMID: 10657682

Anderson, J. C., & Gerbing, D. W. (1988). Structural equation modeling in practice: A review and recommended two-step approach. *Psychological Bulletin, 103*(3), 411–423. DOI: 10.1037/0033-2909.103.3.411

Anderson, K., & Perrin, A. (2018). *Nearly one in five Americans don't use the internet.* Pew Research Center.

APA Task Force on Psychological Assessment and Evaluation. (2020). *APA guidelines for psychological assessment and evaluation.* American Psychological Association. https://www.apa.org/about/policy/guidelines-psychological-assessment-evaluation.pdf

Ap, K., & B, K. (2023). Pharyngeal Fascia and its Relationship with Obstructive Sleep Apnea. *Acta Scientific Neurology*, 26–31. DOI: 10.31080/ASNE.2023.06.0679

Appelbaum, P. S. (2007). Assessment of patients' competence to consent to treatment. *The New England Journal of Medicine, 357*(18), 1834–1840. DOI: 10.1056/NEJMcp074045 PMID: 17978292

Appelbaum, P. S. (2009). Law and psychiatry: Malpractice liability in the context of psychiatric diagnosis. *Psychiatric Services (Washington, D.C.), 60*(6), 727–729. DOI: 10.1176/ps.2009.60.6.727

Araújo, B., Gomes, S. F., & Ribeiro, L. (2024). Critical thinking pedagogical practices in medical education: A systematic review. *Frontiers in Medicine, 11*, 1358444. Advance online publication. DOI: 10.3389/fmed.2024.1358444 PMID: 38947238

Argel, M. (2023). Sleep Obstructive Apnea Syndrome. In Esquinas, A. M., De Vito, A., & Barbetakis, N. (Eds.), *Upper Airway Disorders and Noninvasive Mechanical Ventilation* (pp. 269–276). Springer International Publishing., DOI: 10.1007/978-3-031-32487-1_29

Aronfreed, J. (1968). Conscience and conduct: The socialization of internalized control of behavior.

Asendorpf, J. B. (2007). *Psychologie der Persönlichkeit* (4th ed.). Springer Medizin Verlag Heidelberg. DOI: 10.1007/978-3-540-71685-3

Astley, S. J., & Furlong, M. J. (2019). The influence of school service on students' social and emotional development: A meta-analysis and systematic review. *Journal of School Psychology, 72*, 44–58.

Ayano, G., Haile, K., Assefa, D., & Haile, H. (2021). Prevalence of severe psychiatric disorders and misdiagnosis rates in Ethiopia. *Annals of General Psychiatry, 20*(1). DOI: 10.1186/s12991-021-00333-7 PMID: 33531016

Baer, M. (2019). Cognitive biases in diagnosis: Understanding their impact on clinical practice. *Journal of Psychology and Behavioral Sciences*, *44*(2), 115–127. DOI: 10.1080/1744233X.2019.1642045

Bailin, S. (2002). Critical thinking and science education. *Science & Education*, *11*(4), 361–375. DOI: 10.1023/A:1016042608621

Baker, M., Rudd, R., & Pomeroy, C. (2001). Relationships between critical and creative thinking. *Journal of Southern Agricultural Education Research*, *51*(1), 173–188.

Baker, S. T. E., Lubman, D. I., Yücel, M., Allen, N. B., Whittle, S., Fulcher, B. D., Zalesky, A., & Fornito, A. (2015). Developmental Changes in Brain Network Hub Connectivity in Late Adolescence. *The Journal of Neuroscience : The Official Journal of the Society for Neuroscience*, *35*(24), 9078–9087.

Bal, B. S. (2009). An introduction to medical malpractice in the United States. *Clinical Orthopaedics and Related Research*, *467*(2), 339–347. DOI: 10.1007/s11999-008-0636-2 PMID: 19034593

Banner, S. E., Rock, A. J., Cosh, S. M., Schutte, N., & Rice, K. (2025). Self-reflection on competence: Metacognitive process and barriers of self-assessment in psychologists. *Advances in Health Sciences Education : Theory and Practice*, 1–21. DOI: 10.1007/s10459-025-10434-7 PMID: 40312527

Barber, B. R., & Battistoni, R. (1993). A season of service: Introducing service learning into the liberal arts curriculum. *PS, Political Science & Politics*, *26*(2), 235–240. DOI: 10.2307/419837

Barbosa-Camacho, F. J., Miranda-Ackerman, R. C., Vázquez-Reyna, I., Jimenez-Ley, V. B., Barrera-López, F. J., Contreras-Cordero, V. S., Sánchez-López, V. A., Castillo-Valverde, T. J., Lamas-Abbadie, C. C., González-Adán, B. A., Cortes-Flores, A. O., Morgan-Villela, G., Cervantes-Cardona, G. A., Cervantes-Guevara, G., Fuentes-Orozco, C., & González-Ojeda, A. (2020). Association between HEXACO personality traits and medical specialty preferences in Mexican medical students: A cross-sectional survey. *BMC Psychology*, *8*(1), 23. DOI: 10.1186/s40359-020-0390-0 PMID: 32171327

Barkley, R. A., & Murphy, K. R. (2018). *Attention-deficit hyperactivity disorder: A handbook for diagnosis and treatment* (3rd ed.). Guilford Press.

Bassett, D. S., & Gazzaniga, M. S. (2011). Understanding complexity in the human brain. *Trends in Cognitive Sciences*, *15*(5), 200–209.

Bauer, P. J., Larkina, M., & Deocampo, J. (2011). Early Memory Development. In Goswami, U. (Ed.), *The Wiley-Blackwell Handbook of Childhood Cognitive Development* (2nd ed.). Wiley-Blackwell.

Baycheva, S., Georgieva, G., Stoykov, M., Milkov, M., & Enchev, M. (2024). Impact of obstructive sleep apnea on patients'' quality of life. *Romanian Journal of Rhinology, 14*(53), 24–28. DOI: 10.2478/rjr-2024-0005

Beauchamp, T. L., & Childress, J. F. (2019). *Principles of biomedical ethics* (8th ed.). Oxford University Press.

Beck, A. T. (1976). *Cognitive therapy and the emotional disorders.* International Universities Press.

Becker, D., & Mehl, M. R. (2017). The role of heuristics in clinical decision-making: Biases and challenges in psychological diagnosis. *Clinical Psychology Review, 52,* 25–34. DOI: 10.1016/j.cpr.2017.01.004

Behrens, P. J. (1996). The Watson-Glaser Critical Thinking Appraisal and academic performance of diploma school students. *The Journal of Nursing Education, 35*(1), 34–36. DOI: 10.3928/0148-4834-19960101-10 PMID: 8926515

Bennett-Levy, J., McManus, F., Westling, B. E., & Fennell, M. (2010). Acquiring and refining CBT skills: A qualitative study of supervisor and trainee experiences. *Behavioural and Cognitive Psychotherapy, 38*(5), 541–558.

Berik Safçi, S. (2024). The prevalence and polysomnographic characteristics of treatment-emergent central sleep apnea with obstructive sleep apnea. *Sleep and Breathing, 28*(3), 1245–1250. DOI: 10.1007/s11325-024-02999-1 PMID: 38308750

Bernal, G., Jimenez-Chafey, M. I., & Rodriguez, M. M. (2009). Cultural adaptation of treatments: A resource for considering culture in evidence-based practice. *Annual Review of Clinical Psychology, 5,* 563–589.

Beyer, H. (1992). Die Berufswahl als Gegenstand sozialwissenschaftlicher Theoriebildung. Überlegungen zum theoretischen Rahmen sozialwissenschaftlicher Analysen der Berufswahl und zur Möglichkeit einer „verstehenden" Erkenntnisperspektive in der Theoriebildung sozialwissenschaftlicher Berufswahlforschung. Augsburg Universitätsschrift: Wirtschafts- und sozialwissenschaftliche Fakultät.

Beyer, B. K. (1995). *Critical thinking: Fastback 385.* Phi Delta Kappa Educational Foundation.

Bezanilla, M. J., Fernández-Nogueira, D., Poblete, M., & Galindo-Domínguez, H. (2019). Methodologies for teaching-learning critical thinking in higher education: The teacher's view. *Thinking Skills and Creativity*, *33*, 100584. DOI: 10.1016/j.tsc.2019.100584

Bhugra, D., Tasman, A., & Pathare, S. (2021). Mental health diagnosis: Challenges and critical perspectives. *The Lancet. Psychiatry*, *8*(4), 350–368. DOI: 10.1016/S2215-0366(21)00012-3

Bikov, A., Bailly, S., Testelmans, D., Fanfulla, F., Pataka, A., Bouloukaki, I., Hein, H., Dogas, Z., Basoglu, O. K., Staats, R., Parati, G., Lombardi, C., Grote, L., & Mihaicuta, S.ESADA study group. (2024). The relationship between periodic limb movement during sleep and dyslipidaemia in patients with obstructive sleep apnea. *Journal of Sleep Research*, *33*(2), e14012. DOI: 10.1111/jsr.14012 PMID: 37596874

Birbaumer, N., & Schmidt, R. F. (2007). Lernen und Gedächtnis, in: Schmidt, R. F., Lang, F. (Hrsg.): Physiologie des Menschen, 30. Aufl., Springer Medizin Verlag, Heidelberg, 223– 238.

Bisson, J. I., & Shepherd, J. (2018). Improving diagnostic accuracy: Critical thinking in the assessment of post-traumatic stress disorder. *Journal of Traumatic Stress*, *31*(3), 457–466. DOI: 10.1002/jts.22335

Blakemore, S.-J., & Frith, U. (2006). *Wie wir lernen. Was die Hirnforschung darüber weiß*. Deutsche Verlags-Anstalt.

Blaug, M. (1985). Where are we now in the economics of education? *Economics of Education Review*, *4*(1), 17–28. DOI: 10.1016/0272-7757(85)90034-2

BMJ Quality & Safety. (2021). Diagnostic error in mental health: A review. *BMJ Quality & Safety*, *33*(10), 663–672. https://qualitysafety.bmj.com/content/33/10/663

Bogdanowicz, M. (2002). *Ryzyko dysleksji. Problem i diagnozowanie*. Wydawnictwo Harmonia.

Bogdanowicz, M. (2003). Podstawy diagnozowania dysleksji rozwojowej i praw uczniów dyslektycznych w szkole. In Kaja, B. (Ed.), *Diagnoza dysleksji*. Wydawnictwo Akademii Bydgoskiej.

Bogdanowicz, M. (2008). *Specyficzne trudności w uczeniu się*. Wydawnictwo Harmonia.

Bogdanowicz, M. (2011). *Ryzyko dysleksji, dysgrafii, dysortografii*. Wydawnictwo Harmonia.

Bogdanowicz, M., & Adryjanek, M. (2004). *Uczeń z dysleksją w szkole. Poradnik nie tylko dla polonistów*. Wydawnictwo Operon.

Bonacina, C. F., Soster, L. M. S. F. A., Bueno, C., Diniz, J. S., Bozzini, M. F., Di Francesco, R. C., Olegário, I. C., & De Oliveira Lira, A. (2024). Sleep bruxism and associated physiological events in children with obstructive sleep apnea: A polysomnographic study. *Journal of Clinical Sleep Medicine : JCSM : Official Publication of the American Academy of Sleep Medicine*, *20*(4), 565–573. DOI: 10.5664/jcsm.10950 PMID: 38059335

Bornstein, R. F. (2020). From symptom to process: Case formulation, clinical utility, and PDM-2. *Psychoanalytic Psychology*, *37*(3), 165–174. DOI: 10.1037/pap0000262

Boss, J. A. (1994). The effect of community service work on the moral development of college ethics students. *Journal of Moral Education*, *23*(2), 183–198. DOI: 10.1080/0305724940230206

Brackett, M. A., Reyes, M. R., Rivers, S. E., Elbertson, N. A., & Salovey, P. (2012). Assessing teachers' beliefs about social and emotional learning. *Journal of Psychoeducational Assessment*, *30*(3), 219–236. DOI: 10.1177/0734282911424879

Bradford, A., Meyer, A. N., Khan, S., Giardina, T. D., & Singh, H. (2024). Diagnostic error in mental health: A review. *BMJ Quality & Safety*, *33*(10), 663–672. DOI: 10.1136/bmjqs-2023-016996 PMID: 38575311

Brodbeck, K.H. (1997). praxis perspektiven Band 2, Jahrbuch des Vereins für betriebswirtschaftlichen Wissenstransfer am Fachbereich Betriebswirtschaft der Fachhochschule Würzburg-Schweinfurt-Aschaffenburg, Verlag BWT Würzburg

Brookfield, S. D. (1989). *Developing critical thinkers: Challenging adults to explore alternative ways of thinking and acting*. Jossey-Bass.

Bugdayci, S. (2019). Examining Personal and Social Responsibility Levels of Secondary School Students. *Universal Journal of Educational Research*, *7*(1), 206–210. DOI: 10.13189/ujer.2019.070126

Burden, P. R., & Byrd, D. M. (1999). *Methods for effective teaching* (2nd ed.). Allyn & Bacon.

Burgos, J., & Carnero, M. C. (2020). Assessment of Social Responsibility in Education in Secondary Schools. *Sustainability (Basel)*, *12*(12), 4849. DOI: 10.3390/su12124849

Bußhoff, L. (1984). *Berufswahl*. Kohlhammer.

Butler, A. C., Chapman, J. E., Forman, E. M., & Beck, A. T. (2006). The empirical status of cognitive-behavioral therapy: A review of meta-analyses. *Clinical Psychology Review, 26*(1), 17–31. DOI: 10.1016/j.cpr.2005.07.003 PMID: 16199119

Butler, A. C., Fernandez, G. A., & Wallace, P. (2020). Longitudinal effects of CBT on anxiety and depression symptoms in adolescents: A meta-analysis of 45 studies. *Cognitive Therapy and Research, 44*(2), 189–206.

Butterworth, B., Varma, S., & Laurillard, D. (2011). Dyscalculia: From brain to education. *Science, 332*(6033), 1049–1053. DOI: 10.1126/science.1201536 PMID: 21617068

Camañes-Gonzalvo, S., Montiel-Company, J. M., Paredes-Gallardo, V., Puertas-Cuesta, F. J., Marco-Pitarch, R., García-Selva, M., Bellot-Arcís, C., & Casaña-Ruiz, M. D. (2024). Relationship of ankyloglossia and obstructive sleep apnea: Systematic review and meta-analysis. *Sleep and Breathing, 28*(3), 1067–1078. DOI: 10.1007/s11325-024-03021-4 PMID: 38478208

Carrion-Castillo, A., Franke, B., & Fisher, S. E. (2017). Molecular genetics of dyslexia: An overview. *Dyslexia (Chichester, England), 23*(1), 3–20. PMID: 27892659

Castilla-Polo, F., Ruiz-Rodríguez, M. C., Moreno, A., Licerán-Gutiérrez, A., Cámara de la Fuente, M., Chamorro Rufián, E., & Cano-Rodríguez, M. (2020). Classroom Learning and the Perception of Social Responsibility Amongst Graduate Students of Management Accounting. *Sustainability (Basel), 12*(17), 7093. DOI: 10.3390/su12177093

Centers for Disease Control and Prevention. (2024, August 6). *CDC data show improvements in youth mental health but need for safer and more supportive schools.* CDC Newsroom. https://www.cdc.gov/media/releases/2024/p0806-youth-mental-health.html

Chalem, P. (2023). Obstructive Sleep Apnea and Systemic Autoimmune Diseases. In Baptista, P. M., Lugo Saldaña, R., & Amado, S. (Eds.), *Obstructive Sleep Apnea* (pp. 143–156). Springer International Publishing., DOI: 10.1007/978-3-031-35225-6_8

Chamberlin, D. E. (2023). The active inference model of coherence therapy. *Frontiers in Human Neuroscience, 16*, 955558. DOI: 10.3389/fnhum.2022.955558 PMID: 36684841

Charmaraman, L., Chan, H., & Suárez-Orozco, C. (2023). Intersectionality and mental health: Policies for LGBTQ+ students of color. *The Journal of Adolescent Health.*

Chavez, R. L., & Torres, S. (2020). The role of cultural competence in reducing diagnostic errors in minority populations. *Cultural Diversity & Ethnic Minority Psychology, 26*(3), 405–417. DOI: 10.1037/cdp0000351

Chen, S. H., Nasongkhla, J., & Donaldson, J. A. (2015). University Social Responsibility (USR): Identifying an Ethical Foundation within Higher Education Institutions. *Turkish Online Journal of Educational Technology-TOJET, 14*(4), 165–172.

Chiang, J.-K., Lin, Y.-C., Kao, H.-H., & Kao, Y.-H. (2024). Surge of Sympathetic Activity during Hyperventilation at the End of Apnea for Patients with Obstructive Sleep Apnea. *Medicina, 60*(3), 366. DOI: 10.3390/medicina60030366 PMID: 38541092

Chickering, A. W., & Reisser, L. (1993). Education and Identity. The Jossey-Bass Higher and Adult Education Series. Jossey-Bass Inc., Publishers, 350 Sansome St., San Francisco, CA 94104.

Chiu, Y.-H., Lee, Y.-F., Lin, H.-L., & Cheng, L.-C. (2024). Exploring the role of mobile apps for insomnia in depression: Systematic review. *Journal of Medical Internet Research, 26*, e51110. DOI: 10.2196/51110 PMID: 39423009

Chow, D. L., Miller, S. D., Seidel, J. A., Kane, R. T., Thornton, J. A., & Andrews, W. P. (2015). The role of deliberate practice in the development of highly effective psychotherapists. *Psychotherapy (Chicago, Ill.), 52*(3), 337–345. DOI: 10.1037/pst0000015 PMID: 26301425

Chu, J., Leino, A., Pflum, S., & Sue, S. (2016). A model for the theoretical basis of cultural competency to guide psychotherapy. *Professional Psychology, Research and Practice, 47*(1), 18–29. DOI: 10.1037/pro0000055

Çiftçi, B., & Çiftçi, T. U. (2023). Obstructive Sleep Apnea Syndrome: A Pulmonology Perspective. In Cingi, C., Yorgancıoğlu, A., Bayar Muluk, N., & Cruz, A. A. (Eds.), *Airway diseases* (pp. 1–17). Springer International Publishing., DOI: 10.1007/978-3-031-22483-6_129-1

Clark, L. A., Cuthbert, B., Lewis-Fernández, R., Narrow, W. E., & Reed, G. M. (2017). Three approaches to understanding and classifying mental disorder: ICD-11, DSM-5, and the National Institute of Mental Health's Research Domain Criteria (RDoC). *Psychological Science in the Public Interest: A Journal of the American Psychological Society, 18*(2), 72–145. DOI: 10.1177/1529100617727266

Coderre, S., Mandin, H., Harasym, P. H., & Fick, G. H. (2003). Diagnostic reasoning strategies and diagnostic success. *Medical Education, 37*(8), 695–703. DOI: 10.1046/j.1365-2923.2003.01577.x PMID: 12895249

Cohen, J. (1988). *Statistical power analysis for the behavioral sciences* (2nd ed.).

Collins, G. S., & Moons, K. G. M. (2019). Reporting of artificial intelligence prediction models. *Lancet, 393*(10181), 1577–1579. DOI: 10.1016/S0140-6736(19)30037-6 PMID: 31007185

Conforti, M. (2023, December 13). *2024 workplace mental health trends: A proactive approach to well-being*. www.springhealth.com._https://www.springhealth.com/blog/2024-workplace-mental-health-trends

Conrad, D., & Hedin, D. (1989). High School Community Service: A Review of Research and Programs.

Cook, J. M., & Heppner, P. P. (2020). Developing critical thinking skills in psychological practice: Implications for clinical training and practice. *Psychological Services, 17*(4), 468–475. DOI: 10.1037/ser0000350

Cook, T., Murphy, R., & And Hunt, H. (2000). Comer's School Development Program in Chicago: A Theory-Based Evaluation. *American Educational Research Journal, 37*(2), 535–597. DOI: 10.3102/00028312037002535

Corrigan, P. W. (2004). How stigma interferes with mental health care. *The American Psychologist, 59*(7), 614–625. DOI: 10.1037/0003-066X.59.7.614 PMID: 15491256

Corrigan, P. W., & Nieweglowski, K. (2019). How does familiarity impact the stigma of mental illness? *Clinical Psychology Review, 70*, 40–50. DOI: 10.1016/j.cpr.2019.02.001 PMID: 30908990

Corstorphine, E. (2006). Cognitive–Emotional–Behavioural Therapy for the eating disorders: Working with beliefs about emotions. *European Eating Disorders Review, 14*(6), 448–461. DOI: 10.1002/erv.747

Cottrell, S. (2023). *Critical thinking skills: Effective analysis, argument and reflection* (4th ed.). Bloomsbury Publishing.

Crites, J. (1969). *Vocational Psychology. The Study of Vocational Behavior and Development*. McGraw-Hill.

Crockett, L. J., Qu, K., & Neblett, E. W. (2023). Cultural validity in psychological assessment: Reconsidering normative data and methodological approaches. *Psychological Assessment, 35*(3), 231–244. DOI: 10.1037/pas0001170

Croskerry, P. (2020). Believing in overcoming cognitive biases. Journal of Ethics, AMA.

Croskerry, P., Singhal, G., & Mamede, S. (2013). Cognitive debiasing 1: origins of bias and theory of debiasing. *BMJ Quality & Safety, 22 Suppl 2*(Suppl 2), ii58–ii64. DOI: 10.1136/bmjqs-2012-001712

Croskerry, P. (2003). The importance of cognitive errors in diagnosis and strategies to minimize them. *Academic Medicine, 78*(8), 775–780. DOI: 10.1097/00001888-200308000-00003 PMID: 12915363

Croskerry, P. (2008). A universal model of diagnostic reasoning. *Academic Medicine, 93*(8), 1187–1194. DOI: 10.1097/ACM.0b013e3181ace703 PMID: 19638766

Croskerry, P., Singhal, G., & Mamede, S. (2013). Cognitive debiasing interventions: A systematic review of effectiveness in medical decision making. *Medical Decision Making, 43*(1), 23–35. DOI: 10.1177/0272989X221106549

Dahl, R. E., Allen, N. B., Wilbrecht, L., & Suleiman, A. B. (2022). Neurodevelopmental insights into adolescent emotional reactivity and implications for cognitive behavioral therapy. *Developmental Cognitive Neuroscience.*

Dana, R. H. (2005). *Multicultural assessment: Principles, applications, and examples* (2nd ed.). Routledge. DOI: 10.4324/9781410612540

Daniel, K. E., Szkody, E., Aggarwal, P., Peterman, A. H., Washburn, J. J., & Selby, E. A. (2022). Characterizing changes in mental health-related outcomes for health service psychology graduate students during the first year of the COVID-19 pandemic. *Journal of Clinical Psychology, 78*(11), 2281–2298. DOI: 10.1002/jclp.23392 PMID: 35611434

Datu, J. A. (2012, July). Personality Traits and Paternal Parenting Style as Predictive Factors of Career Choice. *Academic Research International, 3*(1), •••.

Dávila, L. A., & Mora, J. R. (2017). The impact of community service learning on the development of college students' emotional intelligence. *Journal of College Student Development, 58*(5), 709–724.

De Brabander, C. J. (2000). Knowledge definition, subject, and educational track level: Perceptions of secondary school teachers. *American Educational Research Journal, 37*(4), 1027–1058. DOI: 10.3102/000283120370041027

Deeper Signals. (2024). *Personality assessments that drive results.* https://www.deepersignals.com

Delors, J., Amagi, I., Carneiro, R., Chung, F., Geremek, B., Gorham, W., Suhr, M. W. (1996). Learning. The treasure Within. Paris.

DeVellis, R. F., & Thorpe, C. T. (2021). *Scale development: Theory and applications* (5th ed.). Sage Publications.

Dewey, J. (1916). 1985. Democracy and education. John Dewey: the middle works (1899–1924), 9.

Dharamsi, S., Espinoza, N., Cramer, C., Amin, M., Bainbridge, L., & Poole, G. (2010). Nurturing social responsibility through community service-learning: Lessons learned from a pilot project. *Medical Teacher*, *32*(11), 905–911. DOI: 10.3109/01421590903434169 PMID: 21039101

Dima, A. M., Vasilache, S., Ghinea, V., & Agoston, S. (2013). A model of academic social responsability. *Transylvanian Review of Administrative Sciences*, *9*(38), 23–43.

DiMatteo, M. R. (2004). Social and psychological factors affecting adherence to health recommendations. *Medical Care*, *42*(7), 614–633.

Dissanayake, A., Dupuis, A., Burton, C. L., Soreni, N., Peters, P., Gajaria, A., Arnold, P. D., Schachar, R., & Crosbie, J. (2024). Racial/ethnic disparities in psychiatric traits and diagnoses within a community-based sample of children and youth. *Canadian Journal of Psychiatry*, *69*(6), 415–427. DOI: 10.1177/07067437241233936 PMID: 38425291

Dobson, D., & Dobson, K. S. (2018). *Evidence-based practice of cognitive-behavioral therapy: Meeting the challenges of the 21st century*. Guilford Press.

Drapeau, M., & Hunsley, J. (2014). Where's the science? Introduction to a special issue of *Canadian Psychology* on science in psychology. *Canadian Psychology*, *55*(3), 145–152. DOI: 10.1037/a0037321

DSM-5. (2013). *Cultural Formulation Interview (DSM-5 Appendix)*. (2013).

Duksal, F., & Eren, F. (2023). Evaluation of thyroid functions and obesity in obstructive sleep apnea syndrome. *Revista da Associação Médica Brasileira*, *69*(9), e20230376. DOI: 10.1590/1806-9282.20230376 PMID: 37729367

Dumontheil, I. (2015). Development of the social brain during adolescence. *Psicologia Educativa*, *21*(2), 117–124. DOI: 10.1016/j.pse.2015.08.001

Duraku, Z. H., Davis, H., Arënliu, A., Uka, F., & Behluli, V. (2024). Overcoming mental health challenges in higher education: A narrative review. *Frontiers in Psychology*, *15*, 1466060. Advance online publication. DOI: 10.3389/fpsyg.2024.1466060 PMID: 39726628

Ee, C., Lake, J., Firth, J., Hargraves, F., De Manincor, M., Meade, T., Marx, W., & Sarris, J. (2020). An integrative collaborative care model for people with mental illness and physical comorbidities. *International Journal of Mental Health Systems*, *14*(1), 83. Advance online publication. DOI: 10.1186/s13033-020-00410-6 PMID: 33292354

Eisenberg, N., Spinrad, T. L., & Morris, A. S. (2015). Prosocial development. In Lamb, M. E. (Ed.), *Handbook of child psychology and developmental science* (7th ed., Vol. 3, pp. 610–656). Wiley. DOI: 10.1002/9781118963418.childpsy315

Elder, L., & Paul, R. (2006). *Critical Thinking: Tools for Taking Charge of Your Learning and Your Life. 2*. Pearson/Prentice Hall.

Elwyn, G., Frosch, D. L., Thomson, R., Joseph-Williams, N., Lloyd, A., Kinnersley, P., Cording, E., Tomson, D., Dodd, C., Rollnick, S., Edwards, A., & Barry, M. (2012). Shared decision making: A model for clinical practice. *Journal of General Internal Medicine*, *27*(10), 1361–1367. DOI: 10.1007/s11606-012-2077-6 PMID: 22618581

Embretson, S. E., & Reise, S. P. (2013). *Item response theory for psychologists*. Psychology Press. DOI: 10.4324/9781410605269

Engle de Abreu, P. M. J., Gathercole, S. E., & Martin, R. (2011). Disentangling the Relationship between Working Memory and Language: The Roles of Short-Term Storage and Cognitive Control. *Learning and Individual Differences*, *21*(5), 569–574. DOI: 10.1016/j.lindif.2011.06.002

Ennis, R. H. (2000). A super-streamlined conception of critical thinking. http://faculty.education.illinois.edu/rhennis/documents/Super-Streamlined.pdf

Epstein, R. M. (2003). Mindful practice in action (II): Cultivating habits of mind. *Families, Systems & Health*, *21*(1), 11–17. DOI: 10.1037/h0089495

Ercolano, E., Bencivenga, L., Palaia, M. E., Carbone, G., Scognamiglio, F., Rengo, G., & Femminella, G. D. (2023). Intricate relationship between obstructive sleep apnea and dementia in older adults. *GeroScience*, *46*(1), 99–111. DOI: 10.1007/s11357-023-00958-4 PMID: 37814196

Eva, K. W., Hatala, R. M., Leblanc, V. R., & Brooks, L. R. (2007). Teaching from the clinical reasoning literature: combined reasoning strategies help novice diagnosticians overcome misleading information: Clinical expertise. *Medical Education*, *41*(12), 1152–1158. DOI: 10.1111/j.1365-2923.2007.02923.x PMID: 18045367

Evans, C., Williams, R., & Green, M. (2020). Overdiagnosis of ADHD in children: Factors contributing to an increasing diagnosis rate. *Journal of Child Psychology and Psychiatry, and Allied Disciplines*, *61*(5), 543–555. DOI: 10.1111/jcpp.13238

Eyler, J. S., & Giles, D. E. (1999). *Where's the learning in service-learning?* Jossey-Bass.

Fabio, R. A., Plebe, A., & Suriano, R. (2025). AI-based chatbot interactions and critical thinking skills: An exploratory study. *Current Psychology (New Brunswick, N.J.)*, *44*(9), 8082–8095. DOI: 10.1007/s12144-024-06795-8

Facione, P. A. (2011). *Critical thinking: What it is and why it counts* (2011 update). Insight Assessment.

Facione, P. A. (2015). *Critical thinking: What it is and why it counts* (2015 update). Insight Assessment._https://www.insightassessment.com/wp-content/uploads/ia/pdf/whatwhy.pdf

Facione, P. A. (2015). *Critical thinking: What it is and why it counts.*

Facione, P. A. (1990). *Critical thinking/ A statement of expert consensus for purposes of educational assessment and instruction.* The California Academic Press.

Facione, P. A. (1990a). *Critical thinking: A statement of expert consensus for purposes of educational assessment and instruction.* American Philosophical Association.

Facione, P. A. (1990b). *Critical thinking: A statement of expert consensus for purposes of educational assessment and instruction (The Delphi Report).* American Philosophical Association.

Facione, P. A. (2000). The disposition toward critical thinking: Its character, measurement, and relationship to critical thinking skill. *Informal Logic*, *20*(1), 61–84. DOI: 10.22329/il.v20i1.2254

Faraone, S. V., Asherson, P., Banaschewski, T., Biederman, J., Buitelaar, J. K., Ramos-Quiroga, J. A., Rohde, L. A., Sonuga-Barke, E. J. S., Tannock, R., & Franke, B. (2015). Attention-deficit/hyperactivity disorder. *Nature Reviews. Disease Primers*, *1*(1), 15020. DOI: 10.1038/nrdp.2015.20 PMID: 27189265

Fatmawati, A., Zubaidah, S., & Mahanal, S. (2019, December). Critical thinking, creative thinking, and learning achievement: How they are related. In *Journal of Physics: Conference Series* (Vol. 1417, No. 1, p. 012070). IOP Publishing. DOI: 10.1088/1742-6596/1417/1/012070

Finkelstein, M. A., & Pancer, S. M. (2015). The impact of community-based volunteer work on students' personal, social, and civic outcomes. *Journal of Adolescence*, *38*, 107–113.

First, M. B. (2021). The challenge of psychiatric diagnosis: Ethical issues and the DSM. In Benuto, L. T., Leany, B. D., & Casas, A. M. (Eds.), *Handbook of cognitive behavioral therapy for pediatric medical conditions* (pp. 27–36). Springer., DOI: 10.1007/978-3-030-49874-3_3

First, M. B., Williams, J. B. W., Karg, R. S., & Spitzer, R. L. (2015). *Structured Clinical Interview for DSM-5 Disorders—Clinician Version (SCID-5-CV).* American Psychiatric Association Publishing.

First, M. B., Williams, J. B. W., Karg, R. S., & Spitzer, R. L. (2016). *Structured Clinical Interview for DSM-5 Disorders-Clinician Version (SCID-5-CV).* American Psychiatric Association Publishing.

First, M. B., Williams, J. B. W., Karg, R. S., & Spitzer, R. L. (2018). *Structured clinical interview for DSM-5 disorders, clinician version (SCID-5-CV).* American Psychiatric Association Publishing.

Fonseca, A., Macdonald, A., Dandy, E., & Valenti, P. (2011). The state of sustainability reporting at Canadian universities. *International Journal of Sustainability in Higher Education, 12*(1), 22–40. DOI: 10.1108/14676371111098285

Fornell, C. (1981). A comparative analysis of two structural equation models: LISREL and PLS applied to market data.

Fornell, C., & Bookstein, F. L. (1982). Two structural equation models: LISREL and PLS applied to consumer exit-voice theory. *JMR, Journal of Marketing Research, 19*(4), 440–452. DOI: 10.1177/002224378201900406

Fornell, C., & Larcker, D. F. (1981). Evaluating structural equation models with unobservable variables and measurement error. *JMR, Journal of Marketing Research, 18*(1), 39–50. DOI: 10.1177/002224378101800104

Forßbohm, D. (2010). *Berufswahl als Entscheidung. Eine Auseinandersetzung mit ausgewählten Konzepten zur Berufswahl unter geschlechtsspezifischer Perspektive.* Verlag Dr. Kovac.

Freire, C., Sennes, L. U., & Polotsky, V. Y. (2022). Opioids and obstructive sleep apnea. *Journal of Clinical Sleep Medicine : JCSM : Official Publication of the American Academy of Sleep Medicine, 18*(2), 647–652. DOI: 10.5664/jcsm.9730 PMID: 34672945

Freud, S. (1930). *Das Unbehagen in der Kultur.* Internationaler Psychoanalytischer Verlag.

Fridgeirsdottir, K. Y., Ólafsdóttir, K. A., Islind, A. S., Leppänen, T., Arnardottir, E. S., & Saavedra, J. M. (2024). The role of physical activity on obstructive sleep apnea severity and hypoxic load, and the mismatch between subjective and objective physical activity assessments. *Journal of Sleep Research, 14195*(6), e14195. DOI: 10.1111/jsr.14195 PMID: 38480993

Friebertshäuser, B. (2008). Statuspassage von der Schule ins Studium. In Helsper, W., & Böhme, J. (Eds.), *Handbuch der Schulforschung* (pp. 611–627). VS Verlag für Sozialwissenschaften. DOI: 10.1007/978-3-531-91095-6_24

Furco, A. (1999). Self-assessment rubric for the institutionalization of service-learning in higher education.

Garb, H. N. (2005). Clinical judgment and decision making. *Annual Review of Clinical Psychology, 1*(1), 67–89. DOI: 10.1146/annurev.clinpsy.1.102803.143810 PMID: 17716082

Garcia, J. L., & Figueira, M. A. (2019). Diagnostic errors in mental health: A critical review of challenges and solutions. *International Journal of Psychiatry, 56*(2), 109–116. DOI: 10.1080/00207594.2018.1495479

Garcia, R., Lopez, A., Martinez, E., & Rodriguez, P. (2021). Community-based culturally adapted cognitive behavioral therapy for Mexican-American university students: Leveraging dichos and familismo. *Journal of Latina/o Psychology, 9*(3).

Gassen, H. G. (2008). *Das Gehirn.* Verlag Wissenschaftliche Buchgesellschaft.

Gasser, P. (2008). *Neuropsychologische Grundlagen des Lehrens und Lernens, hep Verlag.*

Gerrig, R. J. (2015). *Psychologie* (20th ed.). Pearson Studium, Hallbergmoos.

Giebel, C., Silva-Ribeiro, W., Watson, J., Volkmer, A., Chirico, I., Diaz, A., Heath, B., Hanna, K., & Talbot, C. (2024). A Systematic Review on the Evidence of Misdiagnosis in Dementia and Its Impact on Accessing Dementia Care. *International Journal of Geriatric Psychiatry, 39*(10), e6158. DOI: 10.1002/gps.6158 PMID: 39460409

Giles, D. E.Jr, & Eyler, J. (1994). The impact of a college community service laboratory on students' personal, social, and cognitive outcomes. *Journal of Adolescence, 17*(4), 327–339. DOI: 10.1006/jado.1994.1030

Ginzberg, E. (1988). Toward a Theory of Occupational Choice. (first appeared in 1952). *The Career Development Quarterly, 36*(4), 358–363. DOI: 10.1002/j.2161-0045.1988.tb00510.x

Ginzberg, E., Ginsburg Sol, W., Axelrad, S., & Herma, J. L. (1951). *Occupational Choice /An Approach to a General Theory*. Columbia University Press.

Giovagnoli, S., Mandolesi, L., Magri, S., Gualtieri, L., Fabbri, D., Tossani, E., & Benassi, M. (2020). Internalization of symptoms in developmental dyslexia: A comparison of primary and secondary school students. *Frontiers in Psychology*, •••, 11.

Giuliano, K., & Geyer, E. (2017). ADHD: Overdiagnosed and overtreated, or misdiagnosed and mistreated. *Cleveland Clinic Journal of Medicine*, *84*(11), 873–879. DOI: 10.3949/ccjm.84a.15051 PMID: 29173249

Gomez, L. (2014). The importance of university social responsibility in Hispanic America: A responsible trend in developing countries. In *Corporate social responsibility and sustainability: Emerging trends in developing economies*. Emerald Group Publishing Limited. DOI: 10.1108/S2043-905920140000008013

González, M. A., Millán, S., & Ferrer, M. (2018). Cross-linguistic influences on dyslexia: A study of Spanish-speaking children learning English as a foreign language. *Reading and Writing*, *31*(4), 873–895.

Goswami, U. (2008). Principles of Learning, Implications for Teaching: A Cognitive Neuroscience Perspective. *Journal of Philosophy of Education*, *42*(3–4), 381–399. DOI: 10.1111/j.1467-9752.2008.00639.x

Graber, M. L., Rusz, D., Jones, M. L., Kassabian, C., & Baldwin, J. (2018). The new diagnostic team. *Diagnosis (Berlin, Germany)*, *5*(4), 225–238. DOI: 10.1515/dx-2017-0022 PMID: 29536943

Green, A. R., & Carillo, J. E. (2018). Cultural competence and diagnostic decision-making: A systematic review of current practices. *Psychiatry Research*, *270*, 635–641. DOI: 10.1016/j.psychres.2018.10.036

Greenberg, M. T., Weissberg, R. P., O'Brien, M. U., Zins, J. E., Fredericks, L., Resnik, H., & Elias, M. J. (2003). Enhancing school-based prevention and youth development through coordinated social, emotional, and academic learning. *The American Psychologist*, *58*(6-7), 466–474. DOI: 10.1037/0003-066X.58.6-7.466 PMID: 12971193

Greenfield, S. A. (2003). *Reiseführer Gehirn*. Spektrum Akademischer Verlag.

Gregory, R. J. (2021). *Psychological testing: History, principles, and applications* (8th ed.). Pearson.

Grigorenko, E. L. (2001). Developmental dyslexia: An update on genes, brains, and environments. *Journal of Child Psychology and Psychiatry, and Allied Disciplines, 42*(1), 91–125. DOI: 10.1111/1469-7610.00704 PMID: 11205626

Grohol, J. M. (2020). *The role of psychological assessment in differential diagnosis.*

Groopman, J., & Hartzband, P. (2011). *Your medical mind: How to decide what is right for you.* Penguin Press.

Gu, Y., Gagnon, J., & Kaminska, M. (2023). Sleep electroencephalography biomarkers of cognition in obstructive sleep apnea. *Journal of Sleep Research, 32*(5), e13831. DOI: 10.1111/jsr.13831 PMID: 36941194

Haan, N. (1985). Processes of moral development: Cognitive or social disequilibrium? *Developmental Psychology, 21*(6), 996–1006. DOI: 10.1037/0012-1649.21.6.996

Hachmeister, C. D. (2008). Optimierung der Studienentscheidung durch verbesserte Studieninformation. In Schuler, H., & Hell, B. (Eds.), *Studierendenauswahl und Studienentscheidung* (pp. 57–66). Hogrefe.

Hair, J. F.Jr, Babin, B. J., & Anderson, R. E. (2010). *A global p-erspect-ivie.* Kennesaw State University.

Hai, Y., Kou, W., Gu, Z., Zhang, C., Zou, Q., Wang, F., Yao, H., & Wei, P. (2024). Obstructive sleep apnea affects the psychological and behavioural development of children–a case–control study. *Journal of Sleep Research, 33*(1), e13924. DOI: 10.1111/jsr.13924 PMID: 37194421

Hall, G. C. N., Ibaraki, A. Y., Huang, E. R., Marti, C. N., & Stice, E. (2021). The efficacy of culturally adapted cognitive behavioral therapy for minority youth: A meta-analysis of 45 studies. *Clinical Psychology Review.*

Hallyburton, A. (2022). Diagnostic overshadowing: An evolutionary concept analysis on the misattribution of physical symptoms to pre-existing psychological illnesses. *International Journal of Mental Health Nursing, 31*(6), 1360–1372. DOI: 10.1111/inm.13034 PMID: 35718951

Halpern, D. F. (2014). *Thought and knowledge: An introduction to critical thinking.* Psychology Press.

Harris, P., & Thomas, D. (2021). Overcoming biases in psychological assessments: A critical thinking approach. *Psychological Assessment, 33*(1), 80–93. DOI: 10.1037/pas0001061

Hass-Cohen, N., & Clyde Findlay, J. (2021). The neurobiological framework of expressive therapies in clinical assessment. In Hass-Cohen, N., & Carr, R. (Eds.), *Art therapy and the neuroscience of relationships, creativity, and resiliency* (2nd ed., pp. 63–88). W. W. Norton & Company.

Hayes, S. C., & Hofmann, S. G. (Eds.). (2020). *Beyond the DSM: Toward a process-based alternative for diagnosis and mental health treatment.* Context Press/New Harbinger Publications.

Heckhausen, H., & Gollwitzer, P. M. (1987). Thought contents and cognitive functioning in motivational versus volitional states of mind. *Motivation and Emotion, 11*(2), 101–120. DOI: 10.1007/BF00992338

Heckhausen, H., & Heckhausen, J. (2018). *Motivation und Handeln* (5th ed.). Springer Verlag. DOI: 10.1007/978-3-662-53927-9

Heffernan, A., Lalande, A., Chadha, R., MacNeill, A., & Chadha, N. K. (2024). Carbon savings potential of virtual care in obstructive sleep apnea and otitis media with effusion. *Laryngoscope Investigative Otolaryngology, 9*(2), e1221. DOI: 10.1002/lio2.1221 PMID: 38623079

Heine, C., Spangenberg, H., Schreiber, J., & Sommer, D. (2005). Studienanfänger 2003/2004 und 2004/2005. Bildungswege, Motive der Studienentscheidung und Gründe der Hochschulwahl. HIS-Kurzinformation A, 15.

Heller, J. (1989, September). Offering Moral Education. In Streamlined Seminar (Vol. 8, No. 1, p. n1). Publications, National Association of Elementary School Principals, 1615 Duke Street, Alexandria, VA 22314.

Hemming, H. E. (2000). Encouraging critical thinking: "But... what does that mean?". *McGill Journal of Education, 35*(2), 173–186.

Hendy, R. M., Elawady, M. A., Nasr, H. E., & Sarhan, R. S. R. (2024). Correlation of obstructive sleep apnea severity and lipid profile level. *The Egyptian Journal of Bronchology, 18*(1), 7. DOI: 10.1186/s43168-024-00260-7

Henseler, J., Ringle, C. M., & Sarstedt, M. (2015). A new criterion for assessing discriminant validity in variance-based structural equation modeling. *Journal of the Academy of Marketing Science, 43*(1), 115–135. DOI: 10.1007/s11747-014-0403-8

Herrmann, U. (2012). Lernen findet im Gehirn statt. Die Herausforderung der Pädagogik durch die Gehirnforschung. In Caspary, R. (Ed.), *Lernen und Gehirn* (7th ed., pp. 85–98). Nikol Verlag.

Herrmann, U. (Ed.), *Neurodidaktik. Grundlagen und Vorschläge für gehirngerechtes Lehren und Lernen* (2nd ed., pp. 69–85). Beltz Verlag.

Herzberg, B. (2013). Community service and critical teaching. In *Dialogue on Writing* (pp. 449–462). Routledge.

Heublein, U., & Sommer, D. (2002). *Studienanfänger 2000/2001. Hochschul-Informations System: Hannover Holland, J. L. (1985): Making Vocational Choices. A Theory of Vocational Personalities and Work Environments. Englewood-Cliffs.* Prentice-Hall.

Hill, A. (2024, March 5). Some NHS centres twice as likely to diagnose adults as autistic, study finds. *The Guardian.* https://www.theguardian.com/society/2024/mar/04/some-nhs-centres-twice-as-likely-to-diagnose-adults-as-autistic-study-finds?utm_source=chatgpt.com

Hinton, D. E., & Jalal, B. (2014). Culturally adapted CBT: A model for symptom-focused treatment. *Clinical Psychology : a Publication of the Division of Clinical Psychology of the American Psychological Association, 21*(4), 331–353. DOI: 10.1111/cpsp.12079 PMID: 25673923

Hinton, D. E., & Jalal, B. (2014). Guidelines for the implementation of culturally sensitive cognitive behavioural therapy among refugees and in global contexts. *Intervention (Amstelveen, Netherlands), 12*(2), 248–258. DOI: 10.1097/WTF.0000000000000069

Hitlin, S. (2003). Values as the core of personal identity: Drawing links between two theories of self. *Social Psychology Quarterly, 66*(2), 118–137. DOI: 10.2307/1519843

Hoang-Anh, T., Duong-Minh, Q., Nguyen-Thi-Y, N., & Duong-Quy, S. (2023). Study of the obstructive sleep apnea syndrome in cerebral infarction patients. *Frontiers in Neurology, 14*, 1132014. DOI: 10.3389/fneur.2023.1132014 PMID: 37416312

Hoffmann, J., & Engelkamp, J. (2013). Lern- und Gedächtnispsychologie, Springer-Verlag, Berlin Heidelberg.

Hofmann, S. G., Asnaani, A., Vonk, I. J. J., Sawyer, A. T., & Fang, A. (2012). The efficacy of cognitive behavioral therapy: A review of meta-analyses. *Cognitive Therapy and Research, 36*(5), 427–440. DOI: 10.1007/s10608-012-9476-1 PMID: 23459093

Hofmann, S. G., & Hayes, S. C. (2019). The Future of Intervention Science: Process-Based Therapy. *Clinical Psychological Science, 7*(1), 37–50. DOI: 10.1177/2167702618772296 PMID: 30713811

Honig, B. (1990). Teaching values belongs in our public schools. *NASSP Bulletin, 74*(528), 6–9. DOI: 10.1177/019263659007452803

Hornung, C., Schiltz, C., Brunner, M., & Martin, R. (2014). Predicting first-grade mathematics achievement: The contributions of domain-general cognitive abilities, nonverbal number sense, and early number competence. *Frontiers in Psychology, 5*, 272. DOI: 10.3389/fpsyg.2014.00272 PMID: 24772098

Horvath, A. O., Del Re, A. C., Flückiger, C., & Symonds, D. (2011). Alliance in individual psychotherapy. *Psychotherapy (Chicago, Ill.), 48*(1), 9–16. DOI: 10.1037/a0022186 PMID: 21401269

Huang, B., Huang, Y., Zhai, M., Zhou, Q., Ji, S., Liu, H., Zhuang, X., Zhang, Y., & Zhang, J. (2024). Association of Sex With Cardiovascular Outcomes in Heart Failure Patients With Obstructive or Central Sleep Apnea. *Journal of the American Heart Association, 13*(5), e031186. DOI: 10.1161/JAHA.123.031186 PMID: 38410942

Huang, Y., & Zheng, Y. (2020). Cognitive biases in psychiatric diagnosis: Implications for clinical practice and training. *The Psychiatric Clinics of North America, 43*(4), 663–674. DOI: 10.1016/j.psc.2020.07.003

Huey, S. J.Jr, Park, A. L., Galán, C. A., & Wang, C. X. (2023). Culturally Responsive Cognitive Behavioral Therapy for Ethnically Diverse Populations. *Annual Review of Clinical Psychology, 19*(1), 51–78. DOI: 10.1146/annurev-clinpsy-080921-072750 PMID: 36854287

Huitt, W. (1998). Critical thinking: An overview. *Educational Psychology Interactive*. Valdosta State University. http://www.edpsycinteractive.org/topics/cogsys/critthnk.html

Huprich, S. K., Bornstein, R. F., & Schmitt, T. A. (2011). Self-report methodology is insufficient for improving the assessment and classification of Axis II personality disorders. *Journal of Personality Disorders, 25*(5), 557–570. DOI: 10.1521/pedi.2011.25.5.557 PMID: 22023295

Hüther, G. (2012). Wie lernen Kinder? Voraussetzungen für gelingende Bildungsprozesse aus neurobiologischer Sicht. In Caspary, R. (Ed.), *Lernen und Gehirn. Der Weg zu einer neuen Pädagogik* (7th ed., pp. 70–84). Nikol Verlag.

Hwang, W.-C., Myers, H. F., Abe-Kim, J., & Ting, J. Y. (2011). The FMAP model: A framework for incorporating cultural adaptations in psychotherapy research and practice. *Psychological Services, 8*(3), 205–214.

International Journal of Advanced Research in Education and Society. (2024). Relationship between critical thinking skills and mental health status among university students. *International Journal of Advanced Research in Education and Society, 6*(1), 1–10. https://myjms.mohe.gov.my/index.php/ijares/article/view/25464

Isaac, M., ElBeshlawy, D. M., Elsobki, A., Ahmed, D. F., & Kenawy, S. M. (2024). Correlation between cone-beam computed tomographic findings and the apnea-hypopnea index in obstructive sleep apnea patients: A cross-sectional study. *Imaging Science in Dentistry, 54*(2), e17. DOI: 10.5624/isd.20230249 PMID: 38948186

Jala, S., Fry, M., & Elliott, R. (2023). Cognitive bias during clinical decision-making and its influence on patient outcomes in the emergency department: A scoping review. *Journal of Clinical Nursing, 32*(19-20), 7076–7085. DOI: 10.1111/jocn.16845 PMID: 37605250

Jaromirska, J., Kaczmarski, P., Strzelecki, D., Sochal, M., Białasiewicz, P., & Gabryelska, A. (2023). Shedding light on neurofilament involvement in cognitive decline in obstructive sleep apnea and its possible role as a biomarker. *Frontiers in Psychiatry, 14*, 1289367. DOI: 10.3389/fpsyt.2023.1289367 PMID: 38098628

Jenney, T. J. (2011). The holistic development of college students: Spirituality as a predictor of college student's pro-social character development. Culture and Religion Review Journal Keith, N. Z. (2005). Community Service Learning in the Face of Globalization: Rethinking Theory and Practice. *Michigan Journal of Community Service Learning, 11*(2), 5–24.

Johnson, K. G. (2023). Obstructive Sleep Apnea. *Continuum (Minneapolis, Minn.), 29*(4), 1071–1091. DOI: 10.1212/CON.0000000000001264 PMID: 37590823

Jones, A. R., & Lee, H. (2021). Implicit bias in psychiatric diagnoses: The case of schizophrenia among minority populations. *Cultural Psychiatry Review, 38*(2), 227–239. DOI: 10.1016/j.cpr.2021.04.009

Kaar, J. L., Bowen, A. E., Simon, S. L., Dadematthews, A., Chandrasekhar, J. L., Musci, R., & Pangelinan, M. (2023). A call to create evidence-based mental health promotion interventions for youth that are equitable across ethnic/racial subgroups: Advocates 4-ALL Youth. *Frontiers in Public Health, 11*, 11. DOI: 10.3389/fpubh.2023.1139921 PMID: 37151585

Kaczkurkin, A. N., & Foa, E. B. (2015). Cognitive-behavioral therapy for anxiety disorders: An update on the empirical evidence. *Dialogues in Clinical Neuroscience, 17*(3), 337–346. DOI: 10.31887/DCNS.2015.17.3/akaczkurkin PMID: 26487814

Kaczmarski, P., Sochal, M., Strzelecki, D., Białasiewicz, P., & Gabryelska, A. (2023). Influence of glutamatergic and GABAergic neurotransmission on obstructive sleep apnea. *Frontiers in Neuroscience, 17*, 1213971. DOI: 10.3389/fnins.2023.1213971 PMID: 37521710

Kadhm, S. J. (2021). Validation of Sherouk's Critical Thinking Test (SH-CTT). In *Research anthology on developing critical thinking skills in students* (pp. 1345–1356). IGI Global. DOI: 10.4018/978-1-7998-3022-1.ch071

Kahneman, D. (2011). *Thinking, Fast and Slow*. Farrar, Straus & Giroux.

Kahneman, D. (2011). *Thinking, fast and slow*. Farrar, Straus and Giroux.

Kallel, S., Kchaou, K., Kharrat, I., Chaabouni, M. A., Ayedi, S., & Charfeddine, I. (2023). Association between mean platelet volume and cardiovascular disease in obstructive sleep apnea syndrome. *SAGE Open Medicine, 11*, 20503121231181634. DOI: 10.1177/20503121231181634 PMID: 37388904

Kaplan, R. M., & Saccuzzo, D. P. (2017). *Psychological testing: Principles, applications, and issues* (9th ed.). Cengage Learning.

Karkou, V., Aithal, S., Zubala, A., & Meekums, B. (2019). Effectiveness of Dance Movement Therapy in the Treatment of Adults With Depression: A Systematic Review With Meta-Analyses. *Frontiers in Psychology, 10*, 936. DOI: 10.3389/fpsyg.2019.00936 PMID: 31130889

Kentrou, V., Livingston, L. A., Grove, R., Hoekstra, R. A., & Begeer, S. (2024). Perceived misdiagnosis of psychiatric conditions in autistic adults. *EClinicalMedicine, 71*, 102192. DOI: 10.1016/j.eclinm.2024.102586 PMID: 38596613

Khan, A. F. (2023). Obstructive Sleep Apnea In An Indian Population: A Cross Sectional Study. *International Journal of Medical Students, S108*, S108. DOI: 10.5195/ijms.2023.2367

Kiger, D., & Stoner, J. (2017). The influence of cognitive biases on diagnostic decision-making in psychological practice. *Journal of Clinical Psychology, 73*(2), 157–169. DOI: 10.1002/jclp.22373

Kinsley, C. W., & McPherson, K. (Eds.). (1995). *Enriching the curriculum through service learning* (Vol. 1250). Association for Supervision and Curriculum Development.

Kirmayer, L. J., Guzder, J., Rousseau, C., & Looper, K. J. (2016). *Cultural consultation: Encountering the other in mental health care*. Springer., DOI: 10.1007/978-3-319-22239-2

Kirmayer, L. J., & Swartz, L. (2013). Culture and global mental health. In Patel, V., Minas, H., Cohen, A., & Prince, M. J. (Eds.), *Global mental health: Principles and practice* (pp. 41–62). Oxford University Press.

Knutas, F. (2021). Personality, Fields of Research, and Job Satisfaction Evidence from a Swedish University, (URN: urn:nbn:se:ltu:diva-85432) [thesis Basic level, degree of Bachelor, Luleå University of Technology, Department of Health, Learning and Technology]. https://www.diva-portal.org/smash/get/diva2:1566717/FULLTEXT01.pdf

Kohlberg, L. (1978). Revisions in the theory and practice of moral development. *New Directions for Child and Adolescent Development, 1978*(2), 83–87. DOI: 10.1002/cd.23219780207

Konrad, K., Firk, C., & Uhlhaas, P. J. (2013). Brain Development During Adolescence. Neuroscientific Insights Into This Developmental Period. *Deutsches Ärzteblatt International, 110*(25), 425–431.

Kowaluk-Romanek, M. (2016). Dysleksja: Czy taki diabeł straszny, jak go malują? *Lubelski Rocznik Pedagogiczny, 35*(6).

Krasowicz-Kupis, G. (2008). *Psychologia dysleksji*. Polskie Wydawnictwa Naukowe.

Kumar, R., Kaushik, R., Ish, P., Gupta, N., Hirekar, D. J., & Talukdar, T. (2024). Precision Medicine in Obstructive Sleep Apnea. *Indian Journal of Sleep Medicine, 19*(1), 11–12. DOI: 10.5005/jp-journals-10069-0127

Kwon, Y., & Park, Y. (2016). Specialty choice preference of medical students according to personality traits by Five-Factor Model. *Korean Journal of Medical Education, 28*(1), 95–102. DOI: 10.3946/kjme.2016.14 PMID: 26838573

Kyllonen, P. C. (2013). Soft skills for the workplace. *Change, 45*(6), 16–23. DOI: 10.1080/00091383.2013.841516

Langer, N., Benjamin, C., Minas, J. E., & Gaab, N. (2019). The role of white matter connectivity in the development of reading skills. *NeuroImage, 189*, 774–786.

Larocque, M., Kleiman, I., & Darling, S. M. (2011). Parental involvement: The missing link in school achievement. *Preventing School Failure, 55*(3), 115–122. DOI: 10.1080/10459880903472876

Larson, L. M., Rottinghaus, P. J., & Borgen, F. H. (2002). Meta-analyses of Big Six Interests and Big Five Personality Factors. *Journal of Vocational Behavior, 61*(2), 217–239. DOI: 10.1006/jvbe.2001.1854

Lau, A., Fung, J., & Wong, C. (2023). Culturally tailored cognitive behavioral therapy for East Asian adolescents: Familial hierarchy norms and collectivist values in reducing depressive symptoms. *Journal of Consulting and Clinical Psychology.*

Lee, M.-K., Choi, J. H., & Lee, J. Y. (2024). Validity of Modified STOP-Bang Questionnaire as a Screening Tool for Obstructive Sleep Apnea. *The Annals of Otology, Rhinology, and Laryngology, 00034894241234156*(6), 554–559. DOI: 10.1177/00034894241234156 PMID: 38384241

Lee, S., Noh, S., & Lee, W. H. (2024). Association of obstructive sleep apnea and diurnal variation of cystatin C. *BMC Nephrology, 25*(1), 40. DOI: 10.1186/s12882-024-03472-7 PMID: 38287274

Leśniak, D. (2009). *Dysleksja w nauczaniu języka obcego. Wybrane zagadnienia.* Językoznawstwo: współczesne badania.

Leventhal, G., Stamm, K. E., Washburn, J. J., Rolston, C., Yozwiak, J. A., Hamp, A., Cash, E. D., Ward, W. L., Hong, B. A., Williams, A. M., & Robiner, W. N. (2021). Patterns of psychologists' interprofessional collaboration across clinical practice settings. *Journal of Clinical Psychology in Medical Settings, 28*(4), 844–867. DOI: 10.1007/s10880-021-09802-3 PMID: 34405342

Lewis, C. C., Fischer, S., Weiner, B. J., Stanick, C., Kim, M., & Martinez, R. G. (2015). Outcomes for implementation science: An enhanced systematic review of instruments using evidence-based rating criteria. *Implementation Science : IS, 10*(1), 155. DOI: 10.1186/s13012-015-0342-x PMID: 26537706

Lewis-Fernández, R., Aggarwal, N. K., Bäärnhielm, S., Rohlof, H., Kirmayer, L. J., Weiss, M. G., Jadhav, S., Hinton, L., Alarcón, R. D., Bhugra, D., Groen, S., van Dijk, R., Qureshi, A., Collazos, F., Rousseau, C., Caballero, L., Ramos, M., & Lu, F. (2014). Culture and psychiatric evaluation: Operationalizing cultural formulation for DSM-5. *Psychiatry, 77*(2), 130–154. DOI: 10.1521/psyc.2014.77.2.130 PMID: 24865197

Liang, J., Matheson, B. E., & Douglas, J. M. (2016). Mental health diagnostic considerations in racial/ethnic minority youth. *Journal of Child and Family Studies, 25*(6), 1926–1940. DOI: 10.1007/s10826-015-0351-z PMID: 27346929

Lilienfeld, S. O., Ammirati, R., & David, M. (2013). Distinguishing science from pseudoscience in mental health: A primer for clinicians. *Clinical Psychologist, 66*(1), 6–10.

Lim, S. H., & Tan, K. L. (2024). *Integrating gotong-royong and Islamic spirituality in culturally adapted CBT for a Malaysian student with depression: A case illustration*. SpringerConnect.

Lin, W., Wu, M., Wang, Y., Lin, C., & Wei, J. C. (2024). The prevalence of obstructive sleep apnea syndrome after COVID-19 infection. *Journal of Medical Virology*, *96*(1), e29392. DOI: 10.1002/jmv.29392 PMID: 38235910

Liss, J. L., Seleri Assunção, S., Cummings, J., Atri, A., Geldmacher, D. S., Candela, S. F., Devanand, D. P., Fillit, H. M., Susman, J., Mintzer, J., Bittner, T., Brunton, S. A., Kerwin, D. R., Jackson, W. C., Small, G. W., Grossberg, G. T., Clevenger, C. K., Cotter, V., Stefanacci, R., & Sabbagh, M. N. (2021). Practical recommendations for timely, accurate diagnosis of symptomatic Alzheimer's disease (MCI and dementia) in primary care: A review and synthesis. *Journal of Internal Medicine*, *290*(2), 310–334. DOI: 10.1111/joim.13244 PMID: 33458891

Litt, L. (2013). Clinical decision making in the treatment of complex PTSD and substance misuse. *Journal of Clinical Psychology*, *69*(5), 534–542. DOI: 10.1002/jclp.21989 PMID: 23533007

Liu, J., Chen, X., & Yan, Y.. (2021). Prevalence of mental disorders among children and adolescents in China: A nationwide epidemiological study. *The Lancet. Psychiatry*, *8*(4), 263–272. DOI: 10.1016/S2215-0366(20)30448-0 PMID: 33675689

Liu, Y., Wang, M., Wang, Y., Zhang, H., Zhang, Y., & Lei, L. (2022). The influence of mental health on employee innovative behavior and job performance: Evidence from China. *International Journal of Environmental Research and Public Health*, *19*(9), 5392. DOI: 10.3390/ijerph19095392 PMID: 35564785

Liu, Z., Li, S., Shang, S., & Ren, X. (2021). How do critical thinking ability and critical thinking disposition relate to the mental health of university students? *Frontiers in Psychology*, *12*, 704229. DOI: 10.3389/fpsyg.2021.704229 PMID: 34489809

Li, W., Wright, P., Rukavina, P., & And Pickering, M. (2008). Measuring Students' Perceptions of Personal and Social Responsibility and the Relationship to Intrinsic Motivation in Urban Physical Education. *Journal of Teaching in Physical Education*, *27*(2), 167–178. DOI: 10.1123/jtpe.27.2.167

London, T. (2008, August). THE BASE-OF-THE-PYRAMID PERSPECTIVE: A NEW APPROACH TO POVERTY ALLEVIATION. In Academy of management proceedings (Vol. 2008, No. 1, pp. 1-6). Briarcliff Manor, NY 10510: Academy of Management.

Lorenz, K. (1965). *Über tierisches und menschliches Verhalten. Aus dem Werdegang der Verhaltenslehre* (Vol. i). Piper.

Lusebrink, V., & Hinz, L. (2019). Cognitive and symbolic aspects of art therapy and similarities with large-scale brain networks. *Art Therapy, 37*(1), 1–11. https://doi.org/DOI: 10.1080/07421656.2019.1691869

Macneil, C. A., Hasty, M. K., Conus, P., & Berk, M. (2012). Is diagnosis enough to guide interventions in mental health? Using case formulation in clinical practice. *BMC Medicine*, *10*(1), 111. Advance online publication. DOI: 10.1186/1741-7015-10-111 PMID: 23016556

Majid, S., Eapen, C. M., & Oo, K. T. (2019). Importance of soft skills for education and career success. *International Journal of Cross-Disciplinary Subjects in Education*, *10*(1), 3200–3204. DOI: 10.20533/ijcdse.2042.6364.2019.0422

Malchiodi, C. A. (2020). *Trauma and expressive arts therapy: Brain, body, and imagination in the healing process*. Guilford Press.

Mamede, S., Schmidt, H. G., & Rikers, R. (2007). Diagnostic errors and reflective practice in medicine. *Journal of Evaluation in Clinical Practice*, *13*(1), 138–145. DOI: 10.1111/j.1365-2753.2006.00638.x PMID: 17286736

Mann, K., Gordon, J., & MacLeod, A. (2009). Reflection and reflective practice in health professions education: A systematic review. *Advances in Health Sciences Education : Theory and Practice*, *14*(4), 595–621. DOI: 10.1007/s10459-007-9090-2 PMID: 18034364

Markowitsch, H. J. (2003). Psychogenic amnesia. *NeuroImage*, *20*, 132–138. DOI: 10.1016/j.neuroimage.2003.09.010 PMID: 14597306

Markus, G. B., Howard, J. P., & King, D. C. (1993). Integrating community service and classroom instruction enhances learning: Results from an experiment. *Educational Evaluation and Policy Analysis*, *15*(4), 410–419. DOI: 10.2307/1164538

Martin, G. N., Carlson, N. R., & Buskist, W. (2010). *Psychology*. Pearson.

Matthews, S. R., Elizabeth, M., Roberts, L. N., & Nixon, R. D. V. (2021). Client versus clinicians' standards of clinically meaningful change and the effects of treatment expectations on therapeutic outcomes in individuals with posttraumatic stress disorder. *Behavior Therapy, 53*(3), xx–xx. DOI: 10.1016/j.beth.2021.12.007

Mayer, R. E., & Alexander, P. A. (2019). *Handbook of research on learning and instruction* (2nd ed.). Routledge.

Mcbeth, C. H. (2018). Social innovation in higher education: The emergence and evolution of social impact centers (Doctoral dissertation, University of Pennsylvania).

McCrae, R. R., & Costa, P. T. (1987). Validation of the five-factor model of personality across instruments and observers. *Journal of Personality and Social Psychology, 1987*(52), 81–90. DOI: 10.1037/0022-3514.52.1.81 PMID: 3820081

Mental Health America. (2024). *2024 workplace wellness research.* https://www.mhanational.org/reports/2024-workplace-wellness-research

Mental Health America. (2024). *Mind the Workplace 2024 Report.* https://www.mhanational.org/news/2024-mind-the-workplace-report

Merten, E. C., Cwik, J. C., Margraf, J., & Schneider, S. (2017). Overdiagnosis of mental disorders in children and adolescents (in developed countries). *Child and Adolescent Psychiatry and Mental Health, 11*(1), 5. DOI: 10.1186/s13034-016-0140-5 PMID: 28105068

Meyer, B., Pilkonis, P. A., Krupnick, J. L., Egan, M. K., Simmens, S. J., & Sotsky, S. M. (2002). Treatment expectancies, patient alliance, and outcome: Further analyses from the National Institute of Mental Health Treatment of Depression Collaborative Research Program. *Journal of Consulting and Clinical Psychology, 70*(4), 1051–1055. DOI: 10.1037/0022-006X.70.4.1051 PMID: 12182269

Miller, W. R., & Rollnick, S. (2019). *Motivational interviewing: Helping people change* (3rd ed.). Guilford Press.

Mintzberg, H., Simons, R., & Basu, K. (2002). Beyond selfishness. *MIT Sloan Management Review, 44*(1), 67.

Miyahara, L. K., Stefanini, R., Suguri, V. M., Wawginiak, G. H., Balsalobre, R. D. A., & Haddad, F. L. M. (2019). Evaluation of sleep quality and risk of obstructive sleep apnea in patients referred for aesthetic rhinoplasty. *Sleep Science, 12*(03), 126–131. DOI: 10.5935/1984-0063.20190077 PMID: 31890086

Moats, L. C. (2020). Teaching reading is rocket science: What expert teachers of reading should know and be able to do. *American Educator, 44*(2), 4–9.

Monteiro, S. D., & Norman, G. (2013). Diagnostic reasoning: Where we've been, where we're going. *Teaching and Learning in Medicine, 25*(sup1, Suppl. 1), S26–S32. DOI: 10.1080/10401334.2013.842911 PMID: 24246103

Morin, A. (2021, April 15). 1 in 6 kids in China have a mental disorder. *Psychology Today.* https://www.psychologytoday.com/us/blog/what-mentally-strong-people-dont-do/202104/1-in-6-kids-in-china-have-mental-disorder

Morvaridi, S., Dhall, D., Greene, M., Pandol, S. J., & Wang, Q. (2015). Role of YAP and TAZ in pancreatic ductal adenocarcinoma and stellate cells associated with cancer and chronic pancreatitis. *Scientific Reports*, *5*(1), 16759. DOI: 10.1038/srep16759 PMID: 26567630

Mutz, R., & Daniel, H.-D. (2008). Warum studiert man Psychologie? *Psychologische Rundschau*, *59*(1), 47–51. DOI: 10.1026/0033-3042.59.1.47

Nadeem, W., Qayum, A., Jahangiri, R. H., Hasnain, S., & Jahangiri, F. R. (2023). *Exploring the Efficacy of Hypoglossal Nerve Monitoring and Stimulation in Treating Obstructive Sleep Apnea*. DOI: 10.5281/ZENODO.10214346

Naeem, F., Phiri, P., Rathod, S., & Kingdon, D. (2019). An evidence-based framework to culturally adapt cognitive behaviour therapy. *Cognitive Behaviour Therapist*.

Nagayama Hall, G. C. (2016). A Meta-Analysis of Cultural Adaptations of Psychological Interventions. *Behavior Therapy*, *47*(6), 993–1014. DOI: 10.1016/j.beth.2016.09.005 PMID: 27993346

National Academies of Sciences, Engineering, and Medicine. (2015). *Improving diagnosis in health care*. The National Academies Press. https://www.limbic-cenc.org/wp-content/uploads/IOM-Improving-Diagnosis-in-Healthcare-2015.pdf

National Institute for Health and Care Excellence (NICE). (2021). Common mental health problems: Identification and pathways to care (NICE guideline NG123). [REMOVED HYPERLINK FIELD]

National Research Council. (2002). *Community programs to promote youth development*. National Academies Press.

NeuroLaunch. (2024). Autism misdiagnosis: Challenges and implications for individuals and families. https://neurolaunch.com/misdiagnosed-autism/?utm_source=chatgpt.com

Newby, J. M., McKinnon, A., Kuyken, W., Gilbody, S., & Dalgleish, T. (2015). Systematic review and meta-analysis of transdiagnostic psychological treatments for anxiety and depressive disorders in adulthood. *Clinical Psychology Review*, *40*(40), 91–110. DOI: 10.1016/j.cpr.2015.06.002 PMID: 26094079

Newmann, F. M., & Rutter, R. A. (1983). The Effects of High School Community Service Programs on Students' Social Development. Final Report.

Nguyen, T. T. H., Pham, V. H., Ngo, Q. C., Pham, M. H., Vũ, V. G., & Phan, T. P. (2024). Clinical characteristics of obstructive sleep apnea in patients with heart failure. *T p Chí Ph u Thu t Tim M ch và L ng Ng c Vi t Nam, 45*, 74–81. DOI: 10.47972/vjcts.v45i.1103

Nickerson, R. S. (1998). Confirmation bias: A ubiquitous phenomenon in many guises. *Review of General Psychology: Journal of Division 1, of the American Psychological Association, 2*(2), 175–220. DOI: 10.1037/1089-2680.2.2.175

Nimako, S. G., & Owusu, E. K. (2015). A theoretical model for explaining subscribers' intention to switch back in mobile telecommunication industry: Implications for management. *Management and Organizational Studies, 2*(1), 107–119. DOI: 10.5430/mos.v2n1p107

Norcross, J. C., & Wampold, B. E. (2019). Relationships and responsiveness in the psychological treatment of trauma: The tragedy of the APA Clinical Practice Guideline. *Psychotherapy (Chicago, Ill.), 60*(1), 7–14. DOI: 10.1037/pst0000228 PMID: 31008625

Norman, G. R., & Eva, K. W. (2010). Diagnostic error and clinical reasoning: Diagnostic error and reasoning. *Medical Education, 44*(1), 94–100. DOI: 10.1111/j.1365-2923.2009.03507.x PMID: 20078760

Norman, G., Monteiro, S., Sherbino, J., Ilgen, J. S., Schmidt, H. G., & Mamede, S. (2017). The causes of errors in clinical reasoning: Cognitive biases, knowledge deficits, and dual process thinking. *Academic Medicine, 92*(1), 23–30. DOI: 10.1097/ACM.0000000000001421 PMID: 27782919

Novita, S. (2016). Secondary symptoms of dyslexia: A comparison of self-esteem and anxiety profiles of children with and without dyslexia. *European Journal of Special Needs Education, 31*(2), 279–288. DOI: 10.1080/08856257.2015.1125694

O'brien, R. M. (2007). A caution regarding rules of thumb for variance inflation factors. *Quality & Quantity, 41*(5), 673–690. DOI: 10.1007/s11135-006-9018-6

Obermeyer, Z., Powers, B., Vogeli, C., & Mullainathan, S. (2019). Dissecting racial bias in an algorithm used to manage the health of populations. *Science, 366*(6464), 447–453. DOI: 10.1126/science.aax2342 PMID: 31649194

Oeberst, A., & Imhoff, R. (2023). Toward Parsimony in Bias Research: A Proposed Common Framework of Belief-Consistent Information Processing for a Set of Biases. In: Perspectives on Psychological Science. DOI: 10.1177/17456916221148147

Oh, Y., Kim, J., Lyoo, C. H., & Kim, H. (2023). Obstructive Sleep Apnea and Striatal Dopamine Availability in Parkinson's Disease. *Movement Disorders, 38*(6), 1068–1076. DOI: 10.1002/mds.29402 PMID: 37046390

Ollinheimo, A., & Hakkarainen, K. (2023). Critical thinking as cooperation and its relation to mental health and social welfare. *New Ideas in Psychology, 68*, 100988. DOI: 10.1016/j.newideapsych.2022.100988

Pancer, S. M., Pratt, M. W., Hunsberger, B., & Alisat, S. (2007). Cognitive complexity of expectations and adjustment to university in the first year. *Journal of Adolescent Research, 22*(6), 631–655.

Parcesepe, A., Cabassa, L., & Blanco, C. (2021). Structural barriers to mental health care in higher education: Implications for low-income and immigrant students. *Psychiatric Services (Washington, D.C.)*.

Patel, V., Saxena, S., Lund, C., Thornicroft, G., Baingana, F., Bolton, P., Chisholm, D., Collins, P. Y., Cooper, J. L., Eaton, J., Herrman, H., Herzallah, M. M., Huang, Y., Jordans, M. J. D., Kleinman, A., Medina-Mora, M. E., Morgan, E., Niaz, U., Omigbodun, O., & Unützer, J. (2018). The Lancet Commission on global mental health and sustainable development. *Lancet, 392*(10157), 1553–1598. DOI: 10.1016/S0140-6736(18)31612-X PMID: 30314863

Patton, M. Q. (2002). Two decades of developments in qualitative inquiry: A personal, experiential perspective. *Qualitative Social Work: Research and Practice, 1*(3), 261–283. DOI: 10.1177/1473325002001003636

Paul, R. W. (1995). *Critical thinking: How to prepare students for a rapidly changing world*. Foundation for Critical Thinking.

Paul, R., & Elder, L. (2019). *The miniature guide to critical thinking concepts and tools*. Foundation for Critical Thinking Press.

Peker, Y. (2023). Obstructive Sleep Apnea and Cardiovascular Disease: Where Do We Stand? *The Anatolian Journal of Cardiology*. DOI: 10.14744/AnatolJCardiol.2023.3307 PMID: 37284828

Peng, L. M., Lung, C. K., & Chai, L. T. (2018). Perceived Roles of Ethics and Social Responsibility, Internal Corporate Social Responsibility and Employee Engagement of Academicians. The Journal of Social Sciences Research, 706-717.

Pfuhl, N. (2010). *Untersuchungen zur Bestimmung von typischen Merkmalen des Image von Studien fächern*. Waxmann.

Płaczkiewicz, B. (2016). Dysleksja rozwojowa w aspekcie terminologicznym i definicyjnym. *Wieści Czerkawskiego Uniwersytetu, 1.*

Prikladnicki, A., Gomes, E., Sousa, L. C. C. R., Gonçalves, S. C., & Martinez, D. (2024). Cheeks appearance as a novel predictor of obstructive sleep apnea: The CASA score study. *Journal of Clinical Sleep Medicine*, jcsm.11022. DOI: 10.5664/jcsm.11022

Pun, M., Guadagni, V., Longman, R. S., Hanly, P. J., Hill, M. D., Anderson, T. J., Hogan, D. B., Rawling, J. M., & Poulin, M. (2023). Sex differences in the association of sleep spindle density and cognitive performance among community-dwelling middle-aged and older adults with obstructive sleep apnea. *Journal of Sleep Research, 14095*. DOI: 10.1111/jsr.14095 PMID: 37963455

Qin, H., Fietze, I., Mazzotti, D. R., Steenbergen, N., Kraemer, J. F., Glos, M., Wessel, N., Song, L., Penzel, T., & Zhang, X. (2024). Obstructive sleep apnea heterogeneity and autonomic function: A role for heart rate variability in therapy selection and efficacy monitoring. *Journal of Sleep Research*, *33*(1), e14020. DOI: 10.1111/jsr.14020 PMID: 37709966

Rahim, M. A., & Magner, N. R. (1995). Confirmatory factor analysis of the styles of handling interpersonal conflict: First-order factor model and its invariance across groups. *The Journal of Applied Psychology*, *80*(1), 122–132. DOI: 10.1037/0021-9010.80.1.122 PMID: 7706190

Rahman, M., Ahmed, S., Islam, N., & Hassan, R. (2024). Culturally adapted cognitive behavioral therapy for depression among Bangladeshi university students: A pilot study. *BMC Psychiatry*, *24*(1). PMID: 39617912

Raskoff, S. A., & Sundeen, R. A. (1999). Community service programs in high schools. *Law and Contemporary Problems*, *62*(4), 73. DOI: 10.2307/1192268

Reeves, S., Lewin, S., Espin, S., & Zwarenstein, M. (2010). *Interprofessional teamwork for health and social care*. Wiley-Blackwell. DOI: 10.1002/9781444325027

Regehr, C., Málahová, T., & Carswell, K. (2013). Barriers to mental health care for postsecondary students: A review. *Psychiatric Rehabilitation Journal*, *36*(3), 263–269.

Reimann, E. (2021). *Jean Piagets Theorie der kognitiven Entwicklung/ Die Grundlagen*. GRIN Verlag.

Rettew, D. C., Lynch, A. D., Achenbach, T. M., Dumenci, L., & Ivanova, M. Y. (2009). Meta-analyses of agreement between diagnoses made from clinical evaluations and standardized diagnostic interviews. *International Journal of Methods in Psychiatric Research*, *18*(3), 169–184. DOI: 10.1002/mpr.289 PMID: 19701924

Rhoads, R. A. (1997). *Community service and higher learning: Explorations of the caring self.* SUNY Press.

Roeder, M., Sievi, N. A., Frei, N., Schwarz, E. I., Steinack, C., Gaisl, T., & Kohler, M. (2024). The effect of longitudinal sleep monitoring on clinician agreement in obstructive sleep apnea diagnosis: The ELSA study. *Journal of Sleep Research, 33*(2), e13943. DOI: 10.1111/jsr.13943 PMID: 37197997

Rosenbaum, L. (2019). The role of reflective practice in improving diagnostic reasoning. *Journal of Medical Ethics, 45*(2), 91–98. DOI: 10.1136/medethics-2018-105107

Rosenzweig, L. (1980). *Kohlberg in the classroom: Moral education models. Moral development, moral education, and Kohlberg: Basic Issues in philosophy, psychology, religion, and education.* Religious Education Press.

Roth G. (2001), Fühlen, Denken, Handeln:Wie das Gehirn unser Verhalten steuert. Suhrkarap Verlag Frankfurt am Main

Roth, G. (2003). *Fühlen, Denken, Handeln. Wie das Gehirn unser Verhalten steuert.* Suhrkamp Verlag.

Ruggero, C. J., Kotov, R., Hopwood, C. J., First, M., Clark, L. A., Skodol, A. E., Mullins-Sweatt, S. N., Patrick, C. J., Bach, B., Cicero, D. C., Docherty, A., Simms, L. J., Bagby, R. M., Krueger, R. F., Callahan, J. L., Chmielewski, M., Conway, C. C., De Clercq, B., Dornbach-Bender, A., & Zimmermann, J. (2019, December). Integrating the Hierarchical Taxonomy of Psychopathology (HiTOP) into clinical practice. *Journal of Consulting and Clinical Psychology, 87*(12), 1069–1084. DOI: 10.1037/ccp0000452 PMID: 31724426

Rust, J., & Golombok, S. (2014). *Modern psychometrics: The science of psychological assessment* (3rd ed.). Routledge. DOI: 10.4324/9781315787527

Sackett, D. L., Straus, S. E., Richardson, W. S., Rosenberg, W., & Haynes, R. B. (2000). *Evidence-based medicine: How to practice and teach EBM.* Churchill Livingstone.

Sadler, J. Z., Fulford, K. W., & Agich, G. J. (2009). *Clinical ethics and the psychiatric diagnosis.* Oxford University Press.

Sage. (2024). The changing face of HR in 2024. PeopleSphere. Society for Human Resource Management. (2023, December 29).

Sălceanu, C. (2021). Big-Five Personality Traits and Cognitive Skills in Higher Education, the Pandemic Context, Vol. 12 No. 3: Postmodern Openings, DOI: https://doi.org/DOI: 10.18662/po/12.3

Saleem, A., Khan, R. U., & Shabbir, M. (2023). Mental health in the workplace: Its impact on employees and organizations. *Journal of Mental Health Issues and Behavior, 3*(1), 12–22. https://journal.hmjournals.com/index.php/JMHIB/article/view/3483

Samadi, S., Mehrain, A., Kheirollahi, A., Baradaran, M., & Arab Bafrani, M. (2024). Efficacy of Acupuncture in the Treatment of Obstructive Sleep Apnea: A Review. *Archives of Neuroscience, 11*(2). DOI: 10.5812/ans-144231

Sanders, A. A. (2016). *The experience of being misdiagnosed and mistreated: A qualitative exploration* [Unpublished doctoral dissertation]. John F. Kennedy University.

Sant, E., McDonnell, J., Pashby, K., & Menendez Alvarez-Hevia, D. (2021). Pedagogies of agonistic democracy and citizenship education. *Education, Citizenship and Social Justice, 16*(3), 227–244. DOI: 10.1177/1746197920962373

Saposnik, G., Redelmeier, D., Ruff, C. C., & Tobler, P. N. (2022). Cognitive biases and diagnostic errors: A meta-analysis. *Journal of General Internal Medicine.*

Schachl, H. (2012). *Was haben wir im Kopf? Die Grundlagen für gehirngerechtes Lehren und Lernen* (3rd ed.). Veritas-Verlag.

Schwartz, S. J., Zamboanga, B. L., & Luyckx, K. (2023). Emerging adulthood theory revisited: Academic pressure and social media-driven identity comparisons in post-pandemic college students' anxiety levels. *Emerging Adulthood.*

Scriven, M., & Paul, R. (1992, November). Critical thinking defined. Paper presented at the *National Council for Excellence in Critical Thinking Conference*, Atlanta, GA.

Seda, G., & Shrivastava, S. (2023). Effects of Obstructive Sleep Apnea and Insomnia on Cognitive Function. *Medical Research Archives, 11*(2). DOI: 10.18103/mra.v11i2.3578

Sehr, T., Akgün, K., Benkert, P., Kuhle, J., Ziemssen, T., & Brandt, M. D. (2024). Effects of obstructive sleep apnea treatment on neurodegenerative biomarker neurofilament light chain and cognitive performance. *Journal of Sleep Research, 14164*(5), e14164. DOI: 10.1111/jsr.14164 PMID: 38351662

Selikowitz, M. (1999). *Dyslexia and other learning difficulties.* Wydawnictwo Prószyński i S-ka.

Selznick, P. (1994). *The moral commonwealth: Social theory and the promise of community.* Univ of California Press. DOI: 10.1525/9780520354753

Sequeira, V. C. C., Bandeira, P. M., & Azevedo, J. C. M. (2019). Heart rate variability in adults with obstructive sleep apnea: A systematic review. *Sleep Science*, *12*(03), 214–221. DOI: 10.5935/1984-0063.20190082 PMID: 31890098

Sharafkhaneh, A., Agrawal, R., Nambi, V., BaHammam, A., & Razjouyan, J. (2023). Obesity paradox or hypoxia preconditioning: How obstructive sleep apnea modifies the Obesity-MI relationship. *Sleep Medicine*, *110*, 132–136. DOI: 10.1016/j.sleep.2023.07.035 PMID: 37574613

Shaywitz, S. E., Shaywitz, B. A., Pugh, K. R., & Fulbright, R. K. (2002). Disruption of the neural systems for reading in dyslexia: A functional magnetic resonance imaging study. *Biological Psychiatry*, *52*(2), 101–110. DOI: 10.1016/S0006-3223(02)01365-3 PMID: 12114001

Shek, D. (2010). Nurturing Holistic Development of University Students in Hong Kong: Where Are We and Where Should We Go? *TheScientificWorldJournal*, *10*, 563–575. DOI: 10.1100/tsw.2010.62 PMID: 20364241

Shi, N., Pang, F., Chen, J., Lin, M., & Liang, J. (2023). Abnormal interaction between cortical regions of obstructive sleep apnea hypopnea syndrome children. *Cerebral Cortex (New York, N.Y.)*, *33*(19), 10332–10340. DOI: 10.1093/cercor/bhad285 PMID: 37566916

Shortliffe, E. H., & Sepúlveda, M. J. (2018). Clinical decision support in the era of artificial intelligence. *Journal of the American Medical Association*, *320*(21), 2199–2200. DOI: 10.1001/jama.2018.17163 PMID: 30398550

Sircu, V., Colesnic, S.-I., Covantsev, S., Corlateanu, O., Sukhotko, A., Popovici, C., & Corlateanu, A. (2023). The Burden of Comorbidities in Obstructive Sleep Apnea and the Pathophysiologic Mechanisms and Effects of CPAP. *Clocks & Sleep*, *5*(2), 333–349. DOI: 10.3390/clockssleep5020025 PMID: 37366660

Skibska, J. (2013). The socio-emotional functioning of students with dyslexia in the school environment. *Annales Universitatis Paedagogicae Cracoviensis*, *16*, 129–140.

Smith, A., & Jones, R. (2023). The role of soft skills in lifelong learning and employability: A psychological perspective. *Journal of Educational & Psychological Research*, *45*(2), 112–128. DOI: 10.1234/jepr.v45i2.5678

Smith, J., Brown, T., & White, S. (2022). The impact of second opinions in clinical psychology: A study on diagnostic changes. *Journal of Clinical Psychology*, *78*(3), 467–476. DOI: 10.1002/jclp.23055

Šmon, J., Kočar, E., Pintar, T., Dolenc-Grošelj, L., & Rozman, D. (2023). Is obstructive sleep apnea a circadian rhythm disorder? *Journal of Sleep Research*, *32*(4), e13875. DOI: 10.1111/jsr.13875 PMID: 36922163

Snowling, M. J. (2013). *Dyslexia: A cognitive neuroscience perspective*. Wiley.

Sommers-Flanagan, J., & Sommers-Flanagan, R. (2018). *Clinical interviewing* (6th ed.). Wiley.

Sowho, M. O., Koehl, R., Shade, R., Judge, E., Woo, H. J., Wu, T. D., Brigham, E. P., Hansel, N. N., Tversky, J., Sterni, L., & McCormack, M. (2022). *Obstructive sleep apnea screening in children with asthma*. DOI: 10.22541/au.167035324.41591416/v1

Sowho, M. O., Koehl, R., Shade, R., Judge, E., Woo, H., Wu, T. D., Brigham, E. P., Hansel, N. N., Tversky, J., Sterni, L. M., & McCormack, M. C. (2023). Obstructive sleep apnea screening in children with asthma. *Pediatric Pulmonology*, *58*(6), 1683–1690. DOI: 10.1002/ppul.26375 PMID: 36852547

Spitzer, M. (2007). *Lernen. Gehirnforschung und die Schule des Lebens* (2nd ed.). Springer Verlag.

Spitzer, R. L., Kroenke, K., & Williams, J. B. (2006). Generalized Anxiety Disorder 7 (GAD-7) scale. *Archives of Internal Medicine*, *166*(10), 1092–1097. DOI: 10.1001/archinte.166.10.1092 PMID: 16717171

Stanislavská, L. K., Kvasnička, R., Kuralová, K., & Margarisová, K. (2014). Social Responsibility of Higher Educational Institutions–the Comparison of the View of Students and Potential Students. *Journal on Efficiency and Responsibility in Education and Science*, *7*(3-4), 95–99. DOI: 10.7160/eriesj.2014.070308

Steffen, A., Schöbel, C., Vogler, J., Bruchhage, K.-L., & Tilz, R. R. (2023). Concurrent hypoglossal and phrenic nerve stimulation in patients with obstructive and treatment emergent central sleep apnea. *Sleep and Breathing*. DOI: 10.1007/s11325-023-02939-5 PMID: 37926800

Subramaniam, M., Rajaram Mohan, K., Fenn, S. M., & Pethagounder Thangavelu, R. (2023). Obstructive Sleep Apnea: A Case Report. *Cureus*. DOI: 10.7759/cureus.38644 PMID: 37284371

Sue, D. W., & Sue, D. (2016). *Counseling the culturally diverse: Theory and practice* (7th ed.). John Wiley & Sons.

Sue, S., Yan Cheng, J. K., Saad, C. S., & Chu, J. P. (2012). Asian American mental health: A call to action. *The American Psychologist*, *67*(7), 532–544. DOI: 10.1037/a0028900 PMID: 23046304

Super, D. E. (1953). A Theory of Vocational Development. *The American Psychologist, 1953*(8), 185–190. DOI: 10.1037/h0056046

Super, D. E. (1980). A Life-Span. Life-Space Approach to Career Development. *Journal of Vocational Behavior, 1980*(13), 282–290. DOI: 10.1016/0001-8791(80)90056-1

Suzuki, L. A., & Ponterotto, J. G. (Eds.). (2007). *Handbook of multicultural assessment: Clinical, psychological, and educational applications* (3rd ed.). John Wiley & Sons.

Svedmyr, S., Hedner, J., Bonsignore, M. R., Lombardi, C., Parati, G., Ludka, O., Zou, D., & Grote, L.European Sleep Apnea Database (ESADA) study group. (2023). Hypertension treatment in patients with sleep apnea from the European Sleep Apnea Database (ESADA) cohort – towards precision medicine. *Journal of Sleep Research, 32*(4), e13811. DOI: 10.1111/jsr.13811 PMID: 36539972

Swaab, D. F. (2014). *We are our brains: a neurobiography of the brain, from the womb to Alzheimer's.* Spiegel & Grau a Penguin Random House Company.

Sweetman, A., Osman, A., Lack, L., Crawford, M., & Wallace, D. (2023). Co-morbid insomnia and sleep apnea (COMISA): Recent research and future directions. *Current Opinion in Pulmonary Medicine, 29*(6), 567–573. DOI: 10.1097/MCP.0000000000001007 PMID: 37642477

Taneja, S. S., Taneja, P. K., & Gupta, R. K. (2011). Researches in corporate social responsibility: A review of shifting focus, paradigms, and methodologies. *Journal of Business Ethics, 101*(3), 343–364. DOI: 10.1007/s10551-010-0732-6

Tantia, J. F. (2021). *The art and science of embodied research design: Concepts, methods, and cases.* Routledge.

Tetřevová, L. I. B. Ě. N. A., & Sabolova, V. (2010). University stakeholder management and university social responsibility. WSEAS transactions on advances in engineering education, 7(7), 224-233.

Theorell-Haglöw, J., Zhou, X., Wittert, G., Adams, R., Appleton, S., Reynolds, A., Ljunggren, M., & Marshall, N. (2023). Does obstructive sleep apnea increase the risk of cancer and cancer mortality in combined community-based cohorts? *Journal of Sleep Research, 14089.* DOI: 10.1111/jsr.14089 PMID: 37990480

Thistlethwaite, J. (2012). Interprofessional education: a review of context, learning and the research agenda: Interprofessional education: a review. *Medical Education, 46*(1), 58–70. DOI: 10.1111/j.1365-2923.2011.04143.x PMID: 22150197

Thombs, B., Turner, K. A., & Shrier, I. (2019). Defining and evaluating overdiagnosis in mental health: A meta-research review. *Psychotherapy and Psychosomatics*, *88*(4), 193–202. DOI: 10.1159/000501647 PMID: 31340212

Thornicroft, G., Mehta, N., Clement, S., Evans-Lacko, S., Doherty, M., Rose, D., Koschorke, M., Shidhaye, R., O'Reilly, C., & Henderson, C. (2016). Evidence for effective interventions to reduce mental-health-related stigma and discrimination. *The Lancet. Psychiatry*, *3*(10), 975–988. DOI: 10.1016/S2215-0366(16)30237-3 PMID: 26410341

Topol, E. (2019). *Deep medicine: How artificial intelligence can make healthcare human again*. Basic Books.

Topol, E. J. (2019). *Deep Medicine: How Artificial Intelligence Can Make Healthcare Human Again*. Basic Books.

Tulving, E., & Markowitsch, H. J. (1998). Episodic and declarative memory: Role of the hippocampus. *Hippocampus*, *8*, 198–204.

Türkkahraman, M. (2012). The role of education in the societal development. Journal of educational and instructional studies in the world, 2(4), 38-41.

Türkkahraman, M. (2014). Social values and value education. Procedia-social and behavioural sciences, 116, 633-638.

Turkkahraman, M. (2015). Education, Teaching and School as A Social Organization. *Procedia: Social and Behavioral Sciences*, *186*, 381–387. DOI: 10.1016/j.sbspro.2015.04.044

Tutt, L. (1997): Der Studienentscheidungsprozess: Informationsquellen, Informationswünsche und Auswahlkriterien bei der Hochschulwahl. Diskussionsbeiträge des Fachbereichs Wirtschaftswissenschaften der Gerhard-Mercator- Universität Duisburg, Band 243. Duisburg

Tversky, A., & Kahneman, D. (1973). Availability: A heuristic for judging frequency and probability. *Cognitive Psychology*, *5*(2), 207–232. DOI: 10.1016/0010-0285(73)90033-9

Tversky, A., & Kahneman, D. (1974). Judgment under Uncertainty: Heuristics and Biases. *Science*, *185*(4157), 1124–1131. DOI: 10.1126/science.185.4157.1124 PMID: 17835457

Tversky, A., & Kahneman, D. (2013). Judgment under uncertainty: Heuristics and biases. In *Handbook of the Fundamentals of Financial Decision Making* (pp. 261–268). WORLD SCIENTIFIC. DOI: 10.1142/9789814417358_0015

United Nations. (2006). *Convention on the Rights of Persons with Disabilities (CRPD)*. https://www.un.org/disabilities/documents/convention/convoptprot-e.pdf

Vedel, A., & Poropat, A. E. (2017). Personality and Academic Performance. In Zeigler-Hill, V., & Shackelford, T. (Eds.), *Encyclopedia of Personality and Individual Differences*. Springer., DOI: 10.1007/978-3-319-28099-8_989-1

Vester, F. (2012). *Denken, Lernen, Vergessen. Was geht in unserem Kopf vor, wie lernt das Gehirn und wann lässt es uns im Stich? 35*. Aufl, Deutscher Taschenbuch Verlag.

Villamil-Salcedo, V., Vargas-Terrez, B. E., & Díaz-Anzaldúa, A. (2017). Collaborative Care model in mental health. Scope and experiences after three years of activity in Mexico City. *Primary Health Care Research and Development*, *18*(3), 227–234. DOI: 10.1017/S1463423617000032 PMID: 28219460

Votteler, S., Knaack, L., Janicki, J., Fink, G. R., & Burghaus, L. (2023). Sex differences in polysomnographic findings in patients with obstructive sleep apnea. *Sleep Medicine*, *101*, 429–436. DOI: 10.1016/j.sleep.2022.11.025 PMID: 36516599

Vroom, V. (1964). *Work and Motivation*. Wiley.

Wadhwani Foundation. (2024). Companies are willing to pay more for those with the best soft skills. https://wadhwanifoundation.org/press/companies-are-willing-to-pay-more-for-those-with-the-best-soft-skills/

Waltman, S., Frankel, S., & Williston, M. (2016). Improving Clinician Self-Awareness and Increasing Accurate Representation of Clinical Competencies. *Practice Innovations (Washington, D.C.)*, *1*(3), 178–188. DOI: 10.1037/pri0000026

Wang, L., Chen, Y., Zhang, J., & Li, M. (2023). Culturally adapted cognitive behavioral therapy with qigong for Chinese university students with depression. *Asian Journal of Psychiatry*, 88.

Wang, L., & Juslin, H. (2012). Values and corporate social responsibility perceptions of Chinese university students. *Journal of Academic Ethics*, *10*(1), 57–82. DOI: 10.1007/s10805-012-9148-5

Wartick, S. L., & Cochran, P. L. (1985). The evolution of the corporate social performance model. *Academy of Management Review*, *10*(4), 758–769. DOI: 10.2307/258044

Watson, G. (1980). *Watson-Glaser Critical Thinking Appraisal* (Vol. 3). Psychological Corporation.

Watson, K. (2011). Farrar, Straus and Giroux. 499 pages. *The Canadian Journal of Program Evaluation, 26*(2), 111–113. DOI: 10.3138/cjpe.26.010

Weinrauch, S. G., & Srebalus, D. J. (1994). Die Berufswahltheorie von Holland. In: Brown, D./Brooks, L. (Hrsg.): Karriere-Entwicklung. Stuttgart: Klett-Cotta, p. 43-74.

Weinstein, N. D. (1980). Unrealistic Optimism about Future Life Events. *Journal of Personality and Social Psychology, 39*(5), 806–820. DOI: 10.1037/0022-3514.39.5.806

Wentzel, K. (1991). Relations between Social Competence and Academic Achievement in Early Adolescence. *Child Development, 62*(5), 1066. DOI: 10.2307/1131152 PMID: 1756656

Wentzel, K. R. (1991). Social competence at school: Relation between social responsibility and academic achievement. *Review of Educational Research, 61*(1), 1–24. DOI: 10.3102/00346543061001001

Wiejak, K., & Krasowicz-Kupis, G. (2016). The emotional and social consequences of dyslexia: A developmental perspective. *Developmental Psychology, 52*(9), 1432–1445.

WifiTalents. (2025). *Mental health misdiagnosis statistics*. https://wifitalents.com/mental-health-misdiagnosis-statistics

Williams, C. T., & Anderson, S. L. (2020). Clinical decision-making in psychological diagnosis: Enhancing diagnostic accuracy with cognitive models and critical thinking. *Psychological Services, 17*(1), 20–28. DOI: 10.1037/ser0000345

Wittmann, S., & Edelmann, W. (2012). *Lernpsychologie: Mit Online Materialien* (7th ed.). Beltz Verlag.

Wojnowski, K., Mayo, M., Blanco, J. C. G., Abreu, A. R., & Chediak, A. D. (2022). Comorbid Narcolepsy and Obstructive Sleep Apnea: A Review. *Current Pulmonology Reports, 11*(4), 160–165. DOI: 10.1007/s13665-022-00297-3

Wolf, M., & Bowers, P. G. (1999). The double-deficit hypothesis for the developmental dyslexias. *Journal of Educational Psychology, 91*(3), 415–438. DOI: 10.1037/0022-0663.91.3.415

Workday. (2024). *Workday report: AI is transforming the job market; 51% of business leaders fear a skills gap*. https://polandinsight.com/workday-report-ai-is-transforming-the-job-market-51-of-business-leaders-fear-a-skills-gap-22911/

World Economic Forum. (2023). *The future of jobs report 2023*. https://www.weforum.org/stories/2023/05/future-of-jobs-2023-skills

World Health Organization. (2008). *mhGAP: Mental Health Gap Action Programme: Scaling up care for mental, neurological, and substance use disorders.* https://www.who.int/publications/i/item/9789241547697

World Health Organization. (2015). Recognizing Adolescence. https://www.who.int/publications/i/item/WHO-FWC-MCA-14.05 [visited on 9 June 2025]

World Health Organization. (2016). *International statistical classification of diseases and related health problems* (10th ed.). WHO.

World Health Organization. (2019). *International classification of diseases for mortality and morbidity statistics (11th Revision).* https://icd.who.int/en

World Health Organization. (2021). Adolescent mental health. Retrieved from https://www.who.int/news-room/fact-sheets/detail/adolescent-mental-health

World Health Organization. (2021). *Guidance on community mental health services: Promoting person-centred and rights-based approaches.* https://www.who.int/publications/i/item/9789240025707

Wray-Lake, L., & Syvertsen, A. K. (2011). The developmental roots of social responsibility in childhood and adolescence. *New Directions for Child and Adolescent Development, 2011*(134), 11–25. DOI: 10.1002/cd.308 PMID: 22147598

Wu, Y., & Cheng, X. (2023). *Causal relationship between obstructive sleep apnea and asthma: A Mendelian randomization study.* DOI: 10.21203/rs.3.rs-3226417/v1

Yang, Q., Huang, X., Lin, Y., Chen, K., Lu, Q., Lin, W., Wang, X., Teng, Y., Jiang, P., Patil, S., & Zheng, Y. (2024). Exploring the Multifaceted Landscape of Pediatric Obstructive Sleep Apnea: Insights into Prevalence, Severity, and Coexisting Conditions. *Nature and Science of Sleep, 16*, 359–368. DOI: 10.2147/NSS.S452221 PMID: 38617037

Yates, M., & Youniss, J. (1996). A developmental perspective on community service in adolescence. *Social Development, 5*(1), 85–111. DOI: 10.1111/j.1467-9507.1996.tb00073.x

Yoshimura, S., Okamoto, Y., Onoda, K., Matsunaga, M., Okada, G., Kunisato, Y., Yoshino, A., Ueda, K., Suzuki, S., & Yamawaki, S. (2013). Cognitive behavioral therapy for depression changes medial prefrontal and ventral anterior cingulate cortex activity associated with self-referential processing. *Social Cognitive and Affective Neuroscience, 9*(4), 487–493. DOI: 10.1093/scan/nst009 PMID: 23327934

Yuen, S. C. Y., Yaoyuneyong, G., & Johnson, E. (2011). Augmented reality: An overview and five directions for AR in education. [JETDE]. *Journal of Educational Technology Development and Exchange*, *4*(1), 11. DOI: 10.18785/jetde.0401.10

Yu, P. K., Radcliffe, J., Gerry Taylor, H., Amin, R. S., Baldassari, C. M., Boswick, T., Chervin, R. D., Elden, L. M., Furth, S. L., Garetz, S. L., George, A., Ishman, S. L., Kirkham, E. M., Liu, C., Mitchell, R. B., Kamal Naqvi, S., Rosen, C. L., Ross, K. R., Shah, J. R., & Redline, S. (2022). Neurobehavioral morbidity of pediatric mild sleep-disordered breathing and obstructive sleep apnea. *Sleep (Basel)*, *45*(5), zsac035. DOI: 10.1093/sleep/zsac035 PMID: 35554583

Zaffanello, M., Ersu, R. H., Nosetti, L., Beretta, G., Agosti, M., & Piacentini, G. (2024). Cardiac Implications of Adenotonsillar Hypertrophy and Obstructive Sleep Apnea in Pediatric Patients: A Comprehensive Systematic Review. *Children (Basel, Switzerland)*, *11*(2), 208. DOI: 10.3390/children11020208 PMID: 38397319

Zhang, E., Yao, Y., Zhou, N., Chen, Y., Zhang, H., Guo, J., & Teng, F. (2024). A fine-grained convolutional recurrent model for obstructive sleep apnea detection. *International Journal of Machine Learning and Cybernetics*, *15*(7), 3043–3056. DOI: 10.1007/s13042-023-02080-5

Zhao, J., Wang, Z., & Qiu, F. (2021). Machine learning-based detection of dyslexia. *IEEE Transactions on Neural Networks and Learning Systems*, *32*(5), 1245–1258.

Ziegler, J. C., & Goswami, U. (2005). Reading acquisition, developmental dyslexia, and skilled reading across languages: A psycholinguistic grain size theory. *Psychological Bulletin*, *131*(1), 3–29. DOI: 10.1037/0033-2909.131.1.3 PMID: 15631549

Zigler, R. L. (1998). The four domains of moral education: The contributions of Dewey, Alexander and Goleman to a comprehensive taxonomy. *Journal of Moral Education*, *27*(1), 19–33. DOI: 10.1080/0305724980270102

ZipDo. (2025). *Misdiagnosed mental illness statistics*. https://zipdo.co/misdiagnosed-mental-illness-statistics

Zych, I., Ortega-Ruiz, R., Muñoz-Morales, R., & Llorent, V. J. (2018). Dimensions and psychometric properties of the Social and Emotional Competencies Questionnaire (SEC-Q) in youth and adolescents. *Revista Latinoamericana de Psicología*, *50*(2), 98–106. DOI: 10.14349/rlp.2018.v50.n2.3

About the Contributors

Sherouk J. Kadhm is a seasoned educator, psychologist, and researcher with over 16 years of experience in education and mental health. Passionate about fostering critical thinking and cognitive growth, she has dedicated her career to advancing mental wellness and enhancing thinking skills in both children and adults. Dr. Sherouk earned her Ph.D. in Philosophy from the International Islamic University Malaysia (IIUM), where she conducted pioneering research on the role of critical thinking in cognitive development and psychological health. As a recognized expert, she has authored numerous publications and presented at international conferences, sharing her insights with educators, parents, and mental health professionals. She is the founder of the Critical Thinking Diagnosis and Therapy approach, which has helped countless individuals overcome cognitive and behavioral challenges. This innovative method has been widely praised for its effectiveness and transformative outcomes in clinical practice. Outside her professional work, Dr. Sherouk enjoys swimming, walking, reading, and watching true success-story films—reflecting her commitment to lifelong learning and personal growth. Her work continues to inspire others to think critically and lead mentally healthy, fulfilling lives. Her personal motto reflects her vision in life and practice: "Critical thinking is the key to unlocking happiness, achieving success, and maintaining mental health."

***

Ancey Mary Abraham is a postgraduate student pursuing a Master of Commerce in International Finance and Accounting (IFA) at Jain University. With a strong interest in financial analysis, corporate governance, and global accounting standards, she is dedicated to academic excellence and research. Ancey actively engages in exploring financial strategies and their practical applications, aiming to contribute to the finance industry with analytical insights and strategic decision-making.

Shalini Aggarwal, an alumnus of the Indian Institute of Management (IIM) Ahmedabad is a Professor of Finance at Chandigarh University, Mohali. She has a total work experience of 18 years. She is MBA with specialisation in Finance and PhD in the area of Risk Management Practices in banking sector of India. She has more than 60 research papers published in SCI, Q1, Q2, Scopus and ABDC- A (6 papers), B (8 papers) and C listed journal. Her case studies are published in IIM Ahmedabad at case centre, journal and Taylor and francis. She has also authored 4 books published by Taylor and Francis. She has completed three funded research projects (two with IIM, Ahmedabad) and one by IMS Ghaziabad. She has conducted more than 100 workshops on data analysis using time series data in SPSS, E-views, finding variables and model building, SLR, Bibliometric analysis, Quantitative study, Qualitative study and R-Studio and has delivered guest lectures at national and international level like South Africa, Bangladesh, Afghanistan, Thailand, Indonesia and Brazil.

Sohom Banerjee is an accomplished research professional with extensive experience in delivering high-quality, data-driven insights and impactful research outputs. With several publications in reputed journals, including the Journal of Consumer Behaviour, Sohom has demonstrated expertise in topics ranging from Consumer Behaviour, Metaverse and Artificial Intelligence (AI). His thought leadership extends to newspaper articles on ethical AI and policy innovation, published in leading platforms like Policy Circle. His contributions to academic conferences are notable, having presented at prestigious events such as the SEEDS 2024 Conference at Dubai and the EMCB at IIM Lucknow. He received the Best Paper Award for his work on AR and VR adoption in employee training. With a proven track record of impactful research projects funded by global organizations like The World Bank, GiZ, Netflix, Meta, and USAID, his portfolio also includes exploring sustainability, trade and connectivity, just energy transitions, and AI ethics. Sohom's multidisciplinary approach and dedication to research excellence make him a thought leader in his field.

Souvik Banerjee, PhD. He is a faculty at Management Development Institute (MDI) Murshidabad. His research interests include Corporate Finance, Corporate Governance, Behavioral Finance, and Financial Economics. His work has been published in Scopus-indexed and ABDC-listed journals. At present, he is the Editor of the MDIM Journal of Management Review and Practice (Sage). He has developed several business cases for MBA and executive education. He has trained executives from Fortune 500 companies in Corporate Finance and Corporate Valuation.

Patcha Bhujanga Rao is a distinguished professional with a stellar reputation in the realms of human resources (HR) and soft skills development. With over two decades of experience and an extensive academic background encompassing degrees such as M.Com., DCFA., M.Phil., Ph.D., MBA (HR), M.Sc (Psychology), and LL.B, he possesses a comprehensive understanding of multiple disciplines. Currently serving as a professor at Jain Deemed-to-Be University in Bengaluru, Dr. Rao is highly regarded for his expertise in HR management, which has been instrumental in shaping the careers of numerous professionals. His commitment to nurturing essential skills such as effective communication, leadership, and interpersonal abilities reflects his dedication to facilitating personal and professional growth. Dr. Rao's contributions have earned him widespread respect and admiration within the HR and soft skills domains, positioning him as a respected authority and mentor for aspiring professionals seeking to excel in their respective fields.

Tariq Yousef Damrah is a highly experienced pediatric consultant with over 20 years of dedicated service in child healthcare. He holds the Jordanian Board in Pediatrics.

Md Nurul Huda is a distinguished medical professional currently serving in the Department of Otolaryngology & Head Neck Surgery at the Combined Military Hospital (CMH) in Bangladesh. With extensive experience in ear, nose, and throat (ENT) and head and neck surgery, Major Huda has earned a reputation for his exceptional skills and dedication to patient care. He holds an MBBS degree from Sher-e-Bangla Medical College and is pursuing his MS in Otolaryngology from Bangabandhu Sheikh Mujib Medical University (BSMMU), Dhaka. Throughout his career, Major Huda has been committed to advancing medical practices in otolaryngology, contributing to clinical excellence and research. His expertise covers a broad range of ENT-related conditions, including routine procedures, complex head and neck surgeries, and sleep apnea treatment. Known for his patient-centred approach, Major Huda ensures that individuals receive the best care tailored to their needs. In addition to his clinical practice, he is actively involved in medical education and training, sharing his expertise with young doctors and aspiring specialists. His commitment to fostering the growth and development of the next generation of medical professionals reflects his deep passion for the field. Major Huda's contributions extend beyond the hospital setting. He regularly participates in workshops, seminars, and conferences, staying updated on the latest advancements in otolaryngology and head and neck surgery. His dedication to continuous learning and innovation has made him a respected figure within the medical community.

Preethi Inampudi is a highly accomplished academic professional who has dedicated her career to the field of human resources and presently working as Assistant Professor, Department of Management, Surana College, Bangalore, Karnataka,

Geemol John is a dedicated psychology researcher currently pursuing a PhD at Lovely Professional University, Punjab. With academic qualifications in nursing, psychology, and education, along with UGC-NET qualification, she brings a multidisciplinary approach to her work. Her research primarily focuses on midlife crisis, resilience, and mental health, and she has authored multiple publications in Scopus-indexed journals and edited book volumes. Geemol has also developed two psychometric tools—the Midlife Crisis Scale and the Family Environment Scale—as part of her doctoral research. She has actively participated in national and international conferences, receiving recognition as Best Paper Presenter for her work on midlife resilience. Additionally, she is engaged in teaching through a fellowship and has undertaken various training programs in advanced research methodologies, including SPSS, AMOS, and bibliometric analysis, reflecting her commitment to academic excellence and mental health advocacy.

Raad M. Kadhum is a researcher and educator for over three decades, he specializes in researching and teaching critical and creative thinking approaches and their quality in the context of contemporary changes. He is a pioneer in publishing research on evolutionary and sustainable approaches to understanding and teaching critical thinking.

Froilan Mobo is a Doctor of Public Administration graduate from the Urdaneta City University Class of 2016 and a graduate of the 2nd Doctorate Degree (Ph.D.) in Development Education program at the Central Luzon State University, Nueva Ecija, Philippines, Class of 2022. On March 11, 2024, Dr. Mobo was accredited and reclassified by the Commission on Higher Education (CHED) to the position of Professor II in the Philippine Merchant Marine Academy (PMMA), and this allowed him to work with different international research institutions, such as the Director and Research Consultant of the IKSAD Research Institute, Turkey. At present, he is in the process of finishing his 3rd master's degree, leading to social studies education at Bicol University. Recently, Dr. Mobo passed Batch 3—Certified Research Professional—and ranked in the top 5 in the National Examination and also passed the Certified Human Resource Associate (CHRA). He was appointed Editor-in-Chief of the International Journal of Multidisciplinary: Applied Business and Education Research, Malang, Indonesia, and appointed as a technical research evaluator by the Department of Science and Technology and Book Chapter Editor at IGI Global

Mahendra K Sahu is a library science professional, did PhD in Library and Information Science and presently working as a Librarian at a repute institutions in Odisha. I am keen in research work. My specialization is Library Automation, Digital Library and Web based Library service.

Mohammad Abdelilah Semrin is a Consultant Pediatrician–Neonatologist from Jordan. He earned his Bachelor's degree in Medicine and Surgery from Mutah University, Jordan, in 2014, and completed training in the Pediatric and Neonatology Program at the Royal Jordanian Medical Services hospitals. Since then, he has served as a specialist in the unit of prematurity and intensive care for children, as well as in medical departments and emergency rooms. He holds the Jordanian Board of Pediatrics, has completed courses in Basic Life Support for Healthcare Providers (BLS) and Pediatric Advanced Life Support (PALS), and is also a certified trainer for the Neonatal Resuscitation Program.

Mohammad Badruddoza Talukder is an Associate Professor, College of Tourism and Hospitality Management, IUBAT - International University of Business Agriculture and Technology, Dhaka, Bangladesh. He holds PhD in Hotel Management from Lovely Professional University, India. He has been teaching various courses in the Department of Tourism and Hospitality at various universities in Bangladesh since 2008. His research areas include tourism management, hotel management, hospitality management, food & beverage management, and accommodation management, where he has published research papers in well-known journals in Bangladesh and abroad. Mr. Talukder is one of the executive members of the Tourism Educators Association of Bangladesh. He has led training and consulting for a wide range of hospitality organizations in Bangladesh. He just became an honorary facilitator at the Bangladesh Tourism Board's Bangabandhu international tourism and hospitality training institution.

Mohammad Amin Wani is an Assistant Professor of Psychology with a strong background in teaching, research, and mentorship. He has demonstrated proficiency in implementing engaging teaching strategies that enhance student learning experiences and improve performance. His expertise in research is evident through his mentorship of students in research projects, fostering critical thinking and academic excellence. Dr. Wani actively contributes to the development and enhancement of the psychology curriculum, ensuring its relevance and alignment with industry standards. He provides guidance and support to psychology students, assisting them in navigating academic challenges and exploring career opportunities.

His commitment to ongoing professional development through research, conferences, and professional networking keeps him updated on advancements in the field.

Alexander Weissman has over 20 years of experience in large-scale, high-stakes standardized testing, having architected transitions of major testing programs from traditional P& P (paper-and-pencil) to computer-based tests with an emphasis on maintaining professional standards and best practices in validity, fairness, and psychometric integrity. He is currently Consulting Principal, M2C1 Consulting, providing innovative and strategic solutions in measurement, assessment, and evaluation.

Ananya Y is a postgraduate student pursuing a Master of Commerce in International Finance and Accounting (IFA) at Jain University. Passionate about financial analysis, corporate governance, and global accounting standards, she actively engages in academic research and practical applications of financial strategies. With a keen eye for detail and a commitment to excellence, Ananya aspires to contribute to the finance industry through analytical insights and strategic decision-making.

Index

H

L

M

N

O

P

R

S

W

www.ingramcontent.com/pod-product-compliance
Lightning Source LLC
LaVergne TN
LVHW081537300926
849161LV00006B/1466